A synopsis of

Children's Diseases

A synopsis of

Children's Diseases

John Rendle-Short MA MD(Cantab) FRCP FRACP DCH

Professor of Child Health, University of Queensland

O. P. Gray MB ChB FRCP DCH

Professor of Child Health, University of Wales College of Medicine

J. A. Dodge MD(Wales) FRCP FRCPE DCH

Reader in Child Health, University of Wales College of Medicine

Sixth edition

WRIGHT

1985 Bristol

Published by
John Wright & Sons Ltd, 823–825 Bath Road, Bristol BS4 5NU, England.

First edition, 1954
Second edition, 1957
Third edition, 1961
Fourth edition, 1967
Fifth edition, 1978
Sixth edition, 1985
Spanish edition, 1956

British Library Cataloguing in Publication Data

Rendle-Short, John
    A synopsis of children's diseases.——6th ed.
    1. Children——Diseases
    I. Title   II. Gray, O. P.   III. Dodge, J. A.
    618.92   RJ45

ISBN 0 7236 0743 5

Library of Congress Catalog Card Number: 84–51548

Typeset by
Activity Ltd, Salisbury, Wiltshire

Printed in Great Britain by
John Wright & Sons (Printing) Ltd, at The Stonebridge Press, Bristol BS4 5NU

Preface to the Sixth Edition

This sixth edition of the Synopsis is smaller than the preceding one, and with an altered format is very nearly a new book. To bring a book up to date by the addition of much new material and simultaneously to reduce its size has proved a formidable task. It has only been possible because many diseases have been virtually eliminated by scientific progress. The huge area of social and psychiatric paediatrics, which occupies much of the modern paediatrician's time, has not been dealt with as it does not lend itself to the synoptic approach. Also the authors, who come from different geographical backgrounds, are well aware that social conditions differ from country to country. For these diseases, therefore, smaller, locally produced books are required.

The authors would like to thank Dr K. Verrier Jones for the chapter on 'Renal Diseases' and Doctors C. Wardrop and B. Holland for considerable help with the chapter on 'Blood Disorders'.

John Rendle-Short takes this opportunity to express his profound thanks to Peter Gray and John Dodge for their increasing help in the preparation of recent editions of the Synopsis, and to Messrs John Wright & Sons Ltd for their care in the production of six editions over 30 years.

J.R-S.

Brisbane, Australia

Preface to the First Edition

The importance of children's diseases is unquestioned; it was therefore considered that there was a place for a book of the synopsis type devoted to this speciality, in order to assemble all the relevant facts tidily for easy reference and rapid revision. It is hoped that this book will be of value to those preparing for examinations, whether Finals, the Diploma of Child Health or Membership of the Royal College of Physicians: also for Paediatric House Physicians and General Practitioners. It should not take the place of standard textbooks.

For the guidance of undergraduates, most diseases have been described as common, rare, etc. With few exceptions (e.g. rickets), those conditions marked as rare, or very rare, are of little importance to students taking their final examinations. It must be remembered, however, that whether a disease is described as common or rare depends largely on how many examples of that particular condition the author has seen.

The section on gastro-enteritis is purposely detailed, as the correct management of this disease is the key to the control of infantile dehydration and biochemical upset of whatever aetiology.

The appendix on drug dosage has been inserted especially for the benefit of House Physicians and General Practitioners. The doses have been checked by Mr A. Williams, PhC, MPS, Chief Pharmacist at Llandough Hospital, whose help is gratefully acknowledged. Dr T. Parry, Pathologist to Llandough Hospital, helped with the appendix on normal biochemical values.

Much of the material in this book is drawn from standard textbooks, especially Garrod, Batten and Thursfield's *Diseases of Children* and Mitchell-Nelson's *Textbook of Pediatrics* and grateful thanks are accorded to the writers of these and many other books and articles too numerous to mention individually. It is hoped that the authors will accept this as adequate acknowledgement. In a few instances, references have been given in a footnote, and illustrations taken from articles are acknowledged under each. Messrs Allen and Hanbury kindly supplied the illustration of the Woolwich nipple shield.

I would like to take this opportunity of thanking all those who read the proofs, and especially Professor A. G. Watkins, for much valuable criticism and advice. Several typists assisted me and my thanks are due to them, and particularly Miss W. R. Davies.

Finally to Messrs John Wright & Sons Ltd I express my sincere gratitude for their unfailing patience and help.

J R-S

Contents

Chapter 1

NORMAL DEVELOPMENT

Developmental paediatrics is concerned with the maturational processes of normal and abnormal children from fetus to adulthood.

Growth refers to increase in size, anatomical and structural, measured in such parameters as height, weight, head circumference and bone age.

Development refers to increase in complexity in both structure and function. Its numerous simultaneous progressions are closely related but manifest many individual variations.

All children follow the same pattern of development—'they pass the same milestones', although the age at which they do so differs within certain limits, even in normal children.

Normally, growth and development of body, intellect and personality progress with age, and are fairly predictable in rate and outcome.

Abnormally, they are dissociated, producing widespread inconsistencies of and between somatic, cognitive and affective progressions, with unpredictable final results.

Factors affecting Growth and Development

Heredity determines the limits of each individual child's capacity to achieve optimal structural and functional maturity.

Environment determines the extent to which each individual child can fulfil his potential.

Purpose of developmental paediatrics is to monitor growth and development to:

1. Promote optimal physical, mental and emotional health.

2. Ensure early diagnosis and effective treatment of handicaps of body, mind and personality.

3. Discover the cause of any handicap.

A child's basic needs are for shelter and protective care; food; warmth and clothing; fresh air and sunlight; activity and rest; prevention of illness and injury; training in habits and skills necessary for the maintenance of life.

The psychological needs of both normal and handicapped children are for:

1. Dignity as a human being; different from an animal or machine; self-respect derived from knowledge of being valued as an individual.

2. Love and individual care.

3. Security based on (*a*) a sense of belonging, (*b*) stable interpersonal relationships, (*c*) familiar environment, but (*d*) not smothered with restrictions.

4. Discipline neither too severe nor too lax.

5. A sense of responsibility and opportunity to be of service to others, even though the child himself be handicapped.

6. Opportunity to achieve success in some field of endeavour.

7. Opportunity to learn from experience.

8. Opportunity to achieve personal, and if possible financial independence.

The Importance of Developmental Assessment

Understanding of normal childhood development with its many minor variations is essential for perceiving what is abnormal.

The normal developing child is active in body, intensely curious in mind and seeks a good relationship with adults and children.

Poorly developing children are inactive, not curious and have stunted personal relationships. If this is a chronic state, such children warrant observation and, if necessary, investigation.

1. If major delay occurs in all fields of development it may indicate:

    1.1 Prematurity—a pre-term baby at (say) 3 months post-natal age is not able to perform in the same way as full-term baby of the same age.

    1.2 Mental retardation.

    1.3 Cerebral palsy or other neurological or muscular disorder, e.g. amyotonia congenita.

    1.4 Severe illness causing weakness, e.g. gastro-enteritis.

    1.5 An emotionally deprived child.

    1.6 Sensory deficits, especially visual handicaps, but auditory and language difficulties also delay social behaviour and may lead to mistaken diagnosis of mental retardation.

    1.7 Infantile autism.

2. Delayed development of one area may occur in isolation, e.g.

    2.1 Delayed maturation. Sometimes a particular area of development (notably speech) fails to develop at usual rate. It eventually catches up and the child becomes completely normal in that area.

    2.2 Gross motor delay. Usually indicates physical disorder, e.g. dislocated hip preventing baby sitting.

    2.3 Fine motor delay. May indicate sensory loss or perhaps blindness.

    2.4 Delay in vocalizing or speech. May indicate deafness (*see* p.180).

    2.5 Minimal brain dysfunction (hyperactive syndrome).

    2.6 Specific learning difficulty in older child, dyslexia, etc.

3. Advanced development, occuring as an isolated phenomenon is of no prognostic significance for future intelligence, except cases of advanced speech development which may indicate high intelligence.

4. The greatest difficulty lies in the field of multiple handicaps. For example, it is very difficult to assess intelligence in a baby with athetosis and deafness who may nevertheless have normal intelligence.

Handicapped and Disadvantaged Children

A handicapped child is one who suffers from any continuing disability of body, intellect or personality which is likely to interfere with his normal growth and development or capacity to learn.

Note: All handicapped children, however well provided otherwise, are disadvantaged and deprived in some way, and all disadvantaged and deprived children are handicapped socially even if not physically or intellectually.

A disadvantaged child is one who suffers from a continuing inadequacy of material, affectional, educational or social provisions, or who is subject to detrimental environmental stresses of any kind, which are likely to interfere with the growth and development of his body, intellect or personality, thus preventing him from achieving his inherent potential.

A handicapped child needs early identification of his disabilities and assets, prompt medical and surgical treatment and help and guidance for the parents to enable them to care for the child as long as possible in his own home. Appropriate training, education and vocational guidance and supervision and regular assessment throughout childhood and adolescence are also required. Finally, placement in the community or in special care.

The Child at Risk

The concept of the child at risk is of value as it enables the paediatrician to mark and follow children who have a poor prognosis. If, however, the net is cast too wide, too many children are followed and the exercise becomes unmanageable. Children at risk include those with an adverse family history, prenatal hazards, perinatal dangers, postnatal mishaps and developmental warning signals, e.g. the mother's suspicion that the child is not seeing, hearing, moving his limbs or taking notice like other children of his own age. She is usually right.

Other warning signals are: paediatric findings such as delayed motor development, lack of normal visual alertness, inattention to sound, delayed development of vocalization or speech, lack of interest in people or playthings and abnormal social behaviour of any sort. It is not safe to rely upon a single examination.

Comprehensive assessment of the handicapped child includes:
1. Neurological capabilities, sensory and motor.
2. Intellectual competence.
3. Social behaviour.
4. Paediatric examination, including careful evaluation of the child's visual and auditory capacity and his powers of communication.

Parent Guidance

1. Guidance regarding upbringing of a child to ensure optimum physical and mental health is required by all young parents. This is normally provided by grandparents in extended family. May be supplemented by paediatrician, books, etc.

2. Parents of handicapped children need additional support with knowledgeable instruction concerning everyday management. Special needs:

>2.1 Truthful explanation of any handicapping condition, causation and prognosis.
>
>2.2 Practical instruction in day-to-day care and management.
>
>2.3 Continuing supportive counselling for all the family.
>
>2.4 Referral to the appropriate social or medical agencies including provision of domestic help and financial assistance.

2.5 Realistic forward planning.

2.6 Genetic advice when necessary.

Management

1. Early training depends upon adequate stimulation. The natural teachers are the parents. The natural place is the ordinary family home. The natural tools of learning are playthings.

2. Education is an integral part of the handicapped child's treatment. Schooling must always be of prime consideration in planning medical and surgical procedures. Education may require special schools and facilities (e.g. school for deaf) but integration with normal children should be the aim as far as possible.

3. Vocational guidance must be based on realistic evaluation of the child's physical capacity, mental ability and social circumstances.

Ultimate Aims

'It is necessary for all concerned with the health, education and welfare of handicapped children to bear constantly in mind that childhood itself is a temporary phase in the life of any individual human being. The ultimate goal is to equip him or her in body, mind and personality to become, in adult life, a contented, self-reliant and useful member of the social community to which he or she belongs' (Mary D. Sheridan).

Patterns of Development

(For patterns of development from 4 weeks onwards, *see* Appendix 3).

The Baby at Birth

The baby at birth sleeps most of the time. When awake he is usually crying. He does not register pleasure. He dislikes a bright light shone into his eyes and responds by closing them. He turns towards a diffuse light, e.g. a window. Most of the time he lies immobile. He can flex and extend his legs and arms. When pulled into the sitting position his head falls back. When lying prone the infant cannot lift his head from the couch.

Jaw clonus is usually present, and occasionally ill-sustained ankle clonus.

The hands are held clenched, usually with the thumb between index and middle finger.

Primitive Reflexes. Many reflexes can be elicited in the newborn. Most are of academic interest only. Following may be of clinical importance as:

They are poorly developed or absent in pre-term or ill babies.

If they persist over age of 3 months, a neurological abnormality may be present.

Reflexes

1. Moro Reflex (age: birth–3 months) can be obtained by banging the cot-side, loud noise, etc. However, it is best elicited by holding the baby with the examiner's hand under the back, and if the head is then allowed to drop backward a few centimetres, the reflex should result:

Phase 1. Arms and legs are thrown out as if the baby were startled.

Phase 2. Arms are flexed as in embrace.

2. Grasp Reflex. Disappears at 6–8 months. This is elicited by examiner rubbing his fingers across the baby's palm. The baby grasps the finger firmly and can be lifted up by this means. It is strong in pre-term infants.

3. Asymmetrical Tonic Neck Reflex (ATNR) is elicited by turning the head to one side. The baby extends the arm and leg on that side and flexes on the opposite side. This fades at 36 weeks' gestation and is almost absent in full term, reappears at 1 month but later disappears.

4. Symmetrical Tonic Neck Reflex. Extensor tone in arms and flexor tone in legs when neck extended, reversed when neck flexed, disappears at 8–10 weeks.

5. Walk Reflex. Elicited by holding baby in standing position. Baby places one foot in front of other as though walking.

6. Step Reflex. If dorsum of baby's foot scraped along undersurface of table, he will step up onto table.

7. Rooting Reflex. If newborn baby's cheek is touched, he turns his mouth towards object which touched it. When baby is put to breast, therefore, and nipple touches cheek, baby turns mouth towards it.

Chapter 2   # *PHYSICAL GROWTH*

Serial measurements of weight, height and head circumference are of great value in young children. They should be plotted on a centile chart (*Fig. 2.1*). Actual measurements are of less importance than whether or not serial measurements run parallel to the centiles.

Weight is more commonly used than height as a criterion of growth. Height, or length in an infant, is of equal importance to weight but considerably harder to measure and therefore less accurate. It has the advantage that a child cannot 'lose' height.

For prognosis of adult height, a bone age measurement (obtained by comparison of a radiograph of hand and wrist with accepted standards) is necessary.

Growth does not proceed regularly and uniformly. For the first 18 months of life there is a period of intense growth. From 18 months to 11 years growth occurs more slowly, about 5–6 cm/year.

At puberty there is a further period of active growth.

Tables of weight or height vary considerably according to the country of origin and date when they were compiled. For this reason local tables should be used as far as possible. Nevertheless international centile charts of value since it is the serial measurement which is important rather than spot checks, and they can also be used to relate weight and height to each other in assessment of nutritional state.

Some Factors influencing Physical Growth

1. Birth Weight
Children whose birth weight is low tend to remain relatively smaller than those with higher birth weight.

Fig. 2.1. Height chart for boys. (By permission of J. M. Tanner and R. H. Whitehouse and Castlemead Publications, Hertford.)

Name.. Date of Birth................ Reg.No. ....

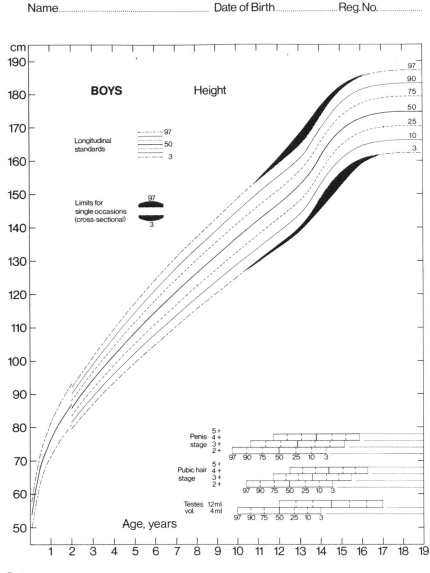

2. Sex
Girls usually smaller than boys.

3. Familial Factors
Large parents tend to have large children.

4. Racial Factors
Some races, e.g. pygmies, tend to be shorter than others.

5. Endocrine Factors
These may influence weight or height: hypothalamic pituitary growth hormone, thyroxine, adrenal and gonadal hormones.

6. Environmental Factors
Children from low socio-economic groups tend to be smaller. All severe or chronic illnesses lead to a poor gain in weight or height.

Weight

The average weight at birth is 3400 g (7½lb), but great variations occur. Weight of 4100 g (9lb) not uncommon. If baby weighs 4600 g (10lb) or more this may indicate that the mother is diabetic or pre-diabetic. The following factors can be used in calculating the expected weight in the first weeks of life: The baby normally loses weight after birth, but should have returned to his birth weight by the tenth day. He should gain approximately 30 g (1oz) per day for the first 100 days of life. Expected weight can thus be calculated as follows: 30 × number of days since birth minus 10 equals weight in grams that child should have gained. This figure added to birth weight gives expected weight.

Fontanelles

The anterior fontanelle is normally closed by 18 months, but there is a wide range of normality. The posterior fontanelle should be closed by 2 months.

Teeth

Time of eruption varies greatly.

Eruption of Temporary (Milk) Teeth. Total number 20.
> Lower central incisors: 6–10 months.
> Upper central and lateral incisors: 8–12 months.
> Lower lateral incisors and first molars: 12–18 months.
> Canines: 18–24 months.
> Second molars: 20–30 months.

Eruption of Permanent Teeth. Total number 32.
> First molars: 6 years.
> Central incisors: 7 years.
> Lateral incisors: 8 years.

Puberty and Adolescence

Puberty occurs earlier in girls than boys. The physical sequence of events is given in Chapter 168.

Psychosocial adjustments in adolescence include achievement of identity and self-image, achievement of adult sexual role, achievement of independence from parents and family, and choice of career. Medically, adolescents are prone to emotional problems, physical trauma, infectious mononucleosis, venereal disease, acne, obesity, anorexia nervosa and behavioural problems such as drug and alcohol abuse.

| Chapter 3 | *MANAGEMENT OF THE NORMAL NEWBORN BABY* |

Immediate Management

1. Umbilical Cord
If conditions permit, the cord should not be clamped immediately. Allow placental transfusion for about 1 min, clamp and then do Apgar Score (*Table* 3.1).

Table 3.1.   Evaluation of newborn baby

Apgar Score:* best scored 60s after birth of entire child and later at 5 min.
0=cardiac arrest and hence poor prognosis; 10=good prognosis.

	Score		
Sign	0	1	2
1. Heart rate	Absent	Slow (<100)	>100
2. Respiratory effort	Absent	Weak cry; hypoventilation	Good; strong cry
3. Muscle tone	Limp	Some flexion of extremities	Well flexed
4. Reflex irritability	No response	Some movement	Cry
(response to stimulation of feet)			
5. Colour	Blue; pale	Body pink; extremities blue	Completely pink

Note: Signs 1 and 2, greatest importance; 3 and 4, less; 5 least importance.
Acronym of Apgar Score:
A—appearance—colour
P—pulse—heart rate
G—grimace—reflex irritability
A—activity—muscle tone
R—respiratory—respiratory effort
*See Apgar V. (1953) Proposal for new method of evaluation of newborn infant. *Anesth. Analg.* (*Cleve.*) **32**, 260; and Apgar V. (1966) The newborn (Apgar) scoring system: reflections and advice. *Pediatr. Clin. North Am.* **13**, 645.

2. Reception
Child should be received into warm, sterile towel, dried and kept under radiant heater if any doubt about condition.

3. Identification
Attach prepared arm/foot band with mother's name and number.

4. Vitamin K₁
Give 1·0 mg orally or intramuscularly.

5. Apgar Score at 1 and 5 minutes
If infant has Apgar score of 7 or less observe closely to determine need for resuscitation. Routine suction of oropharynx not necessary and may be harmful.

Later Management

Baby is observed in nursery for first few hours while mother recuperates. Observe respirations and colour, note whether baby 'mucusy'—if so pass catheter by mouth to check for oesophageal atresia.

Check umbilical cord for number of vessels, swab with 70% alcohol or apply triple dye or antibiotic spray.

Feeding

Considerable psychological help to mother if baby put to breast shortly after birth. Then infant goes to nursery until ready for a feed as judged by experienced nurse—usually within 6 h.

Medical Examination

Made as soon as is convenient after birth on all normal infants.

Objects
To find:
1. Any ill-effects from birth process.
2. Any congenital abnormalities.

Method

a. General Observation.
Look for:
1. Obvious congenital abnormalities, e.g. Down's syndrome (mongolism), spina bifida.
2. Colour

> 2.1 Pallor (white)—a pale infant is a sick infant; pallor due either to shock or anaemia.
> 2.2 Cyanosis (blue)—normal when confined to hands, feet, around mouth; abnormal if generalized and involves mucous membranes.
> 2.3 Jaundice (yellow)—within first 24 h of life, is to be considered as due to haemolytic disease until proved otherwise.
> 2.4 Plethora (red)—polycythaemia.

3. Posture

> 3.1 Normal—infant lies on side; arms and legs flexed at side.
> 3.2 Abnormal—infant lies on back; arms and legs abducted—frog position.

4. Spontaneous movements

> 4.1 Normal—random. Asymmetrical. Note cry, and fine movements of face and individual fingers.
> 4.2 Abnormal—jerky. Symmetrical. May be big movements. Or absence of movement.

5. Reactivity to stimuli

> 5.1 In response to handling, undressing, pinprick, cotton wool stimulation of anterior nares.

5.2 In response to coincidental stimuli, e.g. door banging.

b. Top-to-toe Routine

Note: Routine examination can be by system, but for clinical convenience a good routine is to start at head and work down to toes; turn infant over and work back to head—the top-to-toe and back system.

1. Head

    1.1 Measure circumference.

    1.2 Palpate for swelling—caput or cephalhaematoma—or fracture.

    1.3 Feel fontanelles, especially tension, and over-riding of sutures.

    1.4 Note injury, e.g. from scalp electrode.

2. Face—capillary naevi over upper eyelids, central forehead, nose and upperlip—normal.

3. Eyes

    3.1 Notice any discharge—swab to laboratory if present.

    3.2 Pupil for coloboma—lens for cataract.

    Note: Infant can be made to open eyes by giving a bottle to suck or holding upright.

4. Mouth

    4.1 Open by gentle pressure on mandible—look for cleft palate. Epstein's pearls on palate in midline—normal.

    4.2 If infant bubbly or history of maternal hydramnios—pass tube to exclude oesophageal atresia.

5. Ears—note accessory auricle, fistula or meatal atresia.

6. Jaw—micrognathos.

7. Neck

    7.1 Note: short in infants. Rotate and extend neck to:

    7.2 Feel sternomastoid for haematoma in lower part. Note branchial fistula. Feel clavicle for fracture.

8. Arms and hands—note full range of movements and correct number of digits.

9. Chest

    9.1 Respiratory rate, absence of insuction, coordinated breathing.

    9.2 Auscultation of little value—râles abnormal after first few hours.

    9.3 Note heart sounds and murmurs—feel apex beat. Pulsation in xiphoid region normal in first 48h.

10. Abdomen

    10.1 Note umbilicus especially for infection or embryonic remains.

    10.2 Size of liver—normally 2 cm below costal margin.

    10.3 Feel for abnormal mass—kidneys are often felt normally.

11. External genitalia.

    11.1 Note any ambiguity of genitalia.

    11.2 Testes usually in scrotum.

    11.3 Vaginal skin tag frequent.

12. Hips—check for dislocation, *see* p. 440.
13. Femorals—palpate arteries—easier if legs flexed a little.
14. Legs and feet—note movements to be full; note posture of feet.
Turn infant over.
15. Inspect anus for patency, sphincter control.
16. Inspect and palpate back and neck—note dermal sinus or central naevus over spine.

c. Central Nervous System Evaluation

Already note made of posture, tone, reactivity, spontaneous movements.
Finally note reflexes:
    1. Those normal in neonatal period: Moro; grasping reflex of fingers and toes; extension reflex of fingers and toes; rooting reflex; sucking and swallowing; lateral trunk incurvation; Galant reflex; walking reflex.
    2. Tendon reflexes.

Multiple Births

Important to ascertain whether twins and sets of multiple births are monozygotic (identical) or dizygotic (not identical).

Criteria
    1. Study of placenta—may give confusing results.
        1.1 Dizygotic twins have two separate placentae or single dichorionic placenta.
        1.2 Monozygotic twins usually have monochorionic placenta but may have separate placentae.
    2. Sex, general appearance, hair colour, iris colour, iris pattern, blood group and serum protein pattern must *all* be identical for diagnosis of monozygosity. Environment and disease may modify height, weight and development (physical or mental).
    3. Blood groups. Of factors listed in (2), blood groups are easiest to determine and most important. Following may be tested for: A–B, M–N, P. Lewis, Kell, Duffy and Rh.
    4. Dermal patterns (dermatoglyphics). Extremely alike but never identical in monozygotic twins.
Note: Often possible to say categorically that twins are dizygotic but never possible to say categorically that they are monozygotic. Evidence will merely point to the fact that it is 99 per cent probable that they are monozygotic.

Prognosis
Second twin twice as likely to die as first. Probably from anoxia or cerebral trauma as second twin is often a breech. Aided delivery of second twin may be required.

Chapter 4   THE APPROACH TO CHILDREN

The growth of children, especially that of their brains, is greatest in infancy. Their emotional and cognitive functions develop most rapidly at this time. Adverse factors, i.e. disease and deprivation exert a disproportionately bigger effect during early life which may be irreparable. However, the rate of repair and catch-up growth is greatest in the very young.

Optimum development demands full physical, emotional and psychological support. It is vital that parents understand children and give them adequate time. The importance of both nature and nurture is greatest in infancy.

Full assessment of children must include the total family, its life-style, level of concern and anxieties.

Psychosomatic disease is a large part of contemporary paediatric practice. The child may be a mother's means of consultation about her own problems.

Children learn relationships, develop their faculties and skills through play. The doctor must know how to assess and record play. The school moulds the child's learning, understanding, social and moral values. The doctor must be able to obtain information about the school performance and to relate to the school doctors and teachers.

Children differ in their physical and physiological development and reactions to diseases or drugs. Their different metabolism and emotional activity requires an age-matched clinical, therapeutic, and personal approach. Adolescents may be treated as adults for drug dosage or clinical investigation, but their emotional development requires different handling. The pre-term infant requires a knowledge of immature physiology and a clinical attitude. Normal physiological values (e.g. Hb, blood pressure, ECG, hormone function,) are age-dependent.

History Taking

The history is extremely important. Older children can give their own history and appreciate being addressed. Evaluate the reliability of the mother as a witness; it is wise to assume that the mother is always right until proved otherwise but occasionally her history is deliberately misleading, as in the case of non-accidental injury. The history should include inherited, familial and psychological factors; emphasize the family history, the social milieu, the obstetric and perinatal history, feeding, and immunizations. Every paediatric history must include an assessment of the child's development.

Children are frightened of new situations, especially hospitals; the doctor's first encounter is crucial for relationships for many years to come. The interview starts immediately with the mother and child, with possibly the father, entering the room; the doctor observes some relationships, anxieties and possible developmental delays before they sit down. Shake hands with the parents and if the child appreciates it, with him too. Have toys within easy reach to keep him amused. At the same time, observe how he manipulates the toys and assess some of his motor skills. Allow the mother to say all that she has to say within reason. The child observes the doctor and medical students during this period and forms his own assessment. He quickly learns the way in which the doctor respects his mother. When talking to the child or examining him, it is best to be on his level, either by sitting on a lower chair or occasionally kneeling at his side. Even young children appreciate being talked to. Direct statements are preferable to questions which often threaten the child.

Examination

The examination must be conducted with the utmost gentleness; avoid pain.

Traumatic procedures such as looking at a throat should be left until the end. Warm the hands and stethoscope.

Examination of children is dependent upon mutual trust. With babies less than the age of 9 months this is easily acquired. It is best to get fairly close to them — about 2–3 feet away — and engage their attention with one's face. A smile and appropriate noises are very effective in evoking similar responses. Much of the examination can be proceeded with whilst engaging the child's attention. Thus at about the age of 9 months the infants become apprehensive of adults and often react against a direct approach. Sometimes best not to look directly at a child but to concentrate on parents and to talk to them. Children of 3 and 4 years may respond to the direct approach.

One of the best ways of obtaining a child's trust is to demonstrate to him your relationships with the parents.

If the child sees that the doctor can relate well and respect the mother and father, he will respond in a similar way. If the child cries, try to find out why — is it because he is afraid, in pain, or been hurt or frightened.

Be opportunist when examining children. If the child is asleep, seize the opportunity to examine his abdomen and auscultate the chest. These can be done without moving the sheets. Be flexible and not necessarily adhere to a rigid order of examination. Two or more separate examinations may be needed at times. Spend time winning his confidence.

Use the same method of examination as for adults, either the geographical or top-to-toe method. Leave examination of the throat and the ears until last. Observing the child is of paramount importance especially in the youngest age groups. Listening is more important in the older. Observe the mother–child interaction. In the newborn infant note the frequency of respiration, the amount of intercostal indrawing, the shape of the chest and the symmetry of movements and the child's spontaneous movements inside the incubator. The infant with the exquisitely fine individual finger, face and eye movements is likely to have an intact central nervous system.

The formal examination in the supine position is fine for the older child and very young infant, but the older infant and the toddler object to lying down, and cry. It is often best to examine them in the upright position and at times this may be the only way in which an abdomen can be examined e.g. sitting on the mother's lap and with his back to the doctor. With a little practice it is possible to examine the abdomen very satisfactorily in this position.

Infants and toddlers do not like to be undressed and it is sometimes best therefore to undertake auscultation underneath the vest. Never forget that the ward sister is extremely important in the paediatric world. Her views are of inestimable value both for diagnosis and appraisal of the infant's condition.

Chapter 5   **GENETICS**

Definitions

Alleles. Alternative forms of gene which may occupy same site on homologous chromosomes.

Autosomes. Chromosomes other than sex chromosomes.

Chromosomes. Chromophilic bodies within cell nucleus, visible as homologous pairs in dividing cells. (They consist of double chains of DNA on framework of protein.) Forty-six pairs in normal individual.

Dominant Trait. One which is determined by presence of gene even in heterozygous form.

Gene. Unit of inheritance, occupying specific site (locus) on chromosome (consists of short segment of DNA coded for synthesis of a particular polypeptide).

Heterozygous. Having different alleles at gene locus on each of a pair of homologous chromosomes.

Homozygous. Having same allele at gene locus on each of a pair of homologous chromosomes.

Karyotype. Chromosome constitution of individual (normal 46XX or 46XY).
Displayed photographically with chromosomes in groups according to size:

Group	Chromosome
A	1–3
B	4–5
C	6–12
D	13–15
E	16–18
F	19–20
G	21–22 + Y

Mosaicism. Presence of more than one cell type in single individual (for example, an individual may be mosaic of normal and trisomy 21 cells).

Mutation. Spontaneous or induced change in a gene.

Recessive Trait. One which is determined by presence of gene only in homozygous form.

Sex Chromosomes. Pair of chromosomes responsible for sex determination (XX in females, XY in males).

Sex-linked Trait. One determined by presence of gene on sex chromosomes. In practice such traits are X-linked since none is yet known to be certainly Y-linked.

Translocation. Transfer of a chromosome or segment of chromosome to site on a different chromosome.

Trisomy. Presence of one chromosome additional to the normal homologous pair.

Chromosome Disorders

Down's Syndrome (*Trisomy 21, Mongolism*)
First described in 1866 by Down. Commonest chromosome anomaly.

Aetiology
Subjects have an extra chromosome of G Group (No. 21). Condition arises in one of three ways:

1. Non-Disjunction (94%). Ovum to be fertilized contains 24 chromosomes, i.e. an extra 21 chromosome, which resulted from unequal chromosome distribution at cell division (meiosis) in ovary. This type of abnormality occurs particularly in older women, towards end of reproductive life. Abnormal spermatozoa produced by males are non-competitive with normal sperm, but only one ovum released each month and if abnormal it may be fertilized. Hence only maternal age important in pathogenesis.

2. Mosaicism (3%). Unequal distribution of chromosomes during cell division *after* fertilization. Some cells then have 46 (normal) chromosomes, others 47 (trisomy 21).

Cell population with 45 chromosomes (monosomy 21) should be present but in practice seems to die out. Clinical features of Down's syndrome often milder in mosaics.

3. Translocation (3%). Cells of patient contain 46 chromosomes, one of which is combination of a chromosome 21 and another chromosome, usually group D or G. If normal parent is a carrier of 'balanced' translocation, with 45 discrete chromosomes but material from 46 normal chromosomes, then cell division will always result in unequal chromosome distribution and possibility of fertilized ovum containing extra chromosome material.

Translocation carrier state should be identified if present in young parents of affected child, because of risk of recurrence.

Risk of translocation carrier mother having affected child 10%; less if father carrier. Translocation carriers may be sporadic (50%) or inherited (50%).

Overall recurrence risk if neither parent translocation carrier is 1%.

Incidence
1 in 600 live births. Incidence rises with maternal age to 2% over age 40.

Clinical Features
N.B. None are pathognomonic in isolation, syndrome identified by combination of several of following features (usually without difficulty).

1. General. Hypotonia, hyperflexible joints, small stature, mental retardation, but usually sociable and happy.
2. Facies. Flat face and occiput, small nose.
3. Eyes. Upward slant (mongoloid) to palpebral fissures. Inner epicanthic folds. Speckling of iris, especially in blue-eyed subjects (Brushfield's spots). Fine lens opacities, tendency to blepharitis. Strabismus.
4. Ears. Small, simple, sometimes protruding.
5. Mouth. Hypoplasia of teeth, irregularity common. Tongue fissured ('scrotal'), not enlarged but frequently protruded.
6. Neck. Short, redundant nape evident in newborn.
7. Hands. Short digits, relatively broad hand. Hypoplasia middle phalanx fifth finger, with clinodactyly (incurving tip). Single palmar crease (Simian crease: N.B. present in 1% normal individuals). Dermatoglyphics: Excess ulnar loops on fingertips. Distal location of palmar triradius (*Fig. 5.1*).
8. Feet. Wide space and plantar crease between first and second toes.
9. Skin. Cutis marmorata, dry skin in older individuals. Hair soft and sparse.
10. Heart. Congenital malformation in 40%, particularly septal defects.
11. Genitalia. Cryptorchidism, small genitalia and infertility in males.
12. Gastrointestinal. Duodenal atresia, oesophageal atresia.
13. Blood. Lymphoblastic leukaemia in 1%.

Natural History
If child survives neonatal period and has no cardiac malformation, life expectancy not much reduced. Hypotonia improves but IQ tends to fall with age. Behaviour and emotional problems may appear at adolescence. Prognosis for IQ better if

Fig. 5.1. Distribution of digital patterns in the normal hand and that of Down's syndrome. The solid lines and dotted lines denote the dermal ridge configurations and dashes within the palm represent the creases. (By kind permission of the publishers of *Recognisable Patterns of Human Malformation*.)

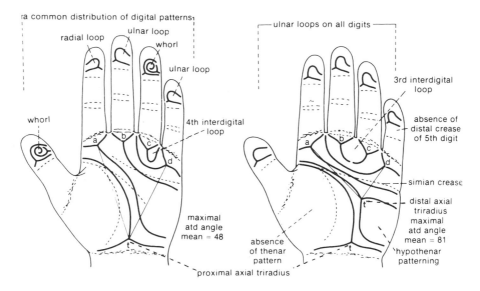

child kept at home, i.e. not in institution, and given developmentally orientated stimulation programme.

Management

1. In early infancy child needs same care as any other baby. Retardation in achieving milestones becomes evident later.

2. Parents need support particularly during first year of life if they are to accept child emotionally.

3. Early training with specific limited objectives helpful to both mother and child, e.g. feeding, dressing, toilet training, etc.

4. Group therapy may be beneficial.

5. Older child needs special school, occasional 'social' admissions to suitable hospital or home to allow parents holiday alone.

6. Medical problems, e.g. frequent respiratory infections, cardiac defect, treated on individual merits.

Trisomy 13 (*Patau's Syndrome*) (*Fig. 5.2*)

Incidence
1 in 5000 live births.

Aetiology
Similar to Down's syndrome. More frequent with advanced maternal age. Patient has additional chromosome 13.

Clinical Features (Not all present in one individual)
General. Failure to thrive, severe mental retardation, minor motor convulsions.

Fig. 5.2. Features of trisomy 13(Patau's syndrome). (By kind permission of *Guy's Hospital Reports*.)

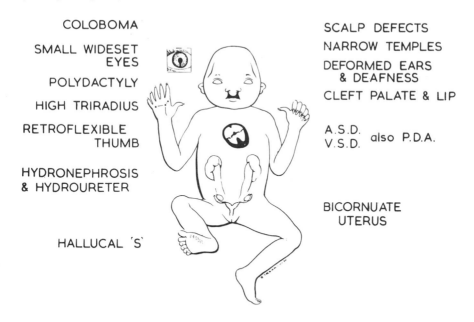

COLOBOMA

SMALL WIDESET EYES

POLYDACTYLY

HIGH TRIRADIUS

RETROFLEXIBLE THUMB

HYDRONEPHROSIS & HYDROURETER

HALLUCAL 'S'

SCALP DEFECTS

NARROW TEMPLES

DEFORMED EARS & DEAFNESS

CLEFT PALATE & LIP

A.S.D. V.S.D. also P.D.A.

BICORNUATE UTERUS

Facies. Midline or bilateral cleft lip and palate, sloping forehead arrhinencephaly (hypoplasia of frontal lobes of brain). Microphthalmia or anophthalmia, colobomas of eye, large nose.
Hands. Polydactyly, hyperconvex fingernails, Simian crease, retroflexible thumb.
Feet. Protuberant heel.
Other. Cardiac defect (80%), particularly septal defects, patent ductus arteriosus. Cryptorchidism. Deafness. Capillary haemangiomas. Single umbilical artery.

Natural History
Forty-four per cent die in first month, only 18% survive first year. Survivors have severe mental defect, failure to thrive and convulsions.

Trisomy 18 (*Edwards' Syndrome*) (*Fig. 5.3*)

Incidence
1 in 3000 live births. Female preponderance 3 : 1.

Aetiology
Similar to Down's syndrome. More frequent with advanced maternal age. Patient has additional chromosome 18.

Clinical Features (Not all present in one individual)
General. Low birth weight, marked failure to thrive, feeble cry. Maternal polyhydramnios. Mental retardation, increased muscle tone. May be postmature.
Facies. Prominent occiput, low set ears, micrognathia, narrow palatal arch.
Hands. Fingers flexed, index finger over middle, small finger over ring. Hypoplasia of nails.

Fig. 5.3. Features of trisomy 18 (Edwards' syndrome). (By kind permission of *Guy's Hospital Reports.*)

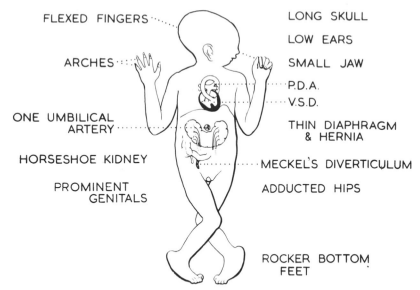

FLEXED FINGERS
ARCHES
ONE UMBILICAL ARTERY
HORSESHOE KIDNEY
PROMINENT GENITALS

LONG SKULL
LOW EARS
SMALL JAW
P.D.A.
V.S.D.
THIN DIAPHRAGM & HERNIA
MECKEL'S DIVERTICULUM
ADDUCTED HIPS
ROCKER BOTTOM FEET

Feet. Rocker bottom feet with vertical talus.
Other. Cardiac defect (VSD or PDA). Cryptorchidism. Hernias. Renal malformations.

Natural History
Thirty per cent die in first month, only 10% survive first year as severely mentally retarded, abnormally small infants.

Other Autosomal Anomalies
Rare but distinct malformation syndromes associated with partial deletion of chromosomes 4, 5 ('Cri-du-chat' syndrome), 18, 21. All have growth failure, severe mental retardation and a variety of malformations.

Turner's Syndrome (*XO Syndrome*)

Incidence
1 in 2500 live female births.

Aetiology
Maldistribution of chromosomes at cell division leading to individual with 45 chromosomes, a single X being only sex chromosome present. Evidence that paternal sex chromosome most likely to be missing, maternal age unimportant. Mosaics XO/XX occasionally found.

Clinical Features
General. Low birth weight, growth retardation. Intelligence usually normal. Oedema of hands and feet in neonate. Perceptive deafness common. Primary amenorrhoea and infertility, except in some mosaics.

Facies. Epicanthic folds, high arched palate, prominent ears.
Trunk and limbs. Webbing of neck, low posterior hairline, redundant nape in infancy. Broad chest, widely spaced nipples. Cubitus valgus of elbow (wide carrying angle). Hyperconvex fingernails.
Gonads. Ovarian dysgenesis or complete absence of germinal tissue. Occasional cystic or malignant change.
Other. Cardiac defect (20%), especially coarctation of aorta. Renal malformations. Pyloric stenosis. May have growth hormone deficiency.

Management
1. Cyclical oestrogen therapy commenced at time of normal puberty. Stature not influenced by growth hormone, anabolic steroids reported beneficial in occasional patient.
2. Cardiac malformations, etc. treated in usual way.
3. Plastic surgery for webbed neck, ears may be indicated.
4. Psychological support often required for problems of small stature, infertility, etc.

Noonan's Syndrome
Rare condition with features of Turner's syndrome in male or female.

Aetiology
No demonstrable chromosome abnormality. Cause unknown. Occasionally familial.

Clinical Features
Short stature, mild mental retardation (40%), facies, ears, neck, chest, elbows as in Turner's syndrome, cardiac defect (50%) especially pulmonary stenosis and septal defects, small genitalia, cryptorchidism, lymphatic abnormalities.

Management
Treatment of individual problems on merit.

Klinefelter's Syndrome (*XXY Syndrome*)

Incidence
1 in 500 live male births.

Aetiology
Antithesis of Turner's syndrome. Affected male has 47 chromosomes, two X chromosomes in addition to normal Y.

Clinical Features
May be mildly mentally retarded. Tall stature, poor musculature, small testes, with normal Leydig cells but atrophy of seminiferous tubules, delayed puberty, gynaecomastia (60%). Infertile. Behaviour and emotional problems common. Not usually detected during childhood.

Management
Methyltestosterone 20–40mg/day may reduce gynaecomastia. Treatment of emotional and educational problems.

XYY SYNDROME
Incidence

1 in 500 live male births.

Aetiology
Male with extra Y chromosome, i.e. 47 XYY.

Clinical Features
Tall stature, aggressive behaviour, tendency to crimes of violence. Rarely detected during childhood.

Management
No medical treatment available. Some XYY individuals avoid social problems and ethics of revealing chromosome status discovered incidentally debatable.

Fragile X Syndrome (*See* p. 360)

Single Gene Disorders

Each gene carries code for synthesis of a single protein. If abnormal, disease state or malformation results (*a*) when gene is dominant, i.e. inherited from one parent, who will also be affected; (*b*) when recessive but present in homozygous form, i.e. inherited from both parents, who are asymptomatic carriers; or (*c*) when recessive but X-linked and transmitted from asymptomatic mother to affected son. Consanguinity increases risk that parents carry same abnormal gene, hence many recessive diseases have high incidence of parental consanguinity. Inborn biochemical errors mostly recessive.

Genetic disorders responsible for many childhood diseases and are dealt with throughout book in relevant sections, e.g. inborn errors of metabolism, congenital malformations, systemic diseases.

Genetic Counselling

Given to advise parents, patient (if appropriate) and relatives of risks of recurrence of illness.

First step is to obtain accurate diagnosis of patient's disease, then accurate family history. For some illnesses, e.g. cystic fibrosis, autosomal recessive risk is well known. For others with partial and complex inheritance, family tree essential. Sometimes empirical risks have to be given in these cases. Where inheritance in doubt, consult text book, e.g. McKusick, V.A. (1983) *Mendelian Inheritance in Man*, Baltimore, Johns Hopkins University Press.

Genetic counselling often carries implication of amniocentesis and abortion of affected infant. Parents' views on abortion vary widely as do state laws. Counsellors should be sensitive to parents' cues about their feelings and be sympathetic and understanding; they should not impose their own views directly or by implication. Manner of presenting risks can influence parents' decisions, e.g. with autosomal recessive risk can be presented as a 1 : 4 chance of recurrence or a 75% chance of a normal child. Factor of great importance is whether illness likely to be fatal in early life, e.g. Tay–Sachs disease, or have a steadily relentless course over years, e.g. Duchenne dystrophy.

Bibliography

Harper P. S. (1984) *Practical Genetic Counselling*, 2nd ed.Bristol, Wright.
McKusick V. A. (1983) *Mendelian Inheritance in Man*. 6th ed. Baltimore, Johns Hopkins University Press.
Smith D. W. (1982) Recognisable patterns of human malformation. 3rd ed. In: *Major Problems in Clinical Pediatrics*. Vol. VII. Philadelphia, Saunders.

Chapter 6   # AETIOLOGY OF CONGENITAL MALFORMATIONS

Definition
Macroscopic abnormalities of structure attributable to faulty development and present at birth. Recognition may be immediately obvious or require the affected organ to be worked (e.g. gut atresia) or complications to reveal the abnormality. Some may escape recognition. Congenital malformations may be caused by one or more different factors, which may interact. In any particular instance, it is often impossible to establish exact cause.

Factors involved
(1) Heredity: (*a*) Chromosomal; (*b*) Genetic; (2) Infections; (3) Mechanical injuries; (4) Endocrine disturbances; (5) Chemical poisons; (6) Radiation hazards; (7) Maternal age and multiparity.

Heredity

1. Chromosomal Abnormalities
Certain chromosomal anomalies have a high incidence of associated congenital malformations, e.g.

Down's Syndrome (Trisomy 21)—Cardiac malformations (A–V canal defects, Fallot's tetralogy), duodenal atresia.

Trisomy 13 (Patau's Syndrome)—Polydactyly, cardiac malformations, microphthalmia, cerebral malformations, cleft lip and palate.

Trisomy 18, (Edwards' Syndrome)—Micrognathia, cardiac malformations, rocker-bottom feet.

Turner's Syndrome (X and variants)—Webbed neck, cardiac malformations (coarctation), pyloric stenosis.

2. Single-gene Defects
2.1 Dominant. Some cataracts, some cleft lip/palate, some polydactyly, neurofibromatosis, some craniosynosto-

sis, Treacher Collins syndrome, cleidocranial dysostosis, Marfan's syndrome.

One in two chance that a child of affected person will be similarly affected.

2.2 Autosomal Recessive. Most inborn biochemical errors are recessive (Chapter 49) and some produce congenital malformations, e.g. Morquio's syndrome (mucopolysaccharidosis IV), adrenogenital syndrome.

One in four chance that future infants will be affected.

Other recessives: Some cleft lip/palate, congenital ichthyosis, Fanconi's pancytopenia with skeletal defects, some cataract.

2.3 X-linked Recessive. Some cataracts, some hydrocephalus, some microcephaly.

One in two chance that carrier female will have affected son or carrier daughter.

2.4. X-linked Dominant (lethal in males). ? Orofacialdigital syndrome, ? incontinentia pigmenti.

2.5 Polygenic—Some cleft lip/palate, pyloric stenosis, spina bifida, dislocated hip.

Infections*

Intra-uterine infections, e.g.

Rubella (p. 81). Cataracts, microphthalmia, cardiac malformations (PDA).

Toxoplasmosis (p. 111). Hydrocephalus, microcephaly.

Cytomegalovirus infection (p. 91). Hydrocephalus, microcephaly.

Herpes simplex. CNS malformations.

Varicella-zoster virus. Multiple defects, skin scars, limb hypoplasia, choroidoretinitis.

Endocrine Disturbances

Excess of sex hormones may act on fetus, e.g. androgens on female leading to pseudohermaphroditism (*see* p. 470).

Maternal long acting thyroid stimulator (LATS) may lead to congenital goitre (*see* p. 476).

Nutritional Disturbances

1. Due to faulty implantation of ovum.
2. Due to maternal dietary deficiency, e.g.
   2.1 Iodine. Leading to congenital goitre or cretinism.
   2.2 Vitamin deficiency. Known to cause cleft palate, etc. in rats. In humans is a probable factor in aetiology of neural tube defects.

*See *Br. Med. Bull.* (1976) **32**, 1.

Mechanical Injuries leading to Deformities

Oligohydramnios can lead to talipes or pulmonary hypoplasia—associated with renal agenesis. Breech delivery more common in congenital dislocation of hip. Congenital amputations may be produced by amniotic bands.

Drugs

Conradi's syndrome occurs after warfarin. Fetal alcohol syndrome occurs in about 10 per cent of women taking more than one ounce of strong liquor daily. Increasing frequency with greater intake. Features: small for dates, persistent growth deficit, short palpebral fissures, epicanthic folds, hypoplasia of maxilla and mandible, thin upper lip, heart and joint abnormalities. Mental deficiency.

Note: No drug should be given to a pregnant woman during early months of pregnancy unless absolutely essential.

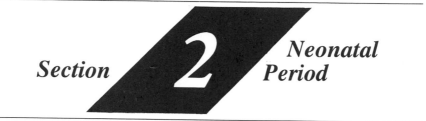

| Chapter 7 | *INFANT MORTALITY AND MORBIDITY* |

Perinatal Mortality and Morbidity

Perinatal mortality rate is the number of stillbirths and first-week deaths per 1000 total births. Rate in 1983 in the UK was about 10—stillbirths and first-week deaths approximately equal. Causes: placental failure (25%), toxaemia and other pregnancy complications (10%), congenital abnormalities (25%), hypoxia (20%). birth injury (5%), infection, haemolytic disease. Most of these conditions cause pre-term birth which is the biggest single factor.

Neonatal Mortality

Figures published refer to number of infants dying during first 4 weeks of extra-utcrinc lifc pcr 1000 live births.

Incidence
Moderate but steady decrease in number of deaths since beginning of century.
    1906–10 rate about 40 per 1000 live births (England and Wales).
    1952 rate was 15·2 per 1000 live births.
    1962 rate was 13·0 per 1000 live births.
    1972 rate was 9·8 per 1000 live births.
    1982 rate was 6·3 per 1000 live births.

Infant Mortality

Figures published refer to number of infants dying during first 12 months of life per 1000 live births.

Incidence
Steady and well-marked decrease in number of deaths since beginning of century.
    1906–10 rate about 118 per 1000 live births (England and Wales).
    1952 rate was 24·1 per 1000 live births.
    1962 rates was 19·6 per 1000 live births.
    1972 rate was 15·6 per 1000 live births.
    1982 rate was 10·8 per 1000 live births.

Cause of Improvement
Largely due to control of infection by antibiotics, and better health and social environment by community. This is shown by following facts:

1. Rate lower in Social Class I than in Class V.*
2. Rate lower in most prosperous and health-conscious countries.
3. Rate lower in more prosperous parts of Great Britain.

For further lowering of infant mortality rate, effort must be directed towards following:

1. Better social conditions, especially adequate housing to prevent over-crowding.
2. Better protection from injury, e.g. burns and poisons.

Chapter 8   # INFANT FEEDING

The natural method is breast feeding, which is possible for more than 90% of women. Modified cow's milk is the next convenient alternative when necessary. Special formulae are required for particular clinical indications, e.g. Cow's milk allergy, phenylketonuria.

Composition of Human and Cow's Milk

Protein
Higher in cow's milk. Mainly casein in cow's milk, which forms a tough curd. Mainly α-lactalbumin (whey protein) in human milk, which is soluble and easily digested. Cow's milk allergy often due to β-lactoglobulin, absent from human milk. Differences in amino-acid content (e.g. relatively low taurine in cow's milk) make utilization of cow's milk protein less efficient and excess is excreted.

Table 8.1.   Approximate percentage composition for mature milk

	Protein					
	Lactalbumin	*Casein*	*Total*	*Fat*	*Carbohydrate*	*Minerals*
Cow's milk	0·5	3·0	3·5	3·5	4·5	0·7
Breast milk	0·7	0·4	1·1	3·5	7·5	0·2

Note: All figures in g/dl milk, but very variable.

Fat
Most variable constituent and fatty acid composition may be modified by maternal diet. Fat content higher in milk obtained at end of breast feed than at the beginning.

Carbohydrate
Occurs as lactose. Jejunal lactase breaks this down into glucose and galactose before absorption.

---

*Social classes used by Registrar-General for statistical purposes: Class I, Upper and professional classes; Class II, Intermediate between I and III; Class III, Skilled workers; Class IV, Intermediate between III and V; Class V, Unskilled workers.

Minerals
Include calcium, phosphorus, iron, copper and zinc. Iron content lower in human than cow's milk, but absorption is better. Calcium content of breast milk lower than cow's milk, but high phosphate content of unmodified cow's milk produces reciprocal depression of serum calcium after absorption and may produce neonatal tetany. Modified (humanized) infant formulae have a $Ca:PO_4$ ratio resembling breast milk.

Vitamins
Neither breast nor cow's milk contains adequate amounts of vitamin D after the first few months. Extra oral vitamin D supplements are needed in babies not exposed to sunshine. Vitamin C content varies with maternal diet. It is usually adequate for the first few months. Goat's milk is deficient in folic acid and unsuitable for feeding young infants unless supplemented.

Caloric Value
About 20 kcal/30 ml for both human and cow's milk.

Antenatal Preparation for Breast Feeding

Talks and group discussions help develop a positive attitude to breast feeding. Ideally the husband should be included as his support is a major factor in determining later success.

Methods of Preparation
Lactation clinic should be routine part of antenatal care.
1. *In early stage of pregnancy* for inspection of breast and nipples.
   For efficient feeding, nipple should be able to be pulled out easily so that baby can draw it well back into mouth. If this is not possible infant will nibble the end and damage it. If nipple inverted, nipple shield should be worn under well-fitting brassière. These shields have hole in centre through which nipple projects, pressure being applied to surrounding breast tissue. Shield may have to be worn throughout pregnancy if nipples poorly developed. Effect is to loosen nipple so that it is no longer inverted.
2. *At about thirtieth week of pregnancy*. Instruction should be given on manual expression of milk. Reasons:

> 2.1 Regular removal of colostrum during pregnancy helps to develop the sinuses and duct system and prevent them becoming blocked with inspissated material, so preventing engorgement of breast when the milk 'comes in' at term.
> 2.2 If mother has been instructed during pregnancy she can easily express milk in postnatal period if necessary, e.g.
> 2.2.1 To relieve breast engorgement.
> 2.2.2 To supply breast milk for bottle feeding if baby cannot be put to breast.
> *Method of Manual Expression* either by compression of whole breast, starting at periphery and working towards areola: this is repeated several times; or by pinching over lactiferous sinuses with thumb and forefinger of hand while other hand supports breast.

Frequency: Manual expression should be performed for about 5 min every day until term.

Physiology of Lactation

Suckling promotes milk secretion via prolactin (anterior pituitary) and milk ejection via oxytocin (posterior pituitary). Therefore, frequent suckling, particularly during the first few days, is the best way to stimulate milk production. Misguided attempts to 'satisfy the baby's hunger' by giving complementary bottle feeds usually result in inhibition of lactation as the contented infant no longer suckles adequately to ensure a good milk supply. Reduced milk output is then followed by more complementary feeds, creating a vicious circle. Release of oxytocin during suckling causes contraction of smooth muscle in the lactiferous ducts, and milk ejection. This may cause mother to feel the 'draught' or 'let down'—a sensation of tingling in both breasts accompanied by flow of milk and sometimes by uterine contractions ('after pains').

Rooting Reflex

If a newborn baby's cheek is touched, he turns his mouth towards object which touched it. When baby put to breast, the nipple touches cheek and, baby turns mouth towards it.

Technique of Breast Feeding

Baby should be put to breast, making use of rooting reflex. With mother's help, the baby should grasp the nipple with his mouth and draw it back so that it comes to lie between base of tongue and soft palate. The whole nipple and as much of areola as possible should be taken. Poor fixing to the nipple with the infant merely nibbling the tip, leads to inadequate feeding and sore nipples. Bringing up wind (burping) during and at the end of the feed is a harmless ritual. The baby is held upright, on the lap or over the shoulder, until swallowed air is eructed.

Frequency of Feeding

Initial feed should be as soon as possible after birth, preferably in labour ward: this assists uterine contraction, mother–child bonding, and effectiveness of lactation. At first colostrum is of small volume, but rich in immunoglobulins. Frequent short periods of suckling on demand more effectively establish lactation than longer feeds at fixed intervals. 'Rooming-in' of mother and baby facilitates demand feeding. Mother and baby will generally adopt a mutually agreed routine after the first few weeks but the principle of demand feeding should continue and a crying baby should be offered the breast. When frequency of feeding falls below 5 or 6 in 24 h, maternal prolactin level falls and monthly cycle (and fertility) is resumed.

Failure of Lactation

Preconceived Failure
A few mothers never intend to feed their young for a variety of reasons. Examples:
1. Memory of pain from previous cracked nipple or breast abscess.

2. Failure to feed successfully on previous occasion.
3. Desire for freedom if someone else available to give bottle.
4. Cosmetic—fear of spoiling figure.
5. Deep psychological revulsion.

Failure during Neonatal Period
1. Inadequate nipples

>1.1 If nipple inverted baby cannot grasp it properly and feeding may be impossible.
>
>1.2 If nipple poorly protracted baby tries to grasp it, but instead of drawing it into mouth properly and thus biting on areola, he bites on nipple, damaging it and causing fissures to form.
>
>1.2.1 During pregnancy nipple should be examined and nipple shield prescribed if necessary.
>
>1.2.2 Proper fixing to the nipple at each feed.
>
>1.2.3 Baby should never be put to breast if mother complains of pain. Nipple should be examined carefully for fissure, which may be minute. If present, baby should not be put to that breast until fissure has healed. Meanwhile milk must be expressed manually and given by bottle. Fissure can be helped to heal by application of lanolin.

2. Engorged breasts. In some women, especially primiparae, milk comes in rapidly and engorgement results.

Clinical Features

Symptoms: Mother complains of considerable aching and pain in breasts which keep her awake at night. Feeding infant often agonizing, as cracked nipple almost inevitable.

On Examination: Breasts hot, hard and oedematous. Individual lobules can be palpated giving 'knotted' feel. Milk does not escape spontaneously nor can it be readily induced to do so. Baby at breast obtains no milk.

Progress without Treatment. During second week engorgement lessens and involution of breast occurs. For a time baby is kept on complementary feeds but flow of milk gradually ceases and by about three weeks breast feeding has usually been abandoned.

Prevention. Routine antenatal expression of colostrum (*see* p. 27) helps to prevent or lessen this complication.

Treatment

>*2.1 Administration of oestrogens*: not usually necessary.
>
>*2.2 Local treatment*: Cold packs may be of value.
>
>*2.3 Manual expression of milk*: Usually not possible when breasts acutely engorged, but should be performed as soon as possible afterwards to prevent involution.

Progress with Treatment. Danger is that involution will proceed unchecked. Breasts must be completely emptied by manual expression until they have recovered sufficiently for baby to be suckled.

Complications of Breast Engorgement

i. *Cracked nipple*: Almost inevitably occurs if infant is put to engorged breast.

ii. *Breast abscess*: May follow from cracked nipple. For signs, symptoms and treatment, *see* surgical textbooks.

Note: Gross breast engorgement as here described is rare. A 'segment' of breast may be involved if a duct is blocked, but the remainder of the breast is normal.

3. Failure of Milk Supply. Usually occurs about ninth day when mother gone home.

3.1 Causes

3.1.1 May be due to (*1*) or (*2*) above.

3.1.2 Due to mother having to recommence housework.

3.1.3 Due to worry at being in sole charge of baby.

3.1.4. Maternal illness.

3.2 Prevention

3.2.1 Some help in home should always be provided when mother resumes her household duties.

3.2.2 Mothers—particularly   primiparae—should   be taught how to look after baby during lying-in period.

3.2.3 Breasts must be completely emptied of milk at each feed. Often manual expression after baby has finished will reveal that some milk remains. This can be given by spoon if baby requires it. *Greatest stimulus to milk production is an empty breast.*

3.2.4 Both breasts must be given at each feed.

3.3 Management and Treatment

3.3.1 *Test weighing*: If baby is not gaining weight adequately, quantity of breast milk he is receiving can be calculated by weighing him before and after each feed. Gain in weight equals quantity of milk ingested.

Precautions: (1) Baby must be weighed in same garments before and after in case he has passed urine or stool during feed.(2) If test weighing performed, baby should theoretically be weighed before and after *all* feeds during a 24-h period as milk yield varies greatly from feed to feed, the early morning feed usually being larger than the others. This greatly reduces the value of test weighing in practice. (3) Test weighing only occasionally required. Should not be repeated for many days as it is time-consuming for nurses and worries mother.

3.3.2 If on expressing it is found that mother only produces small quantity of milk then baby obviously not getting enough.

3.3.3 *Complementary feeds*: If on test weighing it is found that infant is not getting enough milk from breast, calculated amount can be made up by giving expressed breast or cow's milk by spoon or bottle after child has finished at breast.

Important Note: In most women lactation is established slowly and baby receives equivalent of 50ml/kg on fourth day, 110ml by seventh day, and often does not receive 160ml/kg until after tenth day. Baby's weight therefore drops during first few days of life, only slowly rising to reach birthweight again by about tenth day. Complementary feeds should very rarely be given as they will tend to further suppress milk supply: baby's hunger is necessary stimulus to adequate suckling and milk production.

Failure after Neonatal Period
Many mothers who give up breast feeding after neonatal period do so for reasons which have foundations in neonatal period, e.g. cracked nipples or engorged breasts. Other reasons:

1. Minor difficulties. Mother often told by grandmother, nurse or doctor that these will disappear if child put on bottle.
2. Social, e.g. mother has to return to work.
3. Admission of mother or baby to hospital. Should never be cause for stopping breast feeding. If possible mother and baby should be admitted together. If not possible mother's milk should be expressed by hand and given to infant by bottle.

Failure to Thrive at the Breast
Occasionally a sleepy or easily satisfied baby may not suck adequately to stimulate milk secretion, and fails to thrive without protest. Awareness of this possibility leads to diagnosis by observation and test weighing. Management is difficult but includes stimulation of infant during feeds.

Drugs in Breast Milk (*Table* 8.2)
Nearly all drugs may enter breast milk but some only as inactive metabolites. The quantity in the milk is related to such factors as lipid or water solubility, pKa (ionization) and unknown transport mechanisms.

Table 8.2.   Drugs excreted in breast milk

Forbidden drugs	Need supervision	Not excreted
Radioactive drugs	Steroids	Codeine
Tetracyclines	Nalidixic acid	Liquid paraffin
Iodides	Phenytoin	Morphine
Ergot	Barbiturates	
Atropine	Lithium	
Metronidazole	Reserpine	
Cathartics	Sulphonamides	
Antithyroid drugs	Diazepam	
	Anticoagulants (oral)	

Artificial Feeding
Milk from many types of mammals can theoretically be used, e.g. cows, goats, asses. In practice cow's milk mainly employed.

Varieties of Cow's Milk
1. Liquid Milk. N.B. Unmodified cow's milk should not be used for children under the age of 6 months. Main dangers are (*a*) hypernatraemia from high solute load which exceeds the ability of the young kidney to compensate by excretion of concentrated urine, (*b*) sensitization to cow's milk protein with risk of eczema, (*c*) occult blood loss from small intestine, (*d*) in first 2 weeks, high phosphate load depresses the infant's serum calcium and may cause neonatal tetany with convulsions. For older children the following possibilities exist:

> *1.1 Untreated.* Should never under any circumstances be used owing to danger of infection, e.g. from tuberculosis, brucellosis, streptococci, etc.
>
> *1.2 Pasteurized Milk.* Bacteriologically safe if efficiently pasteurized.

1:3 Boiled Milk
1.3.1 Safe from infection.
1.3.2 Boiling denatures protein so that curds are smaller, also alters fat, thus rendering assimilation by infant easier.

2. Dried Milk. Usually obtainable as 'humanized' preparations with protein and sodium content reduced to resemble those of human milk. Fat content varies according to source, and fatty acid composition usually very different from breast milk.

Advantages

2.1 Convenient to use: Method of preparation as per instructions on container.
2.2 Sterile when first opened and remains almost completely so while being used.
2.3 Protein denatured by drying process.
2.4 Easy to carry when travelling and no upset from change of milk occurs. Unopened tin keeps for several months.
2.5 Fact that milk is dried not fluid cuts down cost of transportation.

3. Prepacked liquid formulae. Relatively expensive compared with dried milks but have the advantages of not requiring preparation and consistently correct concentration.

4. Liquid evaporated milk has similar advantages to dried milk powders, but disadvantage that when tin opened it only keeps as well as fresh milk.

5. Liquid sweeted condensed milk contains about 45% added sugar. Should never be used for feeding babies.

Nutrient Requirements of a Milk for Infants

1. Energy. 64–72 kcal/dl.
2. Protein. 1·8–2·8 g/100 kcal   (1·2–1·9 g/dl)   as   good   quality   protein (amino acids similar to human milk).
3. Fat. 4–6 g/100 kcal (2·7–4·1 g/dl) (should be readily absorbed and contain about 3–6% of total calories as linoleic acid).
4. Carbohydrate. 8–12 g/100   kcal   (5·4–8·2 g/dl)   preferably   as   lactose, sucrose or maltodextrin.
5. Sodium, potassium and chloride. The sum of these ions should not be less than 20 mEq/l or greater than 50 mEq/l. (Sodium should not be less than 8 mEq/l and not be more than 12 mEq/l.)
6. Calcium. Minimum of 34 mg/dl.
7. Phosphorus. Minimum of 25 mg/dl and maximum 35 mg/dl. Ca/P ratio not less than 1·2 and not more than 2·0.
8. Vitamins (*see* Chapter 42).

Quantity of Milk

1. Impossible to make exact rules.
2. Most babies fed *ad libitum* take correct amount for satisfactory growth, but some take excess and become obese and a few insufficient and fail to thrive.
3. Range in first month—120–200 ml/kg/day.
   Range in fourth month—120–150 ml/kg/day.
4. Accurate weighing every 2 weeks and use of centile charts recommended.

Preparation of Bottles and Teats for Feeds
1. Chemical. Use of commercial hypochlorite solution to soak bottles and teats satisfactory if following points noted:
> 1.1 Solution readily inactivated by traces of protein (milk), so clean bottles and teats with detergent before complete immersion in solution.
> 1.2 At least 3h immersion in fresh solution (made at least every 24h).
> 1.3 Bottle not 'sterile' so milk must be used immediately or within 24h if stored in a refrigerator.

2. Boiling. Satisfactory if fully submerged and boiled for 15 min.

Preparation of Feed
1. Strict hygiene (but not surgical sterilizing) is essential.
2. Follow manufacturer's instructions (these vary).
3. Never add extra powder or evaporated milk.
4. Measure scoop accurately—do not heap or compress powder.
6. Water used must be pathogen free. Warm water mixes more easily with powder than boiling or cold.
7. Feed accepted at room temperature or 37°C.

Food Supplements

Vitamins
Essential that every baby should have:

1. Vitamin C
For requirements, *see* Chapter 42.

2. Vitamin D
For requirements, *see* Chapter 42. Supplements necessary for low birth weight babies.

3. Other Vitamins
> *3.1. Vitamin A.* Adequate quantity present in milk.
> *3.2. Vitamin B Complex.* Supplements not required for babies on a normal diet. Addition is important when infant is on special milk for metabolic disease.

Vitamins should be continued until baby receiving full mixed diet.

Iron
Adequate intake essential, and supplements may be needed for low birth weight babies with poor iron stores.

Fluoride
Supplement may be given as a prophylaxic against dental caries where water content inadequate.

Weaning

Definition
'To teach sucking child to feed otherwise than from the breast' (*Concise Oxford*

Dictionary), but term commonly used when child, on breast or bottle, commences food other than milk.

Age of Weaning

Most authorities advocate that small additions should be made to diet from 4 to 6 months of age, but great variations occur in what individual baby will take. Appetite should be respected and food must not be forced.

Advantages of Mixed Feeding

1. Less trouble is experienced in weaning if additions to diet made by small increases over long time.
2. Milk alone contains inadequate quantity of iron. Sufficient quantity not obtained until solid food is taken.
3. Enables more calories to be given without increasing volume of feed.

Danger of too Vigorous Weaning

1. Hypernatraemia.
2. Immunological insult.
3. Obesity.

Method

1. Give one food at a time.
2. Cereal, vegetable or meat purée/fruit purée (minimum of sugar) all acceptable. Egg if meat not available.

Chapter 9 PERINATAL INJURY

Birth injury includes damage to the nervous system from asphyxia (before and during delivery) and physical birth trauma.

Physical Birth Trauma

Serious birth trauma now much less common with improvements in obstetric antenatal care and delivery practice.

Superficial Trauma

1. Abrasions and Blisters. Occur on scalp and face after forceps or Ventouse-assisted delivery. Also on buttocks, labia, scrotum and lower limbs in breech presentations.
2. Petechiae and Bruising. Usually confined to head and neck after prolonged labour or cord around neck. Sometimes associated with subconjunctival haemorrhage.
3. Incisions. Rarely after Caesarean section. Sutures sometimes required. Removal of scalp electrodes for fetal monitoring occasionally produce tears.
4. Subcutaneous Fat Necrosis. More common in fat babies following pressure during labour. Secondary infection can occur.

Fractures

Clavicle
Commonest birth fracture. Usually, but not always, caused by difficult delivery, usually detected on routine examination.

Signs
1. Child may not move arm. Moro reflex diminished or absent on affected side. Crepitus may be elicited.
2. Condition often remains unrecognized until lump noticed on clavicle due to development of callus at site of fracture; callus forms within week and may be profuse.
Treatment. None required and prognosis excellent.

Humerus

Usually caused by difficulty in bringing down extended arm. Crack may be heard by obstetrician.
Signs. Arm hangs limp, pseudoparalysis.
Treatment. Immobilization. Light splint often required for about 10 days.
Prognosis. Good.
Note: Associated brachial plexus injury must be looked for (*see below*).

Femur

Very rare. Usually caused by difficulty in bringing down extended leg in breech delivery.
Signs. Crepitus may be felt and leg hangs limp.
Treatment. Immobilization in extension.

Skull

Fissure Fractures. Not uncommon but rarely recognized. Twenty-five per cent of cephalhaematomas have associated fissure fracture. Occasionally complicated by subdural or extradural haemorrhage.
Treatment. None required.
Prognosis. Excellent.

Depressed Fracture. Depressed fracture from pressure of skull by sacral promontory occasionally seen.
Treatment. Majority resolve spontaneously, surgical elevation through burr holes sometimes performed.
Prognosis. Depends whether intracranial haemorrhage is associated (*see* p. 37).

Nerve Injuries

Types:
1. Upper brachial plexus paralysis (Erb's palsy).
2. Lower brachial plexus paralysis (Klumpke's paralysis).
3. Lesions of cervical sympathetic chain (Horner's syndrome) (*see* p. 312).
4. Facial nerve palsy (Bell's palsy). Usually due to pressure of forceps or sacral promontory on extracranial part of VIIth cranial nerve. Recovery may be expected within a few weeks without therapy. If eye cannot be closed methyl cellulose drops should be instilled.
   Note: Rarely facial palsy is due to a congenital defect of the VIIth cranial nucleus with Moebius syndrome. Palsy then permanent.
5. Abducens nerve palsy. Very rare. Can occur after prolonged labour. Resolves in a few weeks.
6. Radial nerve palsy. Rare. Associated with fractured humerus or pressure in

utero. Resulting wrist drop treated with cock-up splint. Complete recovery anticipated.

Visceral Trauma
Rare. Haemorrhage under capsule of liver may occur at birth causing localized haematoma. May rupture into peritoneal cavity with fatal results.

Spinal Cord Injuries
Fractures or dislocations now very rare. Usually caused by stretching cord during traction in breech delivery. Usually occur in cervical or thoracic spinal cord. One cause of 'floppy baby syndrome'.

Sternomastoid Haematoma (sternomastoid tumour)
Cause: Uncertain. Possibly related to undue torsion of sternomastoid during delivery, resulting in haemorrhage within muscle substance.
Signs. Small, hard lump develops in sternomastoid after first few days. Sometimes not noted for a few weeks. Rarely, head tilted to the side on which injury occurs due to fibrosis in muscle.
Treatment. Nil or passive stretching successful in most cases. Rarely, partial or complete section of affected sternomastoid required if severe torticollis develops.

Injuries during Instrumentation

Forceps Delivery
Injury to ear, facial nerve, or skin may occur. May be followed by traumatic fat necrosis days later. Subcutaneous fat is hard and tethered to skin.

Caesarean Section
Over-deep incision of uterus may cut fetus.

Chapter 10	*CRANIAL AND INTRACRANIAL HAEMORRHAGE*

Cephalhaematoma

Definition
Extravasation of blood under scalp. Two types according to tissue planes involved:

1. Subperiosteal
Clinical features. Swelling of scalp occurs. Not usually recognized until second or third day. More than one may be present. Swelling limited by suture lines, usually over parietal region.
Course and prognosis. Edge occasionally becomes calcified. Centre remains soft as blood slowly absorbed. Resembles depressed skull fracture. Sometimes aggravates neonatal jaundice (*see* p. 51).

Treatment. Nil required. Aspiration should never be performed. Mother should be warned that it may take several weeks or months to disappear.

2. Subaponeurotic

Cause. Bleeding between epicranial aponeurosis and periosteum. May follow use of vacuum extractor. Rarely occurs after fetal blood sampling in labour. Infants with haemostatic failure particularly at risk.

Clinical features. Often difficult to diagnose because of generalized scalp oedema. Bleeding usually more severe than in subperiosteal cephalhaematoma. Jaundice intensified.

Treatment. Investigate and treat haemostatic failures.

Intracranial Haemorrhage

Common cause of death or permanent neurological disability, particularly in pre-term infants. Now fortunately less frequent with improvements in perinatal care.

Cause

1. Mechanical birth injury from:

       1.1 High or midcavity forceps or Ventouse-assisted delivery.

       1.2 Breech extraction.

       1.3 Prolonged labour with excessive skull moulding.

       1.4 Precipitate delivery.

2. Perinatal asphyxia: Haemorrhage caused by a combination of high or sudden changes of cerebral venous pressure, capillary weakness and defects of intravascular coagulation. Seen particularly in pre-term infants with hyaline membrane disease when haemorrhage is mainly peri- and intraventricular (*see* p. 69).

Pathology

Site of bleeding determined largely by cause. May be subdural due to laceration of tentorium cerebelli, rupture of great vein of Galen or intracranial venous sinuses. Intraventricular haemorrhage results from ruptured subependymal terminal veins.

Clinical Features

Signs include:

   1. Infant often pale.

   2. Movements. Range from diminished, with poor muscular tone (cerebral depression) to increased with hypertonia, exaggerated clenching of fists and occasional fits (cerebral irritation). Cry may be high pitched. Occasionally a hemisyndrome may exist. Primitive reflexes may be lost.

   3. Occasionally apnoeic attacks.

   4. Anterior fontanelle tension might be increased. Later, sutures may separate.

   5. Sometimes generalized oedema.

Investigations

   1. Radiography of skull sometimes reveals a fracture.

   2. Lumbar puncture not indicated when clinical diagnosis is obvious; may cause coning.

3. Ultrasound examination via fontanelle very helpful.

Differential Diagnosis

Main difficulty in asphyxiated infant is to decide whether haemorrhage or asphyxia is primary cause of illness (low haematocrit might indicate haemorrhage). Clinical features not pathognomonic for a particular intracranial pathology. The following may all give similar clinical picture: intracranial haemorrhage; congenital malformations; asphyxia; cerebral oedema; meningitis (only value of lumbar puncture is to exclude this diagnosis); overwhelming toxaemia from virulent infection; biochemical disturbances (hypoglycaemia, hypocalcaemia, hyper- or hyponatraemia); adrenal haemorrhage.

Management

Depends on severity of damage.

1. Baby should be disturbed as little as possible and nursed in incubator protected from light and sound. Body temperature must be maintained as hypothermia common in brain-damaged babies. Nasogastric feeding or intravenous feeding advisable.

2. Monitor oxygen transcutaneously, respiration, heart rates and blood pressure by appropriate instruments.

3. Adequate sedation (with chloral) in cases of cerebral irritability. If convulsions present, phenobarbitone, diazepam or paraldehyde should be given.

4. Cerebral oedema should be treated with dexamethasone 1 mg by i.m. injection every 8 h for 3 days, thereafter tailing off gradually. Intravenous mannitol can also be given but note possibility of causing fresh haemorrhage.

5. Manual bladder expression usually required.

6. Test for coagulation defects and treat as appropriate.

7. Respiratory support if necessary.

8. Subdural collection displayed by ultrasound or transillumination should be evacuated by needle or neurosurgeon.

Prognosis

1. Massive haemorrhage rarely compatible with life.

2. With small or even moderate haemorrhage, future neurological and psychological prognosis can rarely be predicted with certainty. Following perinatal factors are sometimes helpful pointers:

2.1 Fits and apnoeic attacks considerably worsen prognosis.

2.2 Prolonged cerebral depression associated with worse prognosis than cerebral irritability.

2.3 Neurological dysfunction less than 48 h duration associated with relatively good long-term prognosis.

Note: Cerebral depression must be interpreted with care because of transplacental passage of analgesic drugs with respiratory depressant properties from mother to fetus in labour (e.g. pethidine, diazepam).

3. Following neurological abnormalities may result:

3.1 Cerebral palsy (mainly dyskinetic or hemiplegic variety).

3.2 Cranial nerve palsies.
3.3 Mental retardation.
3.4 Epilepsy.
3.5 Hydrocephalus.

Note: All infants suspected of intracranial haemorrhage or perinatal anoxia require careful long-term follow-up to include development assessment, tests of hearing and vision, and measurements of head circumference.

Chapter 11   # RESPIRATORY DISORDERS

Perinatal Hypoxia

An important cause of perinatal mortality and long-term neurological disability. Asphyxia can affect infant in utero, during delivery, immediately after birth or complicating neonatal respiratory problems, e.g. hyaline membrane disease. The pathophysiological effects are similar irrespective of aetiology.

Physiological Factors connected with Onset of Respiration

1. Fetus is in an environment in which arterial blood supply to brain may have Po_2 of $4.0\,kPa$ ($30\,mmHg$), Pco_2 of $6.7\,kPa$ ($50\,mmHg$) and pH 7.20.

2. Small, rhythmical respiratory movements occur in latter half of intra-uterine life associated with rapid-eye-movement sleep. These shift little fluid.

3. Stimulus to initiate and maintain adequate respiration after birth still poorly understood but likely to include a combination of factors mainly:

   3.1 Massive sensory bombardment of the central nervous system by birth process activating reticular system to 'reset' respiratory centre.

   3.2 Changing sensitivity of carotid chemoreceptor.

4. Respiratory centre particularly susceptible to oxygen lack and certain maternally administered analgesic drugs, e.g. pethidine, diazepam, which depress the ability to respond to sensory input at birth.

Intra-uterine Hypoxia

Aetiology
Placental insufficiency, placenta praevia, accidental haemorrhage, cord prolapse. Poor fetal growth may be noted before labour and fetal movement chart shows fetus less active.

Fetal Hypoxia during Labour

Clinical Features
Monitoring changes in intra-uterine pressure and fetal heart rates show the following problems of 'fetal distress':

1. Sustained fetal heart rate less than 120 or greater than 160 per min; absence of beat to beat variation; late or variable decelerations (Type II dips).
2. Meconium staining of liquor amnii may occur.
3. Sampling of fetal scalp blood for pH measurements may indicate fetal asphyxia (pH 7·25).

Treatment
Expedite delivery—by section if necessary, with paediatrician at hand.

Neonatal Hypoxia

Clinical Features of Hypoxia at Birth

Those from associated brain damage, e.g.

1. Poor respiratory effort.
2. Hypotonia, pallor, absent movements and reactivity.

Fig. 11.1.   Some factors producing fetal and neonatal hypoxia.

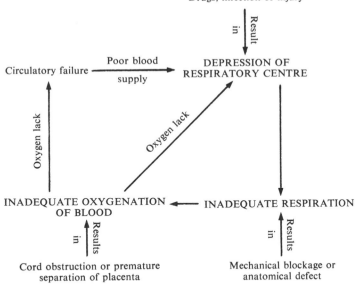

Sequelae
Hypoxia in utero gives rise to:
1. Passage of meconium which may be aspirated at birth.
2. Damage to all organs including brain, with subsequent failure of respiration and heart. Heart failure due to myocardial damage and arrhythmias. Renal failure occurs after hypotension and poor perfusion. Late effects are mental deficiency, cerebral palsy and deafness.

Neonatal Interstitial Emphysema, Pneumomediastinum and Pneumothorax

Not uncommon cause of death in first 48h of life.

Clinical Picture
May follow intubation of trachea, artificial ventilation, meconium aspiration, or arise spontaneously from violent inspiratory efforts. Infant becomes progressively more dyspnoeic when a few hours old. Examination may reveal shift of mediastinum and/or hyper-resonance of chest. Diagnosis confirmed by radiology which may show over-translucent lung, emphysematous bullae, air in mediastinum and pneumothorax.

Treatment
In severe cases paracentesis should be performed to reduce pneumothorax. Catheter attached to underwater seal. Air bubbles out under pressure.

Other Causes of Respiratory Difficulty in Neonatal Period

1. Congenital lobar emphysema—may be due to absent bronchial cartilages—often affects right middle lobe—whole lobe distends, compresses normal lung. Treat by lobectomy.
2. Pulmonary lymphangiectasia—widespread interlacing network of dilated lung lymphatics—may show reticular pattern on X-ray.
3. Left heart failure.
4. Agenesis of lung.
5. Chylous pleural effusion.

Chapter 12   **INFECTIONS IN NEONATAL PERIOD**

Infection still an important cause of mortality and morbidity, usually acquired from birth canal or postnatal environment (*see below*).
Improvement due to:
1. Better understanding of cross-infection.
2. Greater care in handling newborn.
3. More critical use of antibiotics.

Vulnerability of Newborn to Infection
1. Skin, important barrier to infection, but thin and easily damaged. Umbilicus may become gangrenous, colonized.
2. Impaired cellular and humoral defence responses, including:
      2.1 Polymorph defects of chemotaxis, opsonization, phagocytosis and intracellular killing.
      2.2 Lymphocytes—T-cells reduced in number.
3. Newborn lacks IgM and IgA but has maternal IgG which is low in prematures.

Note: Males have less well-developed defence mechanisms than females.

Bacterial Colonization
Infant usually born sterile. Acquisition of bacteria occurs soon after birth with colonization in nose, throat, umbilicus, rectum and perineum, resulting in a flora of saprophytes and pathogenic organisms. May acquire Group B streptococcus from birth canal; *Staphylococcus aureus*, acquired from attendant staff; Gram-negative organisms from nursery apparatus, particularly those containing water (mechanical ventilators, sinks, incubators, humidifiers).

Infection dependent on extent of colonization at various sites by one organism. Mixed colonization less likely to cause serious infection.

Sources of Infection
1. Antenatal

1.1 Transplacental infection, e.g. rubella, herpes, cytomegalovirus, Coxsackie B, influenza A, vaccinia, hepatitis B, syphilis, tuberculosis, toxoplasmosis, malaria, listeria; also sometimes following urinary tract infection in mother.

1.2 Ascending infection, e.g. from prolonged rupture of membranes resulting in non-specific infection or congenital pneumonia.

2. Intranatal
Long difficult labour increases risk of infection.
Neisseria gonorrhoea, Candida albicans, Herpes hominis, Listeria, Chlamydia trachomatis, group B streptococcus occur in (*1*) and (*2*).

3. Postnatal

3.1 Faults in infant predispose to infection, e.g. congenital malformations (nervous system, urinary tract), surgical problems, indwelling umbilical catheters (*see* p. 72).

3.2 Environmental factors, e.g. hands of attendants, intensive care apparatus (particularly those containing water).

Note: Better control of *S. aureus* and Group A β-haemolytic streptococcus has resulted in Gram-negative organisms and Group B β-haemolytic streptococcus assuming much greater importance in neonatal infections.

Clinical Features
High index of suspicion is needed because of vague non-specific symptoms associated with infection which often appear late. Signs include: refusal of feeds, failure to gain weight, vomiting, abdominal distension, apnoeic attacks, convulsions, unexplained jaundice, colour changes, thermolability.

Diagnosis
Thorough clinical examination vital. If diagnosis is not evident, following investigations are needed.
1. Swab cultures from nose, throat, umbilicus and rectum.
2. Blood cultures: peripheral veins should be used because of frequent contamination from umbilical vein.

3. Urine collected by either 'clean catch' method or suprapubic bladder paracentesis. Examine for protein, white cells and bacterial count.

4. Lumbar puncture: technically difficult; must always be performed if there is the slightest suspicion of meningitis.

5. White cell count: particular emphasis on differential count, presence of immature polymorphs (band cells) and appearance of toxic granulation.

6. Haemoglobin and platelets: anaemia often accompanies infection; thrombocytopenia sometimes associated with intra-uterine infections (e.g. rubella, cytomegalovirus) and intravascular coagulation secondary to severe infection.

7. Radiology: chest radiograph for pneumonia. Radiography of bones may show rubella syndrome, syphilis or osteomyelitis.

Note: At present postnatally acquired virus infections are relatively uncommon. However, where bacterial pathogens are not isolated seek viruses.

Prevention of Postnatal Infection

1. Since mothers do not usually carry coagulase-positive staphylococci, 'rooming-in' policy will result in less infection than in a communal nursery cared for by different nurses.

2. Effective handwashing by all attendant staff is most important single measure. Three per cent hexachlorophane emulsion or 4% chlorhexidine most widely used antiseptic soaps.

3. Infant skin care: bathing infants with above solutions reduces staphylococcal skin sepsis. Umbilicus must also be kept clean.

Note

a. Recent reports that hexachlorophane is neurotoxic to animals when applied to skin for long periods has led to its discouragement for routine use in bathing infants. Four per cent chlorhexidine solution is a suitable substitute or a 0·3% hexachlorophane dusting powder after bathing.

b. Widespread use of hexachlorophane may cause increased incidence of Gram-negative sepsis.

4. Routine use of masks and gowns are not an effective means of preventing infection.

5. Isolation of baby (preferably with mother) with obvious superficial sepsis is desirable to prevent widespread dissemination of organisms.

6. Surveillance of bacterial flora of nose, throat, umbilicus and rectum for infants on special care units important. Also swab fixtures (e.g. sinks) and mobile equipment (e.g. ventilators, incubators).

7. Thorough and frequent cleaning of equipment and nursery important to keep a 'clean house'.

8. Antibiotic prophylaxis of infant where bacterial infection might be anticipated (e.g. after prolonged rupture of membranes) is of unproven benefit and incurs risk of antibiotic resistances.

Antibiotic Treatment of Postnatal Infections

1. Antibiotics invariably overprescribed in neonatal period because of difficulty in early diagnosis of infections.

2. Choice of antibiotics largely dependent on prevailing bacterial flora, hence importance of regular surveillance (*see above*). Also, because of frequent failure to isolate responsible organisms combinations of a penicillin with an aminoglycoside (gentamicin) commonly used.

3. With serious infections parenteral therapy required for at least a week followed by oral therapy for a few weeks.

4. Other antibiotics of benefit in neonatal period either singly or in combination, e.g. chloramphenicol (but avoid high dosage).

5. Consider rotation of antibiotics at regular intervals to minimize emergence of resistant strains.

Common Neonatal Infections

Most commonly encountered clinical types of neonatal infection are skin sepsis, conjunctivitis, thrush, umbilical sepsis, gastro-enteritis, pulmonary infections, urinary tract infections, meningitis, septicaemia, osteomyelitis.

1. Skin Sepsis
Commonest variety of staphylococcal infection. May be small pinhead pustules, boil, breast abscess, umbilical infection, paronychia. Pemphigus neonatorum is a staphylococcal disease with superficial blebs which burst and liberate many organisms. The disease is very infectious and serious with risk of septicaemia.

Treatment
Isolate baby. Swab lesions for culture. Local antiseptic cream (e.g. hexachlorophane, chlorhexidine, triple dye) can be applied. Systemic antibiotics in severe infections. When a number of infants in nursery are affected swab staff and apply antiseptic cream (e.g. neomycin) into nares of infants and attendants.

Note: Any superficial infection of the skin can act as a source of systemic infection and should therefore be taken seriously.

2. Conjunctivitis

2.1 'Sticky Eye' Usually due to infection by *S. aureus* or *Chlamydia trachomatis*.
Treatment. Swabbing or local sulphonamide or chloramphenicol.

2.2 Gonococcal Ophthalmia Now much less common but still seen: a cause of permanent blindness from corneal damage.
Treatment. Local and systemic penicillin (check sensitivity).

3. Thrush (Superficial Candidiasis)
Newborn particularly susceptible because of deficient cellular immunity. Acquired from maternal birth passages. Antibiotics contribute to this development.

4. Umbilical Sepsis
Purulent discharge from umbilical cord at the time of separation not uncommon. Erythema of surrounding skin suggests more severe infection. Staphylococcus usually responsible, may cause local cellulitis, portal pyaemia or vein thrombosis—septicaemia.

Treatment
Keep clean, use isopropyl alcohol swabs and/or local antiseptic (triple dye) or antibiotic.

5. Gastro-enteritis
Very uncommon in healthy newborn infants, particularly if breast fed. Sick infants at risk on special care units where enteropathic *Escherichia coli* or rotavirus usually responsible.

Aetiology, clinical features and treatment essentially the same as with older infants (*see* p. 244). Rarely adrenal hyperplasia of the salt-losing variety (*see* p. 472) may present with acute diarrhoea and vomiting.

Note: Occurrence of gastro-enteritis in hospital maternity units poses particular problems because of rapid spread. Strict barrier nursing essential. Antibiotics of little benefit.

6. Pulmonary Infections
Two forms according to mode of infection:

6.1 Intra-uterine (Congenital) Pneumonia Following ruptured membranes; infants have features of pneumonia from birth onwards; now uncommon.

Treatment. Systemic antibiotics. Pathogen should be identified. Vaginal swab cultures may help.

6.2 Postnatal Pneumonia Group B β-haemolytic streptococcus carried by 25 % of women in vagina causes severe illness just before or shortly after birth. Illness is often indistinguishable from respiratory distress syndrome clinically and radiologically in preterm, but white cell changes help differentiate either by marked polymorph leucocytosis or leucopenia. Suspect Group B β-haemolytic streptococcal illness in any infant above 36 weeks' gestation with respiratory difficulty. X-ray shows patchy consolidation in older baby and infant develops metabolic acidosis, disseminated intravascular coagulation, shock and hypoxia. There is persistence of fetal circulation. Pneumonia often follows ventilation. Chlamydia, staphylococci, streptococci and pneumocystis are among many organisms causing neonatal pneumonia.

7. Urinary Tract Infections (*see* also p. 372)
Significant bacteriuria found in 1–2 % of newborn infants. Males more commonly affected. Often asymptomatic. When signs present these are non-specific (*see* p. 42).

May be jaundiced. Sometimes pass large volumes of dilute urine. Diagnosis by urine cultures obtained by suprapubic bladder paracentesis, or 'clean catch' specimen. Bag specimens unreliable because of contamination. Blood culture also required.

Aetiology
Look for congenital abnormalities, e.g. hydronephrosis (*see* p. 393). Vesico-ureteric reflux may exist as only abnormality.

Management
Review for recurrence and radiography.

8. Meningitis (*see also* p. 335)

Most cases occur in first 2 weeks. Babies with meningomyelocele particularly vulnerable. Gram-negative organisms usually responsible but any organism may be found. Classic signs of meningitis usually absent early in disease. Lethargy, poor feeding and other non-specific signs (*see* p. 42) should arouse suspicion. Convulsions and bulging anterior fontanelle late features. Diagnosis confirmed by examination of CSF.

Treatment
Intensive use of appropriate antibiotics. Mortality between 30 and 50%. Sequelae in those who survive include mental retardation, hydrocephaly, hearing loss, neurological and behavioural disorders, epilepsy.

9. Septicaemia
Any sudden severe illness with no obvious explanation should be suspected as due to septicaemia. Death may occur before localizing signs of infection appear. Can also occur as a complication of localized infection (e.g. umbilicus, skin, urinary tract).

Treatment
After blood culture taken, vigorous antibiotic therapy required.
   Note: Coagulase-negative staphylococci frequently grown from blood cultures. Although occasionally contaminants they may indicate genuine low-grade septicaemia.

10. Osteomyelitis
Bones most commonly involved are head of femur, humerus and maxilla. Multiple sites might be involved. Infection blood borne from superficial source of infection. Non-specific signs of infection (*see* p. 42) usually present. Sometimes presents with immobility of limb (pseudoparesis).

Aetiology
Usually *S. aureus*, but Gram-negative organisms assuming greater importance.

Diagnosis
Blood culture essential for antibiotic sensitivites. Radiological examination negative in early stages. Bone changes—rarefaction, subperiosteal calcification—appear after about 10 days.

Treatment
Antibiotics. Surgery sometimes needed.

Chapter 13   # METABOLIC DISORDERS OF THE NEONATAL PERIOD

Carbohydrate Metabolism

1. Neonatal Hypoglycaemia
Is defined as blood glucose level less than 1·1 mmol/l (20 mg/dl) in low birth weight infants (less than 2500 g) or 1·65 mmol/l (30 mg/dl) in term infants on two sequential samples obtained at least 1 h apart during first 3 days of life. After this period 2·2 mmol/l (40 mg/dl) is the critical level and many consider that this limit should be observed in newborn also.

Note: Blood glucose 15% below serum and venous blood 10% lower than capillary or arterial blood.

Infants at Risk
Hypoglycaemia found in following infant categories: normal pre-term (*see* p. 69); light-for-dates (*see* p. 62); of diabetic mothers; with birth asphyxia, hypothermia, respiratory distress syndrome, haemolytic disease; after exchange transfusion with acid-citrate-dextrose (ACD) blood; with polycythaemia. Very rarely initial manifestation of rare illness, e.g. galactosaemia, fructose intolerance, Wiedemann–Beckwith syndrome, islet-cell adenoma or nesidioblastosis, glycogen storage disease, leucine sensitivity.

Note: Wasted term infants with subacute fetal distress (*see* p. 61) even if appropriate weight for gestation, also at risk.

Symptoms
In most instances hypoglycaemia is asymptomatic. If symptoms occur (rare in first 24 h) usually non-specific, include jitteriness; convulsions; apnoeic attacks; poor feeding; hypotonia; drowsiness or coma; tachypnoea; pallor; abnormal eye movements and cry.

Note
1. Symptoms should not be attributed to hypoglycaemia unless they disappear with its correction.
2. Symptoms are non-specific and can occur with other neonatal disorders, e.g. hypocalcaemia, infections, brain damage.

Management
1. *Prevention*. Early and adequate feeding of milk to light-for-dates and pre-term infants. Prevention of hypothermia. Infants at risk should have blood glucose monitored every 4 h for the first few days.
2. *Treatment*

2.1 Asymptomatic. Check adequacy of feeding and give 10–20 ml/kg milk. Continue to monitor blood glucose until normal. If hypoglycaemia lasts more than 2 h consider treating as symptomatic.

2.2 Symptomatic. Give 2 ml/kg 10% dextrose i.v. in 1 min (equivalent to 200 mg/kg glucose) followed by 5ml/kg/h (equivalent to 8mg glucose/kg/min). Increase oral feeds. Monitor hourly—reduce i.v. dextrose when blood glucose satisfactory. If i.v. glucose rates of more than 12 mg/kg/min needed to keep blood glucose satisfactory, look for nesidioblastosis or islet-cell adenoma, glycogen storage disease, amino acidopathy, galactosaemia. Give dexamethasone 0·1 mg/kg i.v. every 6 h or glucagon.

Note: 10 % glucose infusions must be discontinued slowly to prevent rebound hypoglycaemia.

Prognosis
1. *Asymptomatic*. Probably no long-term neurological damage.
2. *Symptomatic*. If untreated, or inadequately treated, all degrees of brain damage can occur. Early and vigorous treatment reduces risk of permanent neurological damage.

2. Infants of Diabetic Mothers
With better ante- and intrapartum control of maternal diabetes neonatal problems are greatly reduced. Overall perinatal mortality a little above that for non-diabetics as congenital abnormalities are more common. These may be reduced following pre-pregnancy counselling and intensive treatment around conception and early weeks thereafter. Poorly treated diabetic's infants are liable to be large for dates, have RDS (*see* p. 64) and hypoglycaemia, hypocalcaemia. Incidence of later juvenile diabetes between 1 and 2 %.

3. Transient Neonatal Diabetes
Very rare. Affected infants usually light-for-dates. Blood glucose sometimes exceeds 55·5mmol/l (1000mg/dl). Symptoms of dehydration and weight loss develop in first few days. Ketonuria usually absent. Treatment with insulin and intravenous fluids. Insulin dependency disappears after several months. Brain damage may be a sequel (probably a consequence of early hypoglycaemia or hypernatraemia). Rarely diabetes is permanent.

Protein Metabolism

1. Plasma Proteins
Usually lower than in older child, particularly pre-term infants. Sometimes responsible for early oedema.

2. Inborn Errors of Amino Acid Metabolism
May be discovered by routine screening or present with failure to thrive, coma or convulsions.

Minerals and Electrolytes

1. Hypocalcaemia
Defined as serum calcium less than 1·75mmol/l (7mg/dl). Ionized calcium less than 0·6mmol/l (2–5mg/dl). Usual laboratory methods measure total

serum calcium (protein bound, ionized and complexed). Ionized calcium physiologically most important but technically difficult to measure as routine procedure.

Physiology
Serum calcium in cord blood about 0·5mmol/l (2mg/dl) higher than maternal blood. In first few days calcium falls to nadir at third day rising to 2·5mmol/l by tenth day.

Symptoms
Like hypoglycaemia these are non-specific and include twitching, jitteriness, various types of convulsions and abnormal E.E.G. and apnoeic attacks. Trousseau's and Chvostek's signs occur in less than 20% of cases. Muscle hypertonia, increased deep reflexes and extreme head retraction often presenting features of late hypocalcaemia (*see below*).

Clinical Syndromes
1. Early hypocalcaemia. Usually associated with the following conditions:
   1.1 Perinatal asphyxia.
   1.2 Extreme prematurity complicated by respiratory distress syndrome.
   1.3 Maternal diabetes.
   1.4 Light-for-dates infants' acidosis.
   1.5 Bicarbonate administration.
   1.6 Exchange transfusion with citrated blood (total calcium might be above normal but ionized component usually low).
   1.7 Rare conditions, including Di George syndrome—with parathyroid, thyroid and thymic aplasia, heart defect, malformed ears, cleft palate, micrognathia; maternal hyperparathyroidism, maternal rickets or maternal anticonvulsants, idiopathic hypoparathyroidism.
2. Late hypocalcaemia (neonatal tetany). Almost exclusively in bottle-fed infants. Now much less common with increased use of low solute modified cow's milk formula, with low phosphate and high calcium : phosphate ratio. Usually presents between 5 and 10 days. Incidence higher in late winter and early spring, possibly related to lack of vitamin D in diet of pregnant mothers. Asian infants and those of multiparae particularly at risk.

Treatment
1. Early hypocalcaemia
   1.1 Treat any underlying condition (e.g. asphyxia, hyaline membrane disease).
   1.2 If symptoms not severe commence oral 10% calcium gluconate, 400mg/kg/day, in four divided doses.
   1.3 If symptoms severe, 10ml of 10% calcium gluconate should be given slowly (1ml/min) via peripheral vein with E.C.G. control or continuous monitoring of heart rate. Subcutaneous leak can produce necrosis. Alternative treatment of i.m. magnesium sulphate 0·2ml/kg of a 50%

solution on 2 occasions separated by 12h—equally effective. Bigger dose acts like curare.

1.4 If symptoms are resistant (very rare) to above therapy, steady intravenous infusion of 10% calcium gluconate can be given, 1–2g (10–20ml)/24h. Magnesium must be checked.

2. *Late hypocalcaemia*. As above. If a high phosphate milk was being given, this should be discontinued.

Note: Magnesium deficiency sometimes coexists with hypocalcaemia. Serum magnesium should be checked at same time, and deficiency corrected (*see below*).

Prognosis
1. Early. That of underlying disorder.
2. Late. Excellent. No permanent neurological sequelae. Sometimes primary dentition shows hypoplastic enamel.

2. Hypomagnesaemia
Magnesium metabolism closely parallels that of calcium. Serum level less than 0·6mmol/l (1·4mg/dl) diagnostic. Commonly associated with late hypocalcaemia. Isolated hypomagnesaemia very rare.

Treatment
As above.

3. Hypernatraemia
Serum sodium greater than 150mmol/l. Very unusual in neonatal period. More common later in infancy (*see* p. 138). Usually related to incorrect constitution of milk formula (e.g. giving added salt instead of sugar or increasing milk concentration). Sometimes follows excessive water loss as in hot climate or fever. May follow treatment of sick infants under radiant heater.

4. Hyponatraemia
Defined as serum sodium less than 120 mmol/l; found in following conditions:

4.1 Very sick infants, particularly those with brain damage. Probably due to inappropriate secretion of antidiuretic hormone.

4.2 Overhydration with intravenous fluids.

4.3 Increased salt loss from diarrhoea or vomiting or congenital adrenal hyperplasia (*see* p. 470).

Note: Sick newborn infants often lose more sodium in their urine which needs replacing. Urine output per day should be checked.

Neonatal Cold Injury

Rare condition caused by accidental exposure of infant to cold. Also seen in Menkes' syndrome.

Symptoms
Increasing apathy, refusal of feeds.

Signs
Baby does not look ill. Rectal temperature may drop to 27°C(80°F). *Note* importance of using low-reading thermometer. Often slight oedema. Skin erythema. Sclerema may be present (*see* p. 458).

Prognosis
Poor. Haemorrhagic pneumonia often found postmortem.

Treatment
Child should be warmed slowly. As warming accelerates metabolic processes, 20% glucose should be given by continuous gastric drip.

Chapter 14   *NEONATAL JAUNDICE*

Bilirubin Metabolism

1. Bilirubin produced in liver and spleen reticulo-endothelial system from:
> 1.1 Breakdown of haemoglobin (75%) 0·5g/day full term infant.
> 1.2 Catabolism of other haem pigments (25%) e.g. myoglobin cytochromes and bone marrow source.

2. One g haemoglobin gives 600 µmol (35mg) bilirubin. Transported in the circulation where it is: (*a*) unconjugated, (*b*) bound to albumin, (*c*) lipid soluble and indirect reacting and (*d*) enters sinusoidal circulation in the liver to be excreted.

3. Bilirubin excreted in the following stages:
> 3.1 Diffuses into hepatocytes and taken up by cytoplasmic protein called ligandin (Y protein) and other glutathione-S-transferases—Z protein. Phenobarbitone increases intracellular ligandin.
> 3.2 Transformed into water-soluble, direct-reacting form, by conjugation with glucuronic acid under the control of microsomal enzyme, bilirubin uridine diphosphate glucuronyl transferase (UDPG-T).
> 3.3 Secreted into bile canaliculi across hepatocyte cell membrane.
> 3.4 Excreted in the bile into the duodenum.

4. In the small bowel conjugated bilirubin is hydrolysed by β-glucuronidase of intestinal mucosa into lipid-soluble bilirubin and glucuronic acid. Reabsorbed to give an enterohepatic circulation of bilirubin, contributing to bilirubin load for liver clearance. Facilitated by limited early bacterial colonization preventing normal bilirubin degradation and increased activity of mucosal β-glucuronidase.

Causes of Jaundice in Newborn Period

1. Overproduction of Bilirubin. Due to:
> *1.1 Haemolytic anaemias,* e.g. haemolytic disease (Rh and ABO incompatibility—*see* p. 402); hereditary spherocyto-

sis; non-spherocytic haemolytic anaemias (e.g. G-6-PD deficiency, vitamin K-induced haemolysis, haemoglobinopathies, infections). Result in:

1.1.1 Liver unable to deal with increased load (often four times normal daily production).

1.1.2 Unconjugated (indirect reacting) bilirubin accumulates in blood. Not excreted by kidneys. Urine and stools normal.

1.1.3 Clinical appearance of jaundice usually within 24h of birth.

1.1.4 Shortened RBC life and higher Hb. Newborns produce twice as much of bilirubin/kg as adults do.

1.2 Polycythaemia. Due to:

1.2.1 Maternal-fetal transplacental bleed.

1.2.2 Feto-fetal transfusion in twins.

1.2.3 Maternal diabetes mellitus.

1.2.4 Delayed clamping of cord.

Jaundice usually appears after 48h. Degree dependent on initial haematocrit.

1.3 Extravasated Blood e.g. from cephalhaematoma, occult haemorrhage. Jaundice appears after 48h. Rarely severe.

Increased Enterohepatic Circulation. Due to:

1.4.1 Inadequate milk intake—increasing intestinal transit time, allowing greater bilirubin absorption.

1.4.2 Swallowed maternal blood.

1.4.3 Intestinal obstruction.

2. Undersecretion of Bilirubin by Liver

2.1 Defect in uptake of unconjugated bilirubin from blood, e.g. Gilbert's disease.

2.2 Defect in conjugating bilirubin to glucuronide, e.g.

2.2.1 Deficiency of UDP-glucuronyl transferase—Crigler–Najjar syndrome. (Mendelian recessive—most die in infancy from kernicterus.)

2.2.2 Inhibition of UDP-glucuronyl transferase by: Drugs (novobiocin), hormones (not yet identified) responsible for prolonged 'physiological' jaundice in breast-fed infants.

2.2.3 Defect in excreting conjugated bilirubin into bile canaliculus, e.g. Dubin-Johnson and Rotor syndromes (autosomal recessives). Very rare. Diagnosed only by specific liver function tests and biopsy. Conjugated bilirubin regurgitates back into blood, appears in urine. Stool usually of normal colour or pale.

2.2.4 Interference with bilirubin transport along biliary tree—obstructive jaundice, e.g. biliary atresia, choledochal cyst, cystic fibrosis (inspissated bile).

3. Combined Bilirubin Overproduction and undersecretion

In some instances aetiology of neonatal jaundice is mixed, e.g. neonatal sepsis, red cell survival time often reduced. Non-specific undersecretion by liver. Infants often lethargic and poor feeders. Careful clinical examination needed to identify possible source of infection. Investigate as for neonatal infections (*see* p. 42).

4. Neonatal Hepatitis Syndrome

Chronic hepatocellular jaundice with obstructive features including pale stools, bilirubinuria, hepatosplenomegaly. Hepatocytes transformed to nucleated giant cells. Inflammatory cell infiltrate in portal tracts and lobules. Causes:

> 4.1 Intra-uterine infections, e.g. rubella, cytomegalovirus, herpes simplex, toxoplasmosis. Hepatitis B jaundice usually part of generalized organ involvement.
> 4.2 Inborn errors of metabolism, e.g. galactosaemia; fructosaemia; tyrosinosis; α_1-antitrypsin deficiency (possibly predisposes to neonatal hepatitis in presence of some additional stimulus such as hepatitis B).

Note: In 50% of neonatal hepatitis no definite aetiological factor can be identified.

5. Bile Duct Atresia (*see* p. 253)

Often impossible to distinguish clinically or biochemically from hepatitis syndrome. Usually presents after second week. Rose Bengal test and duodenal intubation for bile salt concentrations may be helpful in differentiation, and α-feto protein level in blood. Poor prognosis.

6. Physiological Jaundice

Characterized by rise in serum total bilirubin to 120–140 μmol/l(7·8 mg/dl) maximum 250 μmol/l (15 mg/dl) by fifth day of life, falling to normal concentration by tenth day.

Note: Jaundice before 48 h or its persistence after the tenth day needs investigation.

Causes of physiological jaundice include:

> 6.1 Increased production of bilirubin (shortened red blood cell survival, 'shunt' bilirubin, excess production from non-haem pigments, polycythaemia from placental transfusion with delayed clamping of cord).
> 6.2 Impaired uptake of unconjugated bilirubin by hepatic cell membranes due to lack of anion-binding transport proteins.
> 6.3. Functional deficiency of bilirubin UDP glucuronyl transferase.
> 6.4 Increased enterohepatic circulation of unconjugated bilirubin from gut.
>   Relative importance of these factors unknown. In general, physiological jaundice represents an imbalance between

bilirubin production and hepatic excretion. Following factors increase risk of physiological jaundice:

6.4.1 Premature birth.

6.4.2 Artificial induction of labour (possibly by loss of the perinatal induction of conjugating enzymes by fetal corticosteroids).

6.4.3 Breast feeding (inhibitors present in some breast milk).

Note: **Prolonged jaundice** (beyond tenth day) often found in breast-fed infants. Other causes include: hypothyroidism, cystic fibrosis, galactosaemia, biliary atresia, infection (particularly of urinary or biliary tract), congenital heart disease.

Management of Neonatal Jaundice

Every attempt must be made to diagnose cause of neonatal jaundice because:

1. It might be first manifestation of serious underlying pathology.

2. High serum levels of unconjugated bilirubin will cause bilirubin encephalopathy (kernicterus) (*see* p. 406).

Examine for hepatosplenomegaly, purpura, extravasated blood, e.g. cephalhaematoma, infection and dehydration. Tests: Hb, ABO and Rh group. Coombs', WBC and differential, urine culture and reducing substances, infection screen. If negative, do LFTs, viruses, toxoplasmosis, α_1-antitrypsin, sweat test.

Once diagnosis is made, management is mainly directed (*a*) to treatment of any underlying condition and (*b*) lowering bilirubin level. This can be achieved in three ways:

1. Mechanical removal of bilirubin by exchange transfusion at levels above 340 µmol/l in term babies (*see* p. 405).

2. Improving bilirubin excretion by liver by pharmacological means, e.g. phenobarbitone which accelerates activity of glucuronyl transferase and ligandin. Rarely of benefit.

3. Phototherapy for photo-oxidation of bilirubin. Bilirubin absorbs light maximally at wavelength 450–460 nm. Light sources whose spectra include peak emissions in this range (blue, white, daylight) will break down bilirubin into substances which are water soluble, non-toxic, rapidly excreted in bile and do not enter central nervous system. Side-effects include loose green or brown stools, skin rashes and increased water loss. Start at about 220 µmol/l for full term and increase fluid intake.

Note:

1. Eyes must be adequately shielded to avoid damage to lens and retina.

2. Because early jaundice is a potentially valuable sign of possible illness, a full search for the diagnosis must be made.

The pre-term infant expecially liable to kernicterus.

Treatment

1. Phototherapy at half exchange levels.

2. Exchange transfusion at $1 \cdot 0$ mg% (17 µmol/l) for each 100 g body weight, i.e.

750 g infant exchange at 7·5 mg % (130 µmol/l)

1000 g infant exchange at 10 mg (170 µmol/l)

1250 g infant exchange at 12·5 mg % (215 μmol/l)
Exchange earlier if baby hypoxic or acidotic.

Chapter 15 # THE LOW BIRTH WEIGHT BABY

Classification

1. By weight: Infants weighing less than 2500 g at birth are called 'low birth weight infants' irrespective of gestational age.
2. By gestation: Birth weight should be related to gestational age.
        2.1 Pre-term: less than 259 days (37 completed weeks).
        2.2 Term: 259–293 days (37–41 weeks)
        2.3 Post-term: 294 days (42 weeks) or more.
3. Low birth weight infants divided into two main groups:
        3.1 Pre-term infants.
        3.2 Term infants weighing less than 2500 g ('light-for-dates').
    Note: Some pre-term infants also underweight for gestation, as same factors which caused early delivery may impair fetal growth (e.g. severe maternal toxaemia).

Pre-term Infants

Incidence

Approximately 7% of live births. Majority of infants in older gestation groups (>32 weeks). Incidence varies greatly in different socio-economic and racial groups.

Aetiology

1. Unknown in about 25–50% of cases

2. Obstetric Causes

        2.1 Multiple pregnancy.
        2.2 Toxaemia, antepartum haemorrhage from placenta praevia or abruptio placentae.
        2.3 Premature rupture of membranes.
        2.4 Early induction of labour or delivery by Caesarean section (elective or emergency) because of:
        2.4.1 Severe toxaemia, hypertension, diabetes, cardiac disease.
        2.4.2 Certain cases of haemolytic disease.
        2.5 Hydramnios.
        2.6 External version for breech presentation.

3. Maternal Factors

    3.1 Urinary tract infection and bactiuria in pregnancy.
    3.2 Cardiac disease.
    3.3 Incompetent cervix; previous abortion.
    3.4 Longstanding malnutrition.

4. Fetal Disorders

    4.1 Congenital abnormalities.
    4.2 Rhesus incompatibility.

5. Social and Economic Factors. High incidences found in women of low socio-economic groups. Also in women below 20 and over 40 years.

Anatomical Characteristics of Pre-term Babies

No vernix, eyebrows and eye-lashes barely visible; oedema (usually confined to lower limbs) sometimes present. Eyelids fused in very pre-term babies.

1. Subcutaneous Tissue. Scanty; subcutaneous fat appears after about 28 weeks' gestation. Bony structures often abnormally prominent. Buttocks almost absent. Anus appears to pout.

2. Lanugo Hair. Abundant until 28 weeks. Decreases in amount with increasing gestational age.

3. Finger and Toe Nails. Sometimes short, particularly toes.

4. Head. Disproportionately large for baby; sutures sometimes widely separate; bones feel soft.

5. Ears. Cartilage is soft and in very small infants deficient. Ears can be easily folded forwards with slow recoil to original position.

6. Eyes. Often appear prominent.

7. Chest. Appears short compared with abdomen. Prominent rib cage.

8. Abdomen. Thin-walled, soft. Peristalsis easily seen. Liver and kidneys usually palpable.

9. Genitalia. Testes may be in abdomen, inguinal canal or scrotum according to gestational age. Labia minora not covered by labia majora until almost term. Vaginal skin tag may be present, pseudomenstruation occurs.

10. Breasts. Nipples flat; rise from surrounding skin after about 36 weeks, breast tissue develops with gestational age.

11. Joints. Elbows, knees, hips, wrists and ankles lack full range of movement.

Note: Because of correlation between these external characteristics and gestational age some have been used to produce 'scores' for assessment of gestational age at birth. Better scores obtained by combining external and neurological characteristics, e.g. 'Dubowitz Score' *see* p. 511.

Physiological Handicaps of Pre-term Infants

Pre-term infants are physically small, functionally immature and have small stocks of vital substances to meet extra-uterine demands.

1. Inadequate Stores

1.1 Protein. Serum proteins reduced.

1.1.1 Leads to peripheral oedema, common in pre-term infants.

1.1.2 Immunoglobulins low and show limited response to antigenic stimulation: infants therefore more liable to infection. IgG antibodies transplacentally acquired; concentration varies with length of gestation. IgM antibodies containing specific bactericidal antibodies to Gram-negative organisms not transferred.

1.1.3 Plasma clotting factors low because of limited ability of liver to utilize vitamin K. Prothrombin time prolonged for about 2 weeks after birth, hence increased likelihood of haemorrhage.

1.2 Carbohydrate. Poor glycogen stores since fetus accumulates glycogen in liver (and to a lesser extent in cardiac and skeletal muscle) in latter part of gestation. Hypoglycaemia (*see* p. 69) occurs unless early feeding is instituted.

1.3 Fat.

1.3.1 Insufficient stores of subcutaneous (white) fat which is laid down after 28 weeks' gestation. Results in: (*a*) Poor insulation increasing heat loss. (*b*) Limited energy reserves. (Pre-term infants utilize fat earlier because of low glycogen stores.) Important where energy requirements increased, e.g. hyaline membrane disease.

1.3.2 Insufficient brown fat—reduced capacity of non-shivering thermogenesis.

1.4 Minerals

1.4.1 Calcium (also probably magnesium). Seventy-five per cent of calcium accumulated by the fetus after 28 weeks. Rapid postnatal growth demands more calcium than can be provided in milk. Increased liability to rickets (*see also* under Vitamin D Deficiency, p. 124).

1.4.2 Iron. Iron stores acquired mainly as haemoglobin in last 2 months of fetal life. Pre-term infants liable to develop iron deficiency anaemia of prematurity unless postnatal supplements of iron given (*see* p. 400).

Pre-term infant kidneys less able to conserve sodium than full term—may lose at least 3 mmol/kg/24h. Easily becomes hyponatraemic, especially if receiving low Na milk (EBM).

Test urine daily for sodium loss and osmolality to differentiate hyponatraemia due to Na loss from that due to inappropriate ADH secretion. Infants become less active, hypotensive and may have convulsions. Occasionally have ileus. Hypernatraemia seen in babies under phototherapy or radiant heaters—when given too high concentration of i.v. glucose leading to water loss with glycosuria.

1.5 Vitamins. All vitamin stores low at birth, especially C, D and E. Combination of rapid early postnatal growth and poor early absorption from milk renders pre-term infants vulnerable to rickets, folic acid deficiency, vitamin E deficiency and hypoprothrombinaemia (vitamin K deficiency). Infants may be unable to hydroxylate 1-OH vitamin D to 1,25-dihydroxyvitamin D until 34 weeks. The one reason for very low birth weight is babies needing dihydroxyvitamin D.

1.6 Enzymes. Certain enzymes known to be reduced or functionally insufficient, e.g.

1.6.1 Bilirubin-UDP-glucuronyl transferase in liver. Important contributing factor to neonatal hyperbilirubinaemia. Other enzymes needed for uptake, transfer and excretion of bilirubin also probably inadequate for the extra-uterine function.

1.6.2 Red-cell enzymes, particularly those maintaining integrity of cell membrane. Predisposes to early haemolysis.

2. Reduced Vitality. Infants less active than those born at term; sleep more, cry weaker. Moro reflex often poorly developed or absent.

3. Unstable Temperature Control. Body temperature has a natural tendency to fall owing to: (*a*) Larger surface to volume ratio; (*b*) Lack of subcutaneous fat; (*c*) Lowered capacity for heat production (inactivity; small food intake; poor stores of brown fat).

Note: Hyperthermia can also occur due to lack of effective sweating mechanisms.

4. Problems in Digestive System

4.1 Small pre-term babies often have feeble sucking and swallowing with pharyngeal incoordination and absent gag reflex. Predisposes to aspiration of feeds.

4.2 Food in stomach may be regurgitated owing to poor tone of inferior oesophageal sphincter mechanism and small size of stomach.

4.3 Gastric emptying time often prolonged; less in prone than supine position.

4.4 Digestion and absorption of protein remarkably good, even in very immature infants; fat absorption less efficient because of inadequate pancreatic lipase and diminished bile acid pool. Lactose malabsorption sometimes seen due to relative lactase deficiency.

4.5 Musculature of bowel wall often weak and easily distended. Incomplete development of bowel autonomic plexuses in very immature infants. Hence tendency towards constipation.

5. *Problems in Respiratory System*

5.1 Breathing often irregular in rhythm and depth. Periodic breathing (rapid bursts of breathing for 20 s alternating with absence of breathing for 10 s), common in very small infants. Recurrent apnoeic attacks (*see* p. 63) lasting longer than 30 s are serious.

5.2 Milk more likely to be inhaled because of poor pharyngeal control and feeble cough reflex.

5.3 Surfactant deficiency leading to respiratory distress syndrome (p. 64).

5.4 Incomplete structural development of alveoli means that respiratory reserve is inadequate or non-existent, hence minor degrees of atelectasis very serious.

6. *Poor Tolerance to Drugs.*

Pre-term infants lack ability of term infants to deal with certain drugs. Great care must be taken in prescribing correct dosage:

6.1 Chemotherapeutic Agents

6.1.1 Sulphonamides; some, e.g. sulphafurazole, compete with bilirubin for albumin binding so that bilirubin displaced into extravascular space, hence to brain lipid causing bilirubin encephalopathy.

6.1.2 Chloramphenicol; normally excreted via hepatic conjugating enzymes. Because of their functional immaturity active drug accumulates, sometimes causing circulatory collapse (so-called 'grey baby syndrome').

6.1.3 Other antibiotics potentially toxic: (*a*) Colistin, aminoglycosides (e.g. gentamicin, kanamycin, tobramycin) cause renal damage. (*b*) Novobiocin causes hyperbilirubinaemia from inhibition of glucuronyl transferase. (*c*) Aminoglycosides, streptomycin cause deafness and vestibular damage. (*d*) Tetracyclines cause brown staining of teeth and inhibition of bone growth.

6.2 Vitamin K Analogues. Large doses of water-soluble preparations can increase haemolysis leading to severe jaundice. Toxicity not associated with naturally occurring fat-soluble vitamin K_1 (phytomenadione) or synthetic derivatives. Dosage should not exceed 5 mg.

6.3 Oxygen (*see* p. 71). Dangers of bronchopulmonary dysplasia and retrolental fibroplasia likely to be inversely related to degree of prematurity. Safe oxygen concentrations not known.

6.4 Dermatological Preparations, e.g. hexachlorophane. Excessive absorption of 3 % solution has caused spongiform myelinopathy in very immature infants. Alcohol, e.g. Steriswabs easily absorbed from skin—also traumatizes thin skin.

7. Incomplete Development of Reflexes. Rooting, sucking, swallowing and laryngeal reflexes imperfectly developed in infants less than 34 weeks' gestation. Predisposes to aspiration of feed.

8. Problems in Circulatory System

>*8.1 Pulse Rate.* Slightly faster than in term infants. Varies between 100 and 160/min. Marked sinus arrhythmia. Immaturity of autonomic nervous system results in abnormal rhythms. Extrasystoles common in early weeks.
>
>*8.2 Blood Pressure.* Lower than in term infants. Increases with gestation—50 mm systolic at 28 weeks, 80 mm at term. Diastolic proportionately low varying from 30 to 45 mm.
>
>*8.3 Blood Volume.* Relatively more blood in placenta of pre-term infant than in placenta of normal infant. Delayed clamping of cord therefore of value in increasing blood volume.

9. Problems in Haemopoietic System

>*9.1 Red Blood Cells.* Haemoglobin increases with gestation until 36 weeks. Red cells poorly adapted to extra-uterine conditions due to low red cell 2,3-DPG and low P_{50} causes oxygen dissociation curve to be shifted to left; high concentration of fetal haemoglobin; diminished intracorpuscular enzymes. All these increase affinity for oxygen but diminish ability to compensate for asphyxia. Cells may show abnormal shapes (infantile pyknocytosis) and have reduced life span of about 70 days. Physiological fall of haemoglobin over first 2–3 months occurs in absence of iron deficiency—refractory early anaemia of prematurity (REAP). 'Top-up' transfusion occasionally required when infant has signs such as diminished interest in feeding and sucking, less active, or breathless over feeding.
>
>*9.2 White Blood Cells.* At birth polymorphonuclear neutrophils are the predominant white cells. Numbers rise rapidly to reach peak at 12 h (9000–18 000/mm³) falling to a fairly constant value after 72 h (1500–7000/mm³). After 1 week lymphocytes predominate. Neonate responds to infection with increase in total neutrophil count (particularly immature forms) which demonstrate toxic granulation.
>
>*9.3* Haemorrhagic disease of the newborn and thrombocytopenia more common in pre-term infants.

10. Problems in Hepatobiliary System

>*10.1* Jaundice frequent because of functional immaturity of various enzymes (*see* p. 58). Regular bilirubin estimations required at 4–6-hourly intervals if indirect bilirubin rises about 170 µmol/l (10 mg/dl) and record on graph to forecast when concentration likely to reach 340 µmol/l. Infants with a rise greater than 17 µmol/l/h likely to need exchange transfusion. Very pre-term infants will require transfusion at lower concentrations.

10.2 Bile acid pool considerably reduced due to inadequate reabsorption by terminal ileum. Contributes to inefficient utilization of fatty acids and fat-soluble vitamins.

Note: Fats of breast milk less dependent on bile acids for digestion and absorption.

11. Problems in Renal System. Degree of kidney maturity varies with gestational age.

11.1 Low renal blood flow due to low mean arterial pressure, increased renal vascular resistance and increased cell thickness of glomerular membrane. There is enhanced renin/angiotensin activity. Adult values reached between 4 and 5 months.

11.2 Renal tubular function even less mature, resulting in glomerular-tubular imbalance.

Functional renal immaturity leads to:

11.2.1 Less ability to excrete water load (dilution) and conserve water (concentration).

11.2.2 Difficulty in conserving filtered amino acids, sodium phosphate and glucose, and in secreting H^+ ions.

11.2.3 Diminished solute (urea) excretion.

11.2.4 Inefficient excretion of many drugs (e.g. penicillin, gentamicin).

Note: Functional immaturity of kidney protected by two important factors which reduce excretory load on kidney and do not stress water-conserving ability: (*a*) Process of growth (anabolism) which incorporates protein, sodium, phosphorus, calcium and water into growing tissues. (*b*) Feeding human milk which has low solute content.

Small for Gestational Age (Light-for-dates) Infants (SGA)

Term applied to infants with birth weight tenth centile and below. Some confine term to infants whose birth weight is less than fifth centile—corrected for sex, maternal height, birth order.

Aetiology

	Percentage
Normal variations	10
Chromosomal and congenital defects	10
Infections—mother and baby	5
Vascular disease in mother, including diabetes and heart	35
Drugs—alcohol, smoking	5
Other, including multiple pregnancy	35

Risks to Fetus

Perinatal Mortality. Five to ten times greater than infants of optimum birth weight. Reasons are perinatal asphyxia; congenital malformations; aspiration pneumonia; massive pulmonary haemorrhage; infections.

Pathology of Deprived Fetus
Compared with infants of the same weight but at mean of their gestation: (*a*) Weight of heart, kidneys, liver, lungs and thymus moderately decreased; (*b*) Brain weight markedly increased with more mature pattern of cerebral convolutions, but still lighter than brain of normal grown infant of same gestational age, both cell number and myelin content diminished.

Clinical Appearance of Small for Gestational Age Infants

1. Diminished Growth Potential. Signs of chromosome or congenital anomalies might be present or those of intra-uterine infection (e.g. jaundice, hepatospleno-megaly, purpura). External proportions often similar to normally grown pre-term infants of same birth weight.

2. Diminished Growth Support. Grouped according to time of onset of diminished growth support.

> *2.1 Subacute (Dysmature).* Supply-line insufficiency for a few weeks. Disproportion of normal or near-normal length with subnormal weight. Head appears relatively large. Soft-tissue wasting (muscle and subcutaneous fat) with loose, thin skin, often dry, cracked with meconium staining. Sparse head hair, skull sutures often wide with large anterior fontanelle. Alert and hungry at birth. Birth weights of these infants are frequently not reduced sufficiently for them to be recorded as small for gestational age.
>
> *2.2 Chronic.* Growth failure for a few months. Weight, length and head circumference similar to that of appropriately grown pre-term infants of same birth weight. Soft-tissue wasting often not apparent.

Neonatal Behaviour
Functional maturity (e.g. of lungs and nervous system) little affected by poor intra-uterine growth. Tend to lose less weight if fed to their 'expected' weight. Adapt themselves well to extra-uterine environment. Chronically-deprived fetuses often apathetic and have feeding problems.

Neonatal Problems
1. Diminished Growth Potential Infants. Problems of any existing chromosome or congenital anomalies or infections.

2. Diminished Growth Support infants

> 2.1 Hypoglycaemia (due to low fat and glycogen reserves).
>
> 2.2 Perinatal asphyxia common, including meconium aspiration, pneumothorax, pneumomediastinum.
>
> 2.3 High haematocrit (packed cell volume greater than 60 per cent not uncommon).

2.4 Massive pulmonary haemorrhage, poor thermal regulation and sometimes persistent fetal circulation.

Long-term Prognosis
Few reliable studies available. Earlier studies invalid because of failure to distinguish from pre-term infants.
1. *Physical Growth.* Infants with diminished head growth in addition to length and weight restriction tend to be smaller than infants of similar birth weight but shorter gestation, and also than healthy term infants; centile distributions of weight, height and head circumference remain below normal standards.
2. *Neurological and Intellectual Development.* Minimal cerebral dysfunction and general lowering of intelligence described. Interaction with social conditions important.
   Note: Relative role of diminished growth potential and diminished growth support in causing these long-term effects not yet known.

Specific Disorders in Pre-term Infants
Clinical conditions encountered more commonly in pre-term infants:

Respiratory System
1. Difficulty in Initiating and Maintaining Respiration

2. Apnoeic Attacks Cessation of breathing for more than 20s. Rarely associated with twitching. Death may occur. Must be differentiated from periodic respiration commonly found in pre-term infants (*see* p. 59); often start on fifth day; are more common in REM sleep but more prolonged in non-REM sleep. Associated with:
> 2.1 Extreme prematurity; RDS.
> 2.2 Intracranial haemorrhage; cerebral oedema.
> 2.3 Infection, e.g. bronchopneumonia, septicaemia, meningitis.
> 2.4 Regurgitation and/or aspiration of stomach contents.
> 2.5 Nasogastric tube feeding with too large volumes (causing fall in Pao_2).
> 2.6 Excessive handling and temperature fluctuation.
> 2.7 Metabolic disturbances, e.g. hypoglycaemia; hypocalcaemia.
> 2.8 Drugs given to mother during labour, e.g. diazepam.
> 2.9 Asphyxia from any cause.

Treatment. Identify and remedy cause: reduce handling to minimum; check incubator temperature, correct anaemia, give sufficient ambient oxygen, observing TcO_2.
Specific: (i) Physical stimulation (e.g. flicking heel). If no response after 15s: (*a*) Resuscitate with bag and mask (percentage of oxygen should be that usually breathed); 100% oxygen not advisable because of risk of retrolental fibroplasia (*see* p. 71). (*b*) If unsuccessful, intubate and ventilate with intermittent positive pressure. (ii) Monitor infant with apnoea and ECG. (iii) Theophylline

4–8 mg/kg/day in 4 doses. Check plasma level 10–20 μg/ml. Continuous inflating pressure CPAP (low pressure) abolishs attacks if theophylline fails.

3. Atelectasis

> *3.1 Primary*: Common in all newborn infants, particularly pre-term. Due to poor respiratory effort from immaturity, maternal over-sedation, brain damage.
> *3.2 Secondary*: Associated with surfactant deficiency (respiratory distress syndrome), inhalation of meconium, amniotic debris, mucus plugs.

4. Pneumonia An important cause of neonatal death. Infection acquired:

> 4.1 Before birth: Ascending infection from prolonged rupture of membranes.
> 4.2 During delivery: most serious organism is Group B β-haemolytic streptococcus. Can cause septicaemia in early hours or pneumonia later. The earlier the onset the higher the mortality; may be 60% despite all treatment (*see* p. 45).
> 4.3 After birth: (i) Aspiration of milk which later becomes infected; (ii) Can complicate respiratory distress syndrome and mechanical ventilation.

5. Respiratory Distress Syndrome (RDS)/Hyaline Membrane Disease
Definition: A symptom complex affecting mainly pre-term infants and characterized:

> 5.1 Clinically: by progressive respiratory difficulty with a sustained respiratory rate of over 60, chest retraction and insuction, expiratory grunt and cyanosis, all coming on within the first few hours after birth.
> 5.2 Pathologically: by widespread atelectasis with eosinophilic hyaline membranes comprising fibrin, and cellular debris in alveolar ducts and terminal bronchioles.

Infants at Risk: Mostly pre-term infants. Babies of diabetic mothers (if poorly controlled) or born by Caesarean section also at increased risk independent of gestation. Also second of twins and following antepartum haemorrhage. Perinatal asphyxia and hypothermia increase vulnerability.
Incidence: Affects about 0·5% of all babies, increasingly more common as gestation diminishes from virtually zero at term to more than 70% at 28 weeks.
Clinical Features. Symptoms almost invariably develop within first 4 h of postnatal life. (i) Tachypnoea, soft expiratory grunt and dilatation of nares. (ii) Laboured breathing, use of accessory muscles, insuction of lower intercostal spaces, xiphoid cartilage and sternal area with 'seesaw' respiration. (iii) Infant lies on back motionless except for breathing. Arms and legs abducted, knees and elbows flexed to right angle—'frog' position. (iv) Cyanosis develops as condition worsens. Prolonged apnoeic attacks develop. (v) Respiratory rate may reach 120. Peripheral oedema common. Percussion note dull. Diminished breath sounds.
Course. Natural course of illness is run in 3–5 days. Progression from mild to severe takes 24–36 h. Thereafter gradual improvement or death from anoxia, intracranial haemorrhage or pulmonary haemorrhage.

Diagnosis. Radiology of chest typically shows: (i) Diffuse reticulogranular density throughout both lungs ('frosted glass' appearance). (ii) As atelectasis worsens air-filled major bronchi seen in relief through partially opaque lungs—the 'air bronchogram' effect. These are considered abnormal only when they extend beyond cardiac silhouette. (iii) Outline of heart becomes diffuse or obliterated by increased density. (iv) Interstitial pulmonary emphysema, with or without pneumothorax, may develop spontaneously without treatment.

Differential Diagnosis. Chest radiograph is essential to exclude following causes of early respiratory difficulties. (i) Primary atelectasis (*see* p. 64). (ii) Pneumonia (*see* p. 64). Sometimes difficult clinically to differentiate from RDS. X-ray usually helps. History of prolonged rupture of membranes or difficult labour sometimes obtained. (iii) Meconium aspiration. More common in light-for-dates infants (*see* p. 61) with history of intrapartum asphyxia. (iv) Congenital anomalies: Diaphragmatic hernia, pulmonary lymphangiectasia, lobar emphysema, lung cysts. (v) Interstitial emphysema and pneumothorax: More common in light-for-dates infants and infants requiring intubation and ventilation at birth. May also complicate RDS. (vi) **Transient tachypnoea**: More common in term infants. Clinical features: uneventful pregnancy and labour; child develops rapid breathing (>100 per min), very little insuction and no abnormal signs in chest. Sometimes infant hypothermic and grunting and develops tachypnoea on warming. Infants improve over 24–48 h. Condition thought to result from delayed absorption of lung fluid. Characteristic radiological appearance: wet lungs—prominent vascular markings and fluid in pleural fissures. Condition thought to be due to delayed clearing of lung fluid.

Pathophysiology. Fundamental problem is high surface tension at air–liquid interface of alveoli due to immaturity of lung mechanisms responsible for synthesis of surface-active lecithin (surfactant) by Type II alveolar cells. Synthesis sensitive to hypoxaemia, acidosis and hypothermia. These perinatal stresses partly explain irregular incidence of disorder at a given gestational age. Surfactant deficiency leads to atelectasis and diminished lung compliance.

Note: Two enzymatic pathways exist for biosynthesis of lecithin: (*a*). Phosphocholine transferase system: Matures at 35 weeks. Synthesizes primarily dipalmitoyl lecithin. (*b*). Methyl transferase system. Identified as early as 20 weeks. Synthesizes palmitoylmyristoyl lecithin. Enzyme activities rapidly drop with acidaemia, cold and asphyxia.

Critical factor determining whether RDS will develop is ability to continue to synthesize enough surfactant to satisfy demands.

Physiological Complications: (i) Right-to-left shunting of blood (30–60%) through foramen ovale, ductus arteriosus and non-aerated parts of the lungs. (ii) Pulmonary vascular bed hypoperfusion due to high vascular resistance from hypoxia. (iii) Reduction of lung compliance. (iv) Anoxic damage to alveolar cells further reduces surfactant production. (v) Decreased alveolar ventilation with increased work in breathing.

Biochemical Disturbances. Most important in severe cases are: hypoxaemia; hypercapnia; acidaemia—this usually has two components: (i) Respiratory: from poor alveolar ventilation. (ii) Metabolic: from accumulation of organic acids from tissue hypoxia (e.g. lactic acid).

Management a. Prevention Corticosteroids (e.g. betamethasone) to mothers accelerates lung maturity by inducing surfactant production thereby reducing risk of RDS: (i) in uncomplicated premature labour; (ii) where premature delivery is planned because of pregnancy complications (e.g. severe toxaemia). *Note*: Perinatal administration of corticosteroids might be harmful to fetus and mother. Controlled studies of its benefits are awaited.

Surfactant also induced by maternal heroin, aminophylline, thyroxine, beta-adrenergic drugs and prolonged rupture of membranes. Prevention of perinatal asphyxia and hypothermia preserves surfactant.

b. Treatment

A. *General Care and Nursing*: Important to maintain neutral thermal environment and provide sufficient water and calories by peripheral intravenous infusions of 10% glucose and electrolyte. Start milk gavage about third day.

B. *Continuous Monitoring* of Breathing, Heart Rate and Blood Pressure, Oxygen (T_cPo_2) or Arterial Pao_2, Carbon dioxide (Pco_2), pH, to assess progress.

C. *Biochemical Monitoring*: Attention must be given to plasma electrolytes, bilirubin, calcium and glucose. Also regular measurements of blood gases and acid–base and clotting status.

D. *Correction of Acidaemia* with alkali if H^+ rises above 55 nmol/l (pH < 7·25). Accepted practice is to use molar (8·4%) sodium bicarbonate. Sufficient bicarbonate should be given to correct the base deficit: (body weight (kg) $\times$ 0·4 $\times$ base deficit) = number of mmol bicarbonate required). *Rate of infusion should not exceed 1 mmol of sodium bicarbonate per min* to avoid rapid changes in blood volume and blood pressure. Sodium bicarbonate may cause hypernatraemia. THAM useful in ventilated babies as it does not cause hypernatraemia.

Note: Infusion of bicarbonate associated with rapid rise in $Paco_2$ and plasma osmolality, and fall in haematocrit and colloid osmotic pressure due to sudden increase in blood volume. Also drop in CSF pH (Posner effect). Possibility of neurological damage from rapid osmotic changes, hence bicarbonate reserved for treatment of *metabolic* acidosis. Respiratory acidosis treated by assisted ventilation.

E. *Oxygen Therapy* (*see also* p. 71). Transcutaneous monitor should be applied at onset of respiratory distress and sensor site changed every 4 h. If respiratory distress worsens, umbilical arterial catheterization may be necessary. Ambient oxygen concentrations should then be adjusted to maintain umbilical arterial Pao_2 8kPa and 10kPa (60 and 75mmHg). If more than 60% $FiO_2 > 0·6$ oxygen required some form of ventilatory assistance likely to be required.

F. *Ventilatory Assistance*. A number of methods now available to keep lungs inflated and minimize surfactant consumption.

i. *Continuous positive airway pressure* (CPAP) applied via head-box (Gregory Box) endotracheal tubes, nasal tubes, face mask.

Indications for continuous inflating pressure vary between different centres. A reasonable indication is that once FiO_2 above 0·6 is required to sustain an arterial Pao_2 of 8 kPa (60mmHg), treatment should be instituted. Adequate intensive care facilities must be available. In weaning from apparatus priority is given to reducing environmental oxygen to FiO_2 0·4, before slowly reducing positive pressure.

Other indications are pulmonary oedema and recurrent apnoea. Many very small babies electively ventilated immediately after birth.

Note: Hazards include:

a. Pneumothorax (reduced to minimum if pressures do not exceed 6cm water).

b. Circulatory effects (decreased venous return, diminished pulmonary blood flow, reduced cardiac output).

c. Intraventricular haemorrhage with possible later development of hydrocephalus.

d. Excoriation of neck by head-box seal.

e. Brachial plexus palsy from pressure by head-box seal.

f. Hazards of endotracheal intubation.

g. Persistent patent ductus.

h. Panophthalmitis if face mask used.

ii. *Mechanical ventilation*: Indications:

a. Apnoea not responding to CPAP and/or theophylline.

b. Rapid deterioration in clinical condition despite treatment.

c. Arterial PaO_2 less than 5·5 kPa (40 mmHg) while infant is breathing FiO_2 1·0 (100 % oxygen).

Optimum survival rates and minimal incidence of bronchopulmonary dysplasia are associated with the following ventilator characteristics:

a. Square pressure wave.

b. Slow respiratory frequency (30–40 cycles/min).

c. Positive end-expiratory pressure (PEEP) 0·02–0·05 kPa (2–5 cm H_2O).

d. Peak airway pressure no greater than 5 kPa (25 cm H_2O).

e. FiO_2 0·8 range from 0·21 to 1·0.

f. High inspiration: expiration ratio 2 : 1 (1 : 3→3 : 1).

G. *Antibiotics*: Not given routinely but only when there are clinical grounds for suspecting infection (*see* p. 42).

H. *Blood Transfusions*: Newborn's blood contains high proportion of HbF which reacts poorly with 2,3-DPG (diphosphoglycerate) and so dissociation curve shifted to left. P_{50} for blood with adult haemoglobin HbA is 3·6 kPa (27 mmHg) and for blood with fetal haemoglobin is 2·6 kPa (19 mmHg). HbA reacts better with 2,3-DPG and so infants with RDS are helped by transfusions of adult blood—but best give small amounts (10–20 ml). Exchange transfusion tried but probably not helpful.

I. *Parental Visiting*: Parents must be encouraged to visit and hold infants as often as possible.

6. Chronic Pulmonary Disease of Prematurity. A collection of poorly understood conditions characterized by the insidious development of respiratory insufficiency beginning within a few weeks after birth, and manifest by tachypnoea, costal recession and cyanosis in severe cases. More common in infants less than 1500 g.

a. Wilson–Mikity syndrome (*pulmonary dysmaturity*): Infants rarely have history of early dyspnoea requiring oxygen or assisted ventilation. Serial radiographs show diffuse interstitial cystic emphysema. Cause unknown. Possibly due to uneven postnatal development of lung alveoli in infants whose lungs are required to perform a respiratory function before full maturity has occurred.

Prognosis: Early fatality 20–50 %. In surviving infants symptoms disappear after a few months. Chest radiograph becomes normal within 2 years.

b. Chronic pulmonary insufficiency of prematurity: Clinically similar to Wilson–Mikity syndrome but radiograph shows diffuse haziness; possibly due to late development of surfactant deficiency—good outlook.

c. Bronchopulmonary dysplasia, see p. 72.

Differential Diagnosis: Following must be considered: pneumonia, heart failure, severe anaemia, congenital anomalies. Check radiograph. Clinical history should give correct diagnosis.

Treatment: Oxygen may be needed for a long time—give via nasal prongs if necessary; careful feeding to avoid tiring baby.

Note: In these conditions abnormalities seem to be reversible in survivors. Normal pulmonary function can be expected in later childhood.

Infection
As for term infants, *see* Chapter 12, p. 41.

Diagnosis of Infection
Diagnosis often difficult, especially in early stages. Alerting features:

1. *Predisposing factors*. Congenital anomalies, prolonged rupture of membranes, protracted labour, birth asphyxia requiring assisted ventilation.

2. *Behaviour*. Diminished activity; hypotonia; lethargic sucking; refusal of feeds; failure to gain weight; vomiting and/or diarrhoea, abdominal distension, pallor, cyanotic or apnoeic attacks, raised respiratory and pulse rate; jaundice.

Note: Fever is uncommon.

When examining for infection:

1. Look for general (above) and local signs, e.g. skin, umbilicus, conjunctivitis, mastitis, osteomyelitis (inflammatory subcutaneous swelling, pseudoparalysis), meningitis, pneumonia, otitis media.

2. Investigations should include: chest radiograph; blood culture; white cell count (particularly for immature polymorphonuclear leucocyte count), urine culture (clean catch specimen or suprapubic bladder tap); examination and culture of CSF; stool culture; skin, nasal and umbilical swabs; immunoglobulins—serial estimations of IgM sometimes of benefit as non-specific index of infection.

Oedema
Common.

1. Early
Manifest in eyelids, hands, feet, dependent side of face. Sometimes present at birth; more commonly comes on within a day or two, found mainly in sick infants, possible due to low serum albumin or overhydration.

2. Late
Seen in infants fed high solute milks and infants changed rapidly from breast milk to higher solute milks. Associated with rapidly accelerating weight gain. No action usually required, but check salt intake. Consider heart failure, urinary protein loss (congenital nephrotic syndrome, renal vein thrombosis).

3. Localized Oedema
e.g. Trauma (caput succedaneum), infection (osteomyelitis). Oedema of dorsum of hands and feet sometimes found in Turner's syndrome.

4. Cerebral Oedema
Associated with difficult delivery and hypoxia. Due to breakdown of cellular

osmoregulation (cytotoxic type) and/or increased vascular permeability (vaso-genic type). Treatment with dexamethasone or mannitol.

Intracranial Haemorrhage (*see also* p. 36)
More frequent in pre-term than full-term infants. Reasons:
1. Rapid delivery more common.
2. Skull bones softer than full-term infants.
3. Intraventricular haemorrhage often occurs in RDS and extreme prematur-ity.
4. Defective haemostasis.

Sites of Haemorrhage
Intraventricular haemorrhage from rupture of veins in the periventricular germinal matrix which are vulnerable to asphyxia and venous congestion. Subdural haemorrhage mainly in posterior fossa, invariably traumatic in origin.

Sequelae
1. Death in perinatal period.
2. Post-haemorrhagic hydrocephalus.
3. Cerebral palsy, mental retardation and epilepsy.

Metabolic Disorders (*see also* Section 8).

1. Hyperbilirubinaemia

More marked in pre-term infants in the first week. Investigation is the same as with term neonates but bilirubin level at which treatment is commenced is lower.

2. Hypoglycaemia
More common in small for gestational age babies. Blood glucose less than 1·1 mmol/l (20 mg/dl) on two or more occasions. Used to be common when initial feeding delayed. Early and liberal feeding with milk lessens risk. Sick infants more vulnerable—hence importance of carly feeds and parenteral glucose infusions if necessary. Regular blood checks necessary. May be responsible for later brain damage, particularly if symptomatic. Treatment with milk or intravenous glucose. Rarely corticosteroids needed.

3. Hypocalcaemia
Early type (1–3 days) more common in pre-term infants, usually if sick with RDS or after asphyxia or surgery. Symptoms include jitteriness; apnoea; convulsions. Due mainly to elevated levels of corticosteroids, calcitonin and glucagon.

Treatment
Oral or intravenous 10% calcium gluconate (maximum 9 ml/24 h). Check for hypomagnesaemia if no response.

Management of Pre-term Infants

Care of Mother before Delivery
Anticipation of mothers at special risk of delivering prematurely very important

(e.g. toxaemia; hypertension; diabetes; poor obstetric history; rhesus isoimmunization; poor social conditions, etc.). Infants born to these mothers have a higher chance of dying in the perinatal period or of later neurological disability. Delivery should take place in a hospital with intensive care facilities. Transport of 'high-risk' infants to such units after birth less effective.

Note: Antepartum amniocentesis for pulmonary phospholipids (lecithin) important when planning early delivery.

Care during Labour

1. Drugs used for analgesia (e.g. pethidine) and sedation (e.g. diazepam) must be used with care. Epidural anaesthesia results in fewer depressed infants at birth.
2. Experienced person should deliver pre-term babies. Number of people allowed to conduct premature labour should be limited. Forceps often used to protect head during second stage.

Immediate After-care

1. *Delivery*. Must take place in a warm room. Under normal delivery room conditions body temperature can fall rapidly from evaporation water loss unless special precautions taken (2°C in first 15 min can be lost in room temperature of 20–25°C). Doctor (or nurse) specially instructed in neonatal resuscitation should be present to look after baby's needs.
2. *Reception* Infant should be transferred to a heated resuscitation trolley equipped with a radiant heat source to reduce heat loss. Brief examination is necessary to exclude obvious congenital malformations. If very small, transfer immediately to a preheated incubator. Cot in heated ward can be used if infant's weight and condition satisfactory. Baby removed from delivery room when adequate respiration established. If well enough should be shown to mother before removal.

Later After-care

Temperature control. Any pre-term infant who causes concern should be nursed naked, except for nappy (diaper) in an incubator. Advantages of an incubator:
1. Constant observation of whole infant possible with easy accessibility.
2. Environment can be adjusted to optimum for individual need.
3. Less risk of cross-infection.

Great care must be given to temperature of incubator.

Consequences of not providing optimum environmental warmth:
1. Higher mortality rate, because,
2. Oxygen consumption increased in attempt to maintain normal body temperature. Under conditions of hypoxia (PaO_2 less than 6·68 kPa (50 mmHg) oxygen consumption does not increase and body temperature falls. May result in hypoglycaemia, metabolic acidosis, sluggish respiration, lethargy, oedema, intravascular coagulation, neonatal cold injury.
3. Cold stress increases caloric demand, less being available for growth.
4. Lower arterial PO_2 possibly by right-to-left shunting in lungs.

Temperature control of incubator: Incubator temperature must be maintained within thermoneutral range, i.e. that within which oxygen consumption is minimal. The smaller and younger the infant the higher the optimum environmental temperature. Temperature for a very small infant is dangerously hot for a bigger infant. Optimum for 1-kg baby in first 24 h about 35°C; for 3-kg baby about 33 °C. When infant is transferred to a cot and wrapped in blanket, thermoneutral range is maintained at lower environmental temperatures. Infant's rectal temperature should be taken every hour until a steady state is reached at 36–37 °C, then every 3 h. Two methods of controlling incubator temperatures:

1. Servo-control method (skin or rectum). Sometimes more convenient for very small infants requiring minimal handling.

Disadvantages: (*a*) Risk of hyperthermia if sensor is detached; (*b*) Might prevent early diagnosis of sepsis by depriving temperature chart of its normal clinical value.

2. Non-servo-controlled method: temperature regulated manually to maintain normal body temperture.

Humidity. Keep humidity at ambient. High humidity encourages multiplication of Gram-negative organisms, e.g. *Pseudomonas aeruginosa* ('water bugs').

Prevention of Infection (*see* p. 43).

Oxygen Therapy. Most small pre-term infants require to be nursed in incubators with extra oxygen for first few days of life or sometimes longer. Cyanosis and hypoxaemia result from:

1. Hypoventilation (e.g. extreme prematurity).
2. Diffusion defect (e.g. pneumonia).
3. Right-to-left shunting of blood (e.g. congenital heart disease, RDS).

Oxygen used in following situations:

1. Birth asphyxia.
2. Recurrent apnoea.
3. RDS (and other respiratory problems).
4. Miscellaneous (e.g. heart failure, anaemia).

Control: Oxygen therapy must be carefully controlled:

1. By regular monitoring of percentage of oxygen in inspired air (FiO_2) by oxygen analyser.

2. By measuring transcutaneous oxygen ($TcPO_2$). Give sufficient oxygen to keep $TcPO_2$ about 8 kPa (60 mmHg). If transcutaneous oxygen monitor not available monitor either by intra-arterial line or arterialized warmed capillary blood samples but latter less satisfactory.

Effects of too much Oxygen (Hyperoxia)

*1. Toxicity to eyes: **Retrolental Fibroplasia***: Condition affecting retinae of mainly very pre-term infants. Degree of immaturity, length of administration, concentration of PaO_2 all contribute to its development.

Pathology: Initial phase of vascular constriction followed by proliferation of retinal arterioles into vitreous humour. Fibrosis follows with ultimate retinal detachment. Blindness results in 30% affected infants. Enucleation sometimes necessary because of glaucoma.

Infants at risk: Mainly infants with recurrent apnoeic spells needing frequent resuscitation with bag and mask and high FiO_2. Monitoring of PaO_2 often difficult since apnoeic attacks often continue beyond second week.

Note: Infants with RDS at less risk (*a*) because of careful monitoring of PaO_2; (*b*) existence of large right-to-left shunts keeping PaO_2 low despite high FiO_2.

Prevention: (*a*) Oxygen administration to all infants must be carefully controlled; (*b*) PaO_2 should be kept between 8 and 12–5 kPa (60–90 mmHg); (*c*) Infants with recurrent apnoeic attacks must be resuscitated with oxygen concentration in which infant is usually nursed.

Note: (*a*) Care must be taken not to substitute anoxic brain damage for dangers of blindness by giving inadequate oxygen; (*b*) All pre-term infants should have regular ophthalmic examinations whilst in neonatal unit.

2. *Toxicity to lungs*: **Bronchopulmonary Dysplasia** (*see also* p. 67): Now believed to be primarily a traumatic effect on the lung from use of unnecessarily high peak airways pressure and oxygen concentration during assisted mechanical ventilation. Not seen when high inspired FiO_2 (greater than 0·6) breathed (as in RDS) without assisted positive-pressure ventilation. Clinically infant shows tachypnoea, insuction and widespread crepitations and cyanosis. Serial radiology shows initial patchy areas of over-aeration, and later interstitial fibrosis. Pathological appearances include squamous metaplasia of bronchiolar epithelium, basement membrane thickening or fibroblastic proliferation around alveoli. Condition protracted and infant may be oxygen dependent for many months and have to be sent home with continuous oxygen via nasal catheter.

Catheterization of Umbilical Vessels

Umbilical Artery. Used for: Blood gas analysis, measurements of arterial pressures in infants with cardiorespiratory problems. Site catheter tip above aortic bifurcation and below renal arteries.

Umbilical Vein. Used for: exchange transfusion for blood group incompatibility. Intravenous therapy should be given via peripheral vein.

Complications:

a. *Thrombosis*

Umbilical Artery. More common in severely ill infants. Lesions range from small fibrin thrombi at catheter tip to thrombotic occlusion of large arteries.

Umbilical Vein. Usually due to infections of umbilicus or hypertonic fluid infusions (e.g. molar bicarbonate, 20% glucose). Portal vein thrombosis a long-term sequel.

b. *Embolism*

Umbilical Artery. If catheter tip is in lower abdominal aorta emboli can break away to occlude circulation to lower limbs.

Umbilical Vein. Depends on position of catheter tip: (i) In portal system—emboli lodge in liver, sometimes cause septic abscesses. (ii) In right atrium—emboli enter lungs or are shunted across foramen ovale into systemic circulation (paradoxical embolus).

Note: If thrombus forms on catheter it must *never* be cleared by flushing since this might force clot into circulation. Catheter should be removed.

c. *Air Embolus*. Danger greater with sick infants (higher negative inspiratory pressures during inspiration). More common with venous catheters.

d. *Vasospasm*. Arterial catheterization sometimes associated with blanching of leg due to spasm. No sequelae if catheter removed promptly.

e. *Haemorrhage*. Constant threat from arterial catheterization. Careful supervision always required, particularly after catheter withdrawal.

f. *Necrotizing Enterocolitis* (*see* p. 272). Acute inflammation of bowel (mainly large) with necrosis, ulceration and sometimes perforation.

g. Infection from organisms at catheter tip entering blood. Strict aseptic technique mandatory.

Drug Therapy. Routines differ widely. Following scheme is reasonable:
1. Haematinics and vitamins (*see* pp. 74, 75).
2. *Antibiotics.* Overprescribed in neonatal period because of difficulties in diagnosing bacterial infections. If indicated, antibiotic combinations are usually used. Gentamicin and a penicillin or a cephalosporin. *Prophylactic antibiotics not indicated.* Antibiotics used in following instances:
    a. Proven antepartum infection.
    b. Vague, non-specific symptoms which suggest bacterial infection.
    c. Significant skin sepsis.
    d. Purulent conjunctivitis.
    e. Specific infections.

Feeding

Main requirements of feeding in neonatal period are (*a*) to provide for growth, (*b*) to make smooth transition from intra-uterine to extra-uterine life by meeting metabolic requirements of various organ systems.

Adequacy of nutrition judged clinically by weight gain and growth in length and head circumference.

Table 15.1. Nutritional requirements of pre-term infants per 24 h

Nutrient per kg		Minerals per kg		Vitamins per kg†	
Calories	110–140	Sodium	0·5–2 mmol	A	1500–2500 iu
Water	150–200 ml	Potassium	0·5–2 mmol	Thiamine	0·4 mg
Protein	3–6 g*	Chloride	0·5–2 mmol	Pyridoxine	0·25 mg
Carbohydrate	10–15 g	Calcium	4–6 mmol	Riboflavin	0·5 mg
Fat	5–7 g	Phosphorus	2–4 mmol	B_{12}	1·0 mg
		Magnesium	0·5–1 mmol	Niacin	6·0 mg
		Iron	6 mg	Folic acid	0·35 mg
				C	30–50 mg
				D	400 iu
				E	5–100 iu
				K	1·5 mg

*Upper range for very immature infants <32 weeks' gestation.
†Most commercial formulae contain added vitamins but additional supplementation (*see* pp. 74, 75) usually given.

Only small amounts of milk usually tolerated. Arterial PaO_2 frequently falls as much as 4·0 kPa (30 mmHg) after large feeds: can precipitate apnoea.

      Healthy Pre-term Infants. Undiluted breast milk should be given to all pre-term infants initially. Mother's own expressed milk or from a human milk bank. Some very low birth weight babies may require a milk with higher protein. Check adequacy of energy content of breast milk by creamatocrit, discard if less than 4%.

If mother not going to breast feed a milk formula closely resembling breast milk should be given.

      1. Frequency. First feed given early, e.g. hour after birth, gives higher blood glucose, lower serum bilirubin, less dehydration, more rapid return to birth weight.

a. Infants older than 34 weeks' gestation usually fed 3-hourly, i.e. 7 or 8 feedings a day. After a few weeks 4-hourly feeds can be instituted.

b. Younger infants best fed by: (i) hourly feeds; (ii) Continuous intragastric feeding as a milk drip if less than 30 weeks; (iii) Transpyloric feeding (nasojejunal or nasoduodenal) continuous or intermittent probably not helpful.

Note: Stomach should be aspirated every 3 h if continuously fed.

2. *Volume*. Allow nutritional requirements to be reached by end of first week.

a. First day 60 ml milk/kg; if less than 1·5 kg start with 80 ml/kg.

b. Increase by increments of 25 ml/kg to reach 200 ml/kg by day 7. Calculate amounts on birth weight until this is regained, then calculate requirements on actual weight. (*Note*: some modern modified milks for low birth weight infants have a higher calorie value (80 kcal/100 ml) and increased sodium content, enabling total calories to be supplied by 150 ml/kg/day).

c. Thereafter maintain daily intake of 200 ml/kg according to twice-weekly weighings. If infant demands more (by nurses' intuition) milk should be given until satisfied.

Note: Some authorities recommend a more rapid build up of milk intake over first week. Others recommend minimum intake of 330 ml/kg by the tenth day. With these regimens risks of milk aspiration increase and infants may open up ductus and develop heart failure—more prone to necrotizing enterocolitis (NEC).

3. *Technique*. Very small infants (<1500 g, <32 weeks) invariably require tube feeding (gavage) via indwelling polyvinyl nasogastric tube. Infants 1500–2000 g (32–34 weeks) likely to need gavage feeding for a short while. Over 2000 g (>34 weeks) most healthy infants have adequate sucking and swallowing reflexes. Tube-fed infants at any stage can be offered a bottle when they make spontaneous sucking movements or put fingers into mouth.

Tube Feeding

a. Soft, sterile, disposable polyvinyl catheter (size 5) passed via nose into stomach.

b. Distance tube is to be passed first marked off by measuring distance from ear to nose to xiphisternum. Pass catheter to this mark. Check catheter is in stomach by injecting small amount of air and listen over stomach for bubbling. Aspirate contents and test for reaction. Small stomach washout with sterile water often necessary if blood or mucus aspirated.

c. Tube secured by fastening to side of face with a thin strip of adhesive plaster. End of tube is brought out of incubator and occluded between feeds (if intermittent).

d. Milk introduced slowly by gravity or by syringe. Feeding should be immediately stopped if any change in infant's colour, or regurgitation occurs.

Additions to feed

1. *Haematinic Supplements*. Following scheme aims to build up stores which would normlly have accumulated in last trimester.

    a. Infants more than 32 weeks' Gestation

        i. Ferrous sulphate BPC 15 mg b.d. (1 mg/kg of elemental iron). Given from 4 weeks until adequate diet established, usually about 3 months. Lessens severity of later anaemia. Has no effect on early ('physiological') anaemia.

ii. Folic acid 0·5 mg/day from 7 days until approximately 40 weeks' gestational age keeps serum and erythrocyte folate levels within normal range (also prevents hypersegmentation of neutrophils).

b. Infants less than 32 weeks' Gestation

i. Ferrous sulphate and folic acid as above.

ii. Vitamin E deficiency with oedema and haemolytic anaemia may occur in very small infants with poor stores. α-Tocopherol acetate 25 mgms. (water-soluble preparation) per day suitable supplement from 7 days to 32 weeks gestational age.

Note: Vitamin E and oral iron should not be given at the same time of day since iron hinders vitamin E absorption.

2. *Vitamin Supplements*. Multivitamin preparations are given from 7 days to about 4 months, e.g. DHSS Children's Vitamin Drops 15 drops/day to breast-fed infants which provide: Vitamin A, 2100 i.u.; C, 65 mg;D, 850 i.u.

Sick Pre-term Infants. Oral feeding initially inadvisable in following situations: (*a*) RDS; (*b*) Recurrent apnoeic attacks or convulsions; (*c*) Congenital anomalies of gastro-intestinal tract; (*d*) 'Functional' ileus; (*e*) Extreme prematurity.

Intravenous Fluids required initially in above conditions—in most instances only for short period. As soon as feasible, oral feeding should be encouraged., Peripheral veins or long catheter in large vein e.g. subclavian used wherever possible in preference to umbilical vein. Requirements:

A. *Short term, birth–5 days*: Basic needs are for water, calories, sodium and potassium. Sick infants require less water than healthy infants because of greater risk of circulatory overload. Daily supplements of sodium chloride (3 mmol/100 ml/i.v. fluid) sometimes given. Unless obvious loss from diarrhoea, vomiting, intestinal fistulae, potassium rarely needed until after 5 days.

Note: Hypocalcaemia can develop with above routine. After 48 h serum calcium should be regularly monitored and corrected if indicated by intravenous additions.

B. *Long term, 5 days or more* (e.g. for extreme immaturity, severe respiratory distress syndrome, gastrointestinal abnormalities).

More complex intravenous solutions needed containing amino acids, carbohydrates and lipids. Many different combinations available. Additional requirements of electrolytes, minerals, vitamins and trace elements needed. Plasma and/or blood transfusion given at intervals to keep Hb at normal level.

Note: Parenteral feeding should not be embarked upon lightly because of high risks of infection and metabolic complications. Comprehensive laboratory, pharmacological, medical and nursing services must be available.

Psychological Care. Human infant dependent on mother to satisfy early emotional needs. Perinatal events have a profound and lasting effect on mother-infant relationship. Critical stages not fully understood but following periods likely to be important:

i. Antenatal—Planning, confirming and expecting pregnancy; feeling fetal movements; accepting fetus as an individual.

ii. Natal—Birth and seeing baby.

iii. Postnatal—Physical contact and looking at and after baby.

Handicaps of pre-term infants: Often interference with normal pattern of maternal-infant 'bonding'. Reasons: (i) Baby 'remote' from mother in incubator; (ii) Special Care Baby Units with complicated machinery awe mothers so that visits are less frequent; (iii) In some units, fortunately few, mother handles baby less often owing to (supposed) risk of infection; (iv) Mother often has to return home leaving baby in hospital, and worries about child's present illness and survival prospects.

Consequences: Mothers often have feelings of anxiety and inadequacy. Affectionate ties difficult to establish. Babies may be consciously, or subconsciously, rejected. Long periods of separation may be one of important factors in child abuse and later behavioural disorders.

Practical considerations: (*a*) Before mother comes to Neonatal Unit, condition of her baby and use of equipment should be described in detail by doctor or nurse; (*b*) Mothers (and fathers) should be encouraged to visit baby as much as possible and, where possible, to nurse baby (even in an incubator) provided baby not seriously ill; (*c*) Parents must be kept fully informed of baby's progress; (*d*) Nursing staff must offer maximum support; (*e*) Baby should be discharged as early as possible; (*f*) Continued support after infant's discharge by special Health Visitor most valuable; (*g*) Mother should be given colour photograph of baby to keep at her bedside.

Prognosis of Low Birth Weight Infants

Mortality
Chances of survival greatly improved over past 10–15 years, particularly infants less than 1500 g at birth. Factors responsible are:
1. Size of infant. Mortality rate varies inversely with birth weight and gestational age because of postnatal disorders (e.g. RDS).
2. Obstetric practice and efficiency of immediate resuscitation.
3. Availability of Intensive Care. Lowest mortality figures occur in Neonatal Intensive Care Units with trained nurses and medical staff and modern equipment.
4. Complications of pregnancy and labour. Breech delivery associated with higher mortality.
5. Congenital malformations and multiple pregnancy.
6. Maternal factors, e.g. Social class, age, previous obstetric history.
7. Smoking in pregnancy.

Primary Causes of Death
Conditions which lead to stillbirth or first-week deaths:
1. Toxaemia, hypertension, rhesus incompatibility.
2. *Prenatal*—asphyxia, birth injury.
3. *Postnatal*—RDS, infections, congenital malformations, intracranial haemorrhage.

Final Causes of Death

1. Pre-term Infants
Intraventricular haemorrhage, anoxia, infection.

2. Small for Gestational Age Infants
Birth asphyxia, pneumonia, massive pulmonary haemorrhage, congenital malformations.

Morbidity
Falling morbidity rates associated with improved quality of survivors.

1. Pre-term Infants
a. Neurological sequelae. All forms of cerebral palsy, particularly spastic diplegia, choreoathetosis and epilepsy now less common than formerly in pre-term survivors. Visual and hearing defects also less frequent.
b. Mental development. Definite improvement in mean IQ of special care unit survivors compared with earlier studies.
   Note: Social class an important determinant of psychoneurological development.
c. Developmental milestones. Very small infants late in reaching various milestones, e.g. smiling, sitting, walking, etc. but usually catch up by 18 months.
d. Physical growth. Later growth in height and weight of very immature infants after about 2 years is normal, if matched for socio-economic factors.
e. Psycho-emotional sequelae. Prolonged maternal-infant separation may result in mothering disorders.

Factors Influencing Long-term Prognosis.
These are multiple. Most important are:
   1. Improvements in antenatal and intrapartum obstetric practice producing fewer asphyxiated or traumatized infants.
   2. Early active resuscitation of asphyxiated infants.
   3. More efficient management of RDS.
   4. Greater emphasis on early nutrition lowers incidence of hypoglycaemia and encourages better brain growth.
   5. Prevention of hypothermia.
   6. Better control of oxygen therapy by monitoring arterial oxygen tensions.
   Note: As incidence of major handicap has fallen, more 'minor' problems such as learning and behaviour disorders have emerged. Socio-economic factors have important role. Regular developmental assessment in infancy and early childhood detects minor disturbances at early age so that remedial therapy improves chances of fulfilling potential.

2. Small for Gestational Age
Prognosis depends upon cause. Damage to fetus early, e.g. by infection or maternal alcohol is likely to lead to permanent growth and intellectual retardation. Fetuses who are growth retarded in late pregnancy have prospect of good catch-up growth which is the better the more recent the growth retardation in utero. The order in which intra-uterine growth is retarded is weight then length then head circumference. Catch-up growth is effective in the reverse order. The extent of growth retardation in these parameters is an indicator of the degree and duration of the retarding process.

Postmaturity

Infants going beyond term are at risk of placental insufficiency with reduction in food and oxygen transportation. Infants liable to perinatal hypoxia, hence doubling of perinatal mortality at 43 weeks. Infants may appear to have little subcutaneous fat, cracked wrinkled loose skin, long meconium-stained nails and hard skull. Two rare causes are placental sulphatase deficiency and congenital adrenal enzyme deficiency.

Section 3 / Infectious Diseases — Viral

Chapter 16   *MEASLES (Morbilli)*

Definition

Common highly infectious endemic disease caused by RNA virus 140 nm diameter; characterized by enanthem—Koplik's spots in mouth during prodromal period, and exanthem—generalized blotchy rash with profuse watering of eyes and nose. Rare before 9 months owing to passive immunity from mother. Commonest age 4–8 years. Epidemics every 2 years. Transmission by droplet infection. Highly infectious; one attack normally conveys immunity for life. Incubation period 8–16 days.

Table 16.1   Infectivity of childhood fevers

Disease	Incubation period in days	Period of infectivity	
		From	*To*
Scarlet fever	1–5	Onset of sore throat	Swabs negative
Diphtheria	2–5	Onset of symptoms	Swabs negative
Whooping cough	7–10	2 days before symptoms	5 weeks after start of cough
Measles	8–16	6 days before rash	5 days after temperature normal
Rubella	10–21	1 day before rash	2 days after appearance of rash
Chickenpox	15–18	1 day before rash	6 days after appearance of rash
Mumps	12–26	2 days before swelling	Until swelling gone
Infectious mononucleosis	5–14	Onset of symptoms	Until symptoms gone
Poliomyelitis	7–14	3 days before symptoms	Unknown. May be weeks

Clinical Features

1. Prodromal phase, 1–6 days.

Symptoms. Fever, anorexia, photophobia, cough. Epistaxis may occur.

Signs. Running eyes, nose and nasopharynx.

Koplik's spots. Pathognomonic. Tiny white specks on erythematous background. On inner side of cheek opposite lower molar teeth. Also described on palpebral conjunctiva. Fade with appearance of rash.

2. Phase of eruption

> *2.1 Rash*. Occurs first as blotchy eruption behind ear. Rapidly spreads to involve whole body. Initially pale pink, macules discrete, itchy; soon becomes darker and macules coalesce. Rarely purpuric. Lasts 5–6 days.
>
> *2.2 Temperature, Pulse and Respiration*. All raised.
>
> *2.3 Catarrhal Signs*. Increase; rhonchi and coarse crepitations may be heard.

3. Convalescence. Rash fades, leaving post-measles staining—purple-brown coloration of skin. Slight desquamation.

Special types

1. Attenuated. Occurs if hyperimmune prophylactic serum given to at-risk children.

2. Severe. Occurs in infants, debilitated children and previously uninfected (virgin) population.

Complications

1. Upper respiratory

> *1.1 Otitis Media*. Due to secondary bacterial infection.
>
> *1.2 Laryngitis*. Mainly during prodromal phase. Mild degree very common. Severe degrees occur in infants.

2. Lung

> *2.1 Immediate*. Bronchopneumonia, especially in young or debilitated children.
>
> *2.2 Remote*
>
> 2.2.1 Collapse and Infection. Often in combination. Used to be common starting point of bronchiectasis.
>
> 2.2.2 Tuberculosis. Measles may lead to temporary Mantoux reversion from positive to negative. Spread of primary lesion may occur.

3. Alimentary

> *3.1 Stomatitis*.
>
> *3.2 Gastro-enteritis*. In babies under 2 years; more common the younger the infant. May precipitate kwashiorkor in developing countries.

4. Ophthalmic. Infection may lead to purulent conjunctivitis.

5. Encephalomyelitis. Rare but majority of children have abnormal EEGs with excess slow waves during illness.

Usually about 4–7 days from eruption.

> *5.1 Clinical Features*. Child becomes drowsy. Complains of headache. Temperature rises. Slight meningeal signs may appear.
>
> Following may occur:
>
> 5.1.1 Convulsions—if repeated, prognosis is poor.
>
> 5.1.2 Coma with decerebrate rigidity. Death may occur but recovery is possible, even after many days. Often residual central nervous system or mental disability.
>
> 5.1.3 Cerebellar ataxia ⎫ May rarely occur as isolated phe-
> 5.1.4 Myelitis ⎬ nomena.

5.2 Cerebrospinal Fluid. Cell count raised, mainly lympho-cytes (7–500/mm^3). Protein may also be increased.

6. Subacute Sclerosing Panencephalitis. A rare progressive illness occurring many years after measles. Child has progressive dementia, mutism, myoclonic jerks, pyramidal and extra-pyramidal signs. EEG shows characteristic periodic complexes; high levels of measles antibodies in blood and CSF. Measles virus recoverable from brain. May be due to immunoincompetent T cells and brain cells containing virus.

Differential Diagnosis of Measles

Exanthem. Following conditions have somewhat similar rashes: Rubella; glandular fever; drug rashes—especially due to penicillin or sulphonamides—erythema multiforme.

Prophylaxis

Measles vaccine. At present two types:

1. Live attenuated measles virus vaccine. Can be further modified by administration of measles-immune globulin.

Results. Produces attack of measles, which although usually mild, occasionally is not.

2. Measles-specific antiserum or pooled gammaglobulin occasionally used to prevent an attack in susceptible individual.

Chapter 17   # RUBELLA (German Measles)

Definition

Common specific infectious fever characterized by long incubation period, mild constitutional symptoms, typical rash and enlargement of lymph nodes in neck. Incubation 10–21 days, droplet transmission.

Clinical features

Little prodrome. Eruptive phase:

1. Rash (exanthem)

  1.1 Character: Pink macules about 1–3 mm diameter.
  1.2 Order of appearance: Behind ears, face, trunk, limbs.
  1.3 Duration: 24–48 h. Fades in order of appearance.
  1.4 Desquamation: Rare, but may occur in more severe varieties.

2. Enanthem. Petechiae sometimes observed on palate.

3. Constitutional symptoms. Usually slight if present. Resemble very mild form of measles.

4. Lymphadenitis. Posterior cervical and occipital lymph nodes always enlarged, may be tender. Occasionally other nodes also involved. Spleen rarely palpable.

Investigations

Virus culture. From nasopharynx, possibly 7 days before or after enanthem.
Rubella titre. Rising haemagglutinin inhibition (HAI) titre.

Complications
1. *Transient Arthralgia* or even arthritis. ESR raised.
2. *Muscular pains*
3. *Thrombocytopenic Purpura*

Differential Diagnosis
May be difficult. Rashes of measles, scarlet fever, glandular fever, toxic erythema, drug rashes most commonly confused.

Prognosis
Excellent.

Prophylaxis
Susceptible girls should receive vaccine in adolescence. Hyperimmune gamma-globulin sometimes given to woman exposed to rubella in early pregnancy (*see below*).

Congenital Rubella Syndrome

If mother contracts rubella during pregnancy risk that infant will be born malformed or die in utero.

Risk of Embryopathy
The younger the fetus at time of rubella the greater the risk.

Risk greater in epidemic than in inter-epidemic years. Severity of maternal rubella not a factor. In affected infant, virus may persist in throat swab for 1 year or more; longer in optic lens. Infant may be infectious and a hazard to pregnant women.

Types of Deformities
1. Deafness. Fifty per cent of affected children. May be only partial and corrected with hearing aid.
2. Congenital heart defect. Fifty per cent. Particularly if mother infected in 5th–8th week of fetal life.
Type of lesion: Patent ductus arteriosus; pulmonary stenosis (which may involve main, right or left pulmonary arteries); ventricular septal defect; aortic stenosis. *Note*: Many of these operable.
3. Eye defects. Thirty per cent. Especially cataract and microphthalmos. Often unilateral. Distinctive choroidoretinitis.
4. Other lesions
> 4.1 Mental retardation (only 1·5% severely affected).
> 4.2 Thrombocytopenic purpura. Not uncommon. May be fatal (*see* p. 417).
> 4.3 Haemolytic anaemia.
> 4.4 Bone lesions. Of considerable diagnostic value. Radiologically: demineralization of metaphysis with multiple areas of translucency and irregular cartilage at shaft junction. Changes best observed at lower end of femur. Changes seen at age of a few days. May be gone by 6 months.
> 4.5 Stillbirth, prematurity and poor postnatal growth described. Frequency uncertain.

4.6 Also possible: cleft palate; diaphragmatic hernia; cryptorchidism.

Note: Virus may remain dormant in brain for years, becoming active during adolescence to produce a slowly progressive encephalitis with ataxia (Progressive Rubella Panencephalopathy, PRP).

Chapter 18	*ROSEOLA INFANTUM (Exanthem subitum; Sixth disease; Pseudo-rubella)*

Clinical Features
Fever 3–5 days: commonly temperature 39–40·5°C (102–105°F). Little malaise. Affects infants between 3 and 6 months.

Rash
1. Appears as pyrexia falls.
2. Character. Small discrete, rose-pink macules. Fade on pressure.
3. Position. Trunk, neck, proximal part of limbs. Face escapes.
4. Duration. 1–3 days.
Associated Signs. Catarrhal pharyngitis; cervical lymphadenopathy.

Blood picture. Neutrophil leucopenia with relative lymphocytosis.

Differential Diagnosis
Upper respiratory infection; drug rashes, rubella, measles, glandular fever.

Chapter 19	*CHICKENPOX (Varicella)*

Definition
Common mild infectious disease caused by virus, with characteristic vesicular rash predominantly centripetal in distribution.

Aetiology
Age. Rare before 1 year, but can occur in newborn.
Cause. Filterable virus. Elementary bodies similar to Paschen bodies of smallpox can be obtained from vesicles.

Epidemiology (see also Table 16.1 p. 79).
Incubation 11–21 days, droplet spread, very infective.

Clinical Features
Exanthem
1. Presents with vesicles which itch usually in following order: back, chest, abdomen, face, limbs.
2. Distribution mainly centripetal; usually spares palms of hands and soles of feet. Rash tends to affect protected parts, e.g. axilla.
3. Stages of macule, papule, vesicle pass rapidly within a few hours. Pustule and crust formation occurs more slowly.

4. Appears in crops. Thus all stages may be present at one time..

5. Most frequent lesion is vesicle, which is: (i) Superficial. Resembles drop of glycerine on skin. (ii) May be oval rather than round. (ii) Unilocular. (iv) Often not surrounded by areola.

General Malaise. Usually mild.

Special Types

All very rare:
1. *Varicella Haemorrhagica*
2. *Varicella Bullosa*
3. *Varicella Gangrenosa*
4. *Congenital Varicella.* (Mortality rate 20%.)

Complications

1. *Secondary infection* rarely with staphylococci.

2. *Encephalomyelitis.* Perivascular demyelinization occurs as in measles. Signs usually develop during first half of second week.

> *Types*
> 2.1 Mainly cerebellar and less prominently cerebral: ataxia, nystagmus, vertigo and pyramidal signs may be present.
> 2.2 Meningeal.

3. *Chickenpox pneumonia* rare in children; also laryngitis; pancarditis, hepatitis, nephritis, myositis. Reye's syndrome due to varicella occasionally.

4. *Steroid therapy.* If child happens to be receiving steroids when he develops chickenpox or herpes zoster, disease may be more severe. Haemorrhagic lesions occur. Deaths have been reported.

5. *In leukaemia* disease severe.

6. *Pregnancy.* Disease serious. Mother may die. Infant can be born with skin; CNS lesions and choroidoretinitis.

Differential Diagnosis

1. *Smallpox*

2. *Papular urticaria* (lichen urticatus). Easily confused. Commoner in toddlers; rash does not pass through characteristic sequence; lesion looks and feels as though it contained tiny central seed pearl; distribution—mainly on limbs and buttocks; does not occur in mouth, never in scalp; intensely itchy.

3. *Scabies.* Characteristic burrows can be found.

Herpes Zoster

Uncommon condition in children. Probably caused by varicella virus which remains in posterior root ganglion. Skin lesion develops in sensory distribution area of that nerve. May be recurrent. May occur with chickenpox, usually affects trunk but can involve cranial nerves V and VII (Ramsay Hunt syndrome.).

Chapter 20   *MUMPS (Epidemic Parotitis)*

Definition
Common infectious disease characterized by fever and painful swelling of salivary glands. Complications of orchitis, meningitis and pancreatitis rare in children.

Aetiology
A paramyxovirus—a RNA virus of 95–135 nm diameter. Commonly occurs at age 5–10 years.
Transmission. Droplet infection from obvious or occult case.
Infectivity. Low. Infectious from a few days before symptoms up to a fortnight after onset of parotitis.
Immunity.   Usually lifelong.
Incubation period. 12–26 days.

Clinical Features
Onset. Enlargement and tenderness of parotid, often unilateral for first few days. Parotid duct (Stensen's) appears reddened. Parotid swelling in front of ear over masseter muscle. *Also fills up recess situated behind lobe of ear in front of mastoid process.*
Trismus may be extreme. Painful to bite.
Skin overlying gland becomes shiny and red but suppuration very rarely occurs.
Duration of swelling: very variable. Commonly 2–4 weeks.
Initial pyrexia common.
Note: Infection subclinical in 40% cases.

Complications
   1. Orchitis and pancreatitis. Common and important in adults, but rarely occur in children before puberty.
   2. Nervous system
                    2.1 *Cerebrospinal Fluid.* Symptomless pleocytosis usual.
                    2.2 *Meningitis* fairly common.
                    2.3 *Meningo-encephalitis.* Rare.
                    2.4 *Polyneuritis*, muscle paralysis similar to polio rare.
   May give rise to local paralysis especially of cranial nerves VII and VIII. Permanent deafness can result.
   3. Myocarditis. Has been recorded in severe epidemics.
   4. Pancreatitis, arthritis, thyroiditis rare.

Differential Diagnosis
   1. From swelling of other structures, e.g.
                    1.1 Pre-auricular lymph nodes.
                    1.2 Painless oedema of neck in severe diphtheria.
   Note: Characteristic extension of parotid tissue into recess behind ear lacking.
   2. From other swellings of parotid, e.g. recurrent parotitis; uveoparotid (Mikulicz) syndrome; sarcoidosis, leukaemia; drug reaction to phenylbutazone or organic iodides used for IVP.

Chapter 21	*INFECTIOUS MONONUCLEOSIS*
	(Glandular Fever)

Definition

Not uncommon, acute infectious disease characterized by protean clinical manifestations, including enlargement of lymph nodes and often spleen, fever, sore throat and morbilliform rash; and characterized haematologically by lymphocytosis with a characteristic mononuclear cell in peripheral blood and sometimes heterophil antibody reaction of serum.

Age. Can occur at any age. Even reported in newborn. Eighty-five per cent of cases occur under age of 12 years.

Cause. Epstein–Barr virus (EBV).

Infectivity. Low.

Incubation period. 5–14 days.

Clinical Features

Three main clinical types described:

1. Lymph-node ('glandular') enlargement. Commonest type in children. Usually acute onset with general malaise, fever, vomiting, epistaxis, rarely abdominal pain.

Nodes Involved. Those in neck almost always. Axillary, epitrochlears, inguinal, occasionally. May be 2·5 cm or so in diameter. Often a little tender, never suppurate. Swelling may not be present until days or weeks after onset of disease. May last for months or years. Spleen often enlarged. Liver less commonly. Jaundice occurs rarely.

2. Anginose. Tonsillar lymph-node enlargement common. Sore throat may be prominent feature with membrane and ulceration. Secondary infection with haemolytic streptococci or Vincent's organisms occur.

3. Febrile. Prolonged pyrexia may be prominent feature.

Additional features

a. Enanthem. Multiple pin-point petechiae seen around junction of hard and soft palate. Usually more than 5 seen. May occur from 2nd to 25th day of disease. Similar petechiae may be seen in rubella or adenopharyngoconjunctival fever.

b. Rash. Uncommon in children unless treated with ampicillin, in which case rash usual. Very variable in type; may be morbilliform or scarlatiniform, rarely purpuric. Usually maximal on body.

c. One per cent may develop lymphocytic meningitis, encephalomyelitis, polyneuritis and mononeuritis.

d. Long-lasting Mental Depression (up to a year) may result.

Investigations

1. White blood count. In early stages polymorphonuclear leucocytosis may occur, followed by leucopenia or lymphocytosis. Characteristic mononuclear cell appears, probably T-cell lymphocytes, occasionally agranulocytosis, thrombocytopenia occur and haemolytic anaemia.

2. Heterophil antibody reaction (Paul–Bunnell test). Serum of patient contains specific agglutinin for washed sheep's red cells. Positive reaction very suggestive of infectious mononucleosis. Many antibodies develop, e.g. to muscle and against blood system hence haemolytic anaemia. Negative reaction does not rule out diagnosis as reaction often not present in initial stage of disease. May be related to development of immunity.

Note: If these investigations negative, tests for toxoplasmosis and cytomegalovirus should be performed automatically on same specimen of blood as clinical findings are so similar.

Differential Diagnosis
Often very difficult unless characteristic mononuclear cell seen or heterophile antibody reaction positive.
1. Other lymph-node enlargements. Acquired toxoplasmosis, Hodgkin's disease, reticuloses, leukaemia.
2. Other causes of sore throat. Haemolytic streptococcal sore throat, viral sore throat, agranulocytosis.
3. Other exanthemas. Measles, German measles, Stevens–Johnson syndrome.

Prognisis
Rarely fatal in children. Convalescence may take months; relapses common, eventual complete recovery.

Treatment.
Symptomatic.

Chapter 22   HERPES SIMPLEX INFECTIONS

Herpesvirus hominis (HVH) is widespread in human beings but does not often give rise to clinical manifestations. Two types of infection—primary in the susceptible individual, and recurrent—when a latent virus is activated by extrinsic or intrinsic factors.

Clinical Syndromes
1. Gingivostomatitis. Usually occurs in children age 1–4 years.
   1.1 Symptoms. Child feverish, irritable, refuses food. Child has severe pain in mouth.
   1.2 Signs. Small vesicles appear in mouth and lips. These soon rupture to form grey ulcers with hyperaemic margin. Tongue frequently involved. Regional lymph nodes become enlarged and tender.
   1.3 Course. Self-limiting, lasts 5–14 days.
   1.4 Treatment. Little value, apart from oral hygiene. Antiviral treatment with Acylovir.
2. Herpes febrilis (Herpes labialis). Common recurrent condition in children and adults. Affected person carries virus latent in skin, often affects mucocutaneous junction. Some other infection enables it to flourish, producing typical vesicular lesion in that site.

2.1 Infections particularly associated with herpes febrilis: coryza, pneumonia, malaria, meningococcal meningitis, leptospirosis.

2.2 Common Sites. Around mouth, elsewhere on face, fingers, genitalia. Can occur in weakened skin, e.g. from drooling or trauma.

3. *Eczema Herpeticum* (Kaposi's Varicelliform Eruption). Rare syndrome in which atopic eczema becomes secondarily infected with herpes simplex virus.

3.1 Symptoms and Signs. Baby with eczema suddenly develops high fever and irritability. Crops of vesicles appear on eczematous skin. Occasionally also normal skin.

3.2 Course. Self-limiting, lasts 5–14 days. Child may be very ill. Disease may be fatal.

3.3 Treatment. Symptomatic. Acyclovir may help. Gammaglobulin given prophylactically in incubation period or at onset may prevent disease.

4. *Generalized herpes simplex infection.* Very rare syndrome almost confined to newborn. Type II virus acquired from birth canal. Onset between 5 and 10 days. Baby becomes very ill with fever, jaundice, thrombocytopenic purpura, enlarged liver and spleen. Usually herpetic skin lesions present; may be very extensive. Sometimes fatal outcome.

5. *Genital herpes* occurs in adolescents, usually Type II. A venereal disease.

6. *Herpes encephalitis.* Commonest non-epidemic encephalitis. Occurs in all age groups. High mortality rate. Often affects temporal lobe and can then mimic tumour. Diagnosis by brain biopsy—virus can be identified in brain cells. Possible help from Acyclovir, idoxuridine, cytosine arabinoside, or dexamethasone.

Diagnosis
Can be confirmed by isolation of virus, by identification from specimens using immunofluorescent technique and by development of specific neutralizing antibodies.

Chapter 23   *POLIOMYELITIS (Anterior Poliomyelitis; Infantile Paralysis)*

Definition
Epidemic or sporadic virus infection, preventable by immunization. Characterized in paralytic form by fever and flaccid paralysis of muscles, abortive forms common; pathologically by degeneration of anterior horn cells.

Aetiology
1. *Causative organism.* Poliovirus, a RNA virus; serotypes 1, 2 and 3. Virus can be demonstrated in faeces and sometimes nasopharynx of cases and carriers. Virus able to remain alive in water or milk for months.

2. *Method of infection.* Via alimentary tract. Virus multiplies in gastro-intestinal tract and related lymphoid tissue and travels up axis cylinders of peripheral nerves to nervous system. Transient viraemia. Predisposing factors to paralysis

include vigorous exercise in incubation stage, and intramuscular injection (when the injected limb may become paralysed).

Epidemiology
Incubation period 5–18 days. Transmission by food, fingers, flies, faeces. *Note*:
1. One attack usually confers immunity. Second attacks have been reported. Immunity type-specific.
2. Many attacks are abortive and pass unrecognized.
3. Carrier rate high.

Pathology
1. Acute. Anterior horn cells of spinal cord and grey matter of medulla show pathological changes varying from perivascular cuffing to complete destruction of cells.
2. Chronic. Muscle wasting and atrophy. Secondary bone changes—osteoporosis and secondary scoliosis—common. Damaged neurones in CNS replaced by scar tissue.

Clinical Features
Three types of disease occur:
1. Abortive form. Commonest. Non-specific illness with fever, sore throat, headache, abdominal pain, vomiting. Condition passes unrecognized except during epidemic.
2. Non-paralytic form. Similar to abortive form but symptoms more severe and meningeal irritation present.
3. Paralytic form. Uncommon. Classically clinical features of paralytic form can be divided into:

> *3.1 First Phase.* General malaise, pyrexia, sore throat, anorexia, aching limbs. During 24–48 h.
> *3.2 Latent Period.* May follow, of 7–10 days.
> *3.3 Second (Paralytic) Phase.* May be severe or mild.
> *3.3.1 Severe*: Pyrexia, malaise, meningism, muscle pain followed by paralysis.
> *3.3.2 Mild*: Slight malaise followed by sudden weakness and tenderness of limb muscles.

Muscle groups particularly involved
1. Leg muscles. Common. Especially anterior tibial and peroneal group.
2. Arm muscles. Especially shoulder girdle. Muscles of hands less commonly involved.
3. Muscles of respiration. Diaphragm and/or intercostal muscles involved in severe cases. Prognosis then poor.
4. Muscles supplied by cranial nerves. May be primarily involved—so-called 'bulbar poliomyelitis'.

Complications
Include gastric dilatation, melaena, hypertension, pulmonary oedema.

Investigations
1. CSF. Very important, especially in abortive cases to confirm diagnosis.

a. Cells. 10–300/cmm. May be polymorphonuclear leucocytes at first, later lymphocytes. Numbers fall during second week.
b. Protein. Normal at first. Rises to 1·0–2·0 g/l during second week.
c. Sugar. Normal.
2. White blood count. May be raised.
3. Faeces. For virus culture.
4. Neutralizing antibodies. Show rising titre.

Prognosis
Varies with severity. Bulbar type carries poor prognosis. If death occurs, usually due to central respiratory failure or secondary respiratory infection.

Course
In cases which survive *some degree of recovery always occurs*. Begins about 1 week after temperature drops. Continues for year or more.
Residual paralysis. Paralysed muscles during acute phase, and those which later fail to recover, show typical lower motor neurone type of paralysis.

Differential Diagnosis of Sudden Paralysis
1. Polyneuritis (Guillain–Barré syndrome, see p. 312). Paralysis symmetrical, pyramidal signs may appear, few cells in CSF.
2. Peripheral neuritis, e.g. lead; toxic, etc.
3. Tetanus
4. Intraspinal neoplasms.
5. Injuries from falls, etc. Child must be observed and encouraged to use limb.
Note: Children always walk self-consciously and awkwardly when watched.
6. Osteomyelitis. Child may not move limb because of pain—'pseudo-paralysis'.

Prevention
Immunization
1. By mouth (Sabin vaccine). Live attenuated poliomyelitis virus given by mouth. Virus spreads through community. Of particular value for mass immunization to cut short epidemic. Three doses of oral vaccine advisable.
2. By parenteral injection (Salk vaccine). Now rarely used. During epidemic triple vaccine inoculations and tonsillectomy should cease.
    For schedule for administration of prophylactic immunizations, *see* p. 520.

Treatment in acute state
1. General. Patients require careful nursing. Warm packs may relieve pain in limbs which should be supported in position of rest. Active movement of any kind must be allowed as this encourages paralysis. Sedatives may be used. Catheterization required for retention of urine.
2. Bulbar paralysis. Essential to prevent aspiration of mucus or vomit into lungs. Immediately palatal paralysis recognized child must be placed in semi-prone position with head to one side and foot of bed raised to angle of at least 15°. Child must be turned from side to side every few hours. Mucus must be sucked from throat.
3. Respiratory and bulbar paralysis
Method of treatment. Positive-pressure respiratory with tracheostomy and suction.

Treatment of paralysis. Purpose of treatment:
1. To prevent stretching of damaged muscles and subsequent contractures.
2. To maintain circulation and nutrition of muscles and skin.
3. Severe cases may require tenotomy; arthrodesis, walking irons.

Chapter 24   CYTOMEGALOVIRUS DISEASE

Rare DNA virus disease of infants or (rarer) older children manifested in newborn by evidence of erythroblastosis with jaundice, haemolytic anaemia and an increased serum bilirubin but with a negative Coombs' test. Excessive extramedullary haematopoiesis occurs. In addition, purpura and bleeding occur due to thrombocytopenia. Virus widespread in body. Most serious lesion is encephalitis followed by mental retardation, fits, cerebral palsy and intracranial calcification. Does not always cause clinical disease. One per cent of newborns excrete virus. Older children may have pneumonia, gastroenteritis or encephalomyelitis. Illness mimics glandular fever.

Diagnosis
Diagnosis made by finding raised titre in blood or by isolating virus. Urine and other body fluids may show inclusion bodies. May be cerebral calcification.

Treatment
Exchange transfusions and corticosteroids may be of value in newborn. Transfer factor infusions may help.

Chapter 25   DENGUE FEVER

Common viral disease in S.E. Asia and other tropical areas caused by several arboviruses, transmitted by mosquitoes.

Clinical Features
Mild infections in young infants may be atypical but in older children there is sudden onset of pyrexia (39–41°) with severe headache and back pain, myalgia, arthralgia, nausea and vomiting, anorexia, lymphadenopathy. A transient skin rash in the first 2 days is followed by a generalized morbilliform rash a few days later, which may desquamate. The pyrexia is characteristically biphasic, falling when the rash appears but rising again a few days later.

A severe form, dengue haemorrhagic fever, is characterized by disseminated intravascular coagulation (DIC) with epistaxis, purpura and gastrointestinal bleeding, and circulatory shock.

Laboratory Investigations
1. Neutropenia is usual.

2. Thrombocytopenia is found in dengue haemorrhagic fever, and the tourniquet test is positive.

3. In cases with shock, hypoproteinaemia occurs and the haematocrit is elevated.

4. ECG changes include bradycardia, low voltage, ectopic ventricular beats and S-T depression.

5. Serological studies show a rise in specific antibodies titres to dengue viruses, while the virus itself may be isolated from blood monocytes or serum.

Management
Symptomatic only: antipyretics, analgesics (avoiding salicylates if there is bleeding), fluid and electrolyte replacement and, if necessary, blood transfusion.

Chapter 26   **KAWASAKI DISEASE**
                  (*Mucocutaneous lymph node syndrome*)

An uncommon disease of unknown aetiology (?viral, ?toxic) affecting most frequently infants and children under 5 years of age.

Clinical Features
At least 5 of the following clinical criteria are required for diagnosis:
1. Fever lasting longer than 5 days without obvious cause.
2. Bilateral conjunctival congestion.
3. Erythema, dryness and fissuring of lips, 'strawberry tongue' and diffuse pharyngeal erythema.
4. Erythema and often oedema of hands and feet, followed by desquamation of skin of fingertips.
5. A variable rash on the trunk.
6. Non-suppurative cervical lymph node enlargement, with at least one node 1·5 cm diameter or more.

Other important symptoms or findings which may occur include diarrhoea, evidence of myocarditis or pericarditis, arthralgia/arthritis, aseptic meningitis, anterior uveitis, mild hepatitis. Rare complications include thromboarteritis ('infantile polyarteritis nodosa') and coronary thrombosis, which may be fatal, in 1–2% of cases.

Laboratory Investigations
Non-specific changes include leucocytosis, raised ESR and α_2-globulin, and thrombocytosis.

Management
Symptomatic only, as cause is unknown. Ischaemic ECG changes, fever persisting for more than 2 weeks with an ESR above 100 mm/h are indications for anticoagulation, and perhaps coronary angiography.

Prognosis
Mild cases recover clinically within a few weeks but if evidence of carditis follow-up should continue for a year or more as ventricular aneurysms may occur.

4

| Chapter 27 | *HAEMOLYTIC STREPTOCOCCAL INFECTIONS* |

α-Haemolytic streptococcus (*S. viridans*). Saprophyte normally found in mouth. Causes subacute bacterial endocarditis and infection of intravenous catheters.

β-Haemolytic streptococcus (*S. pyogenes*). Two varieties: Group A. Responsible for classic β-haemolytic streptococcal infection as below. Group B. May be acquired from vagina during birth, may cause neonatal septicaemia and meningitis.

Clinical Manifestations of β-Haemolytic Streptococcal Infection
1. Immediate
        1.1 Local. Due to invasive properties of organism.
        1.2 Septicaemia. Due to blood-borne dissemination.
        1.3 Toxic. Due to erythrogenic toxin.
2. Late. Allergic phenomena (*see* p. 97).

Clinical Features of Throat Infection
Onset. Acute. Shivering, and often vomiting. Temperature may be high—40·5 °C (105 °F). Pulse rate rapid.
Course. Pain in throat may be absent (especially in young children) or severe. As local symptoms develop, systemic disturbance decreases. Temperature usually falls to normal in 3–5 days (more rapidly with treatment). May persist up to fortnight in severe cases. Cervical lymphadenitis common usually during acute phase of disease. Tonsillar lymph node at angle of jaw affected. May be uni- or bilateral.
Appearance of throat. Varies from slight injection of tonsils and pharynx to generalized fiery redness of pharynx, tonsils and buccal mucous membrane. Tongue abnormalities especially obvious in scarlet fever: First day: *Strawberry tongue*: covered with white fur through which swollen red papillae project. Third day: Peeling: white fur peels off in patches. Fifth to seventh day: Fur completely gone, leaving bright red surface with papillae still visible ('*raspberry tongue*').
    Follicular Tonsillitis. Tonsils studded with white areas of exudate.
    Membranous Tonsillitis. May arise as above or appear without previous follicular eruption. Can be removed easily. Causes only slight bleeding.
Other modes of presentation
    1. Pyrexia of unknown origin. Very common presentation especially in young children.

2. General malaise with enlargement of cervical lymph nodes.
3. As one of its complications (*see below*).

Special Clinical Features of Scarlet Fever
Site of infection either throat or surgical wound; burn, chickenpox, etc.
Rash
1. Most commonly occurs 1 day after start of symptoms.
2. Commences on neck and chest. Spreads to trunk, limbs, face. Not palms of hands, soles of feet, or scalp.
3. Appears classically as pin-point erythema on an erythematous base. Pressure produces blanching. Characteristic pallor of circumoral region, not pathognomonic. Seen with many rashes.
4. *Pastia's sign*: Linear petechial markings in folds and creases of skin, especially cubital fossa and base of neck.
5. Duration: Few hours to about 7 days.
6. Desquamation: Usually commences centrally and works centrifugally. Small pieces of epidermis flake off; rarely occurs in larger areas. May last several weeks. Peeling skin not infectious.
Antistreptolysin titre of blood. Rises 2–3 weeks after onset of sore throat. Diagnostic over 1 in 200. May rise to 1 in 1000.

Differential Diagnosis
1. Pharyngitis and tonsillitis
> *1.1 Virus Infection*. Throat red but no exudate.
> *1.2 Vincent's Infection*. Ulceration of tonsil; not tender. Foul smell.
> *1.3 Infectious Mononucleosis*. May involve pharynx as well as tonsils, generalized enlargement of lymph nodes; palatal petechiae.
> *1.4 Agranulocytosis*. Ulceration on pharynx or in mouth rarely acute. Associated with acute leukaemia or its therapy.
> *1.5 Diphtheria*. Exudate fuses into membrane, may spread to involve pharyngeal wall. Painless oedema of neck in severe cases.

2. Rash in scarlet fever
> *2.1 Rubella*. Macular rash; enlarged cervical lymph nodes; sore throat not marked.
> *2.2 Measles*. Koplik's spots; blotchy appearance of rash.
> *2.3 Infectious Mononucleosis*. Distinction may be impossible. Blood film and Monospot diagnostic.
> *2.4 Drug Eruptions*, e.g. ampicillin or sulphonamides, etc.
> *2.5 Roseola Infantum*. In young children only. Rash appears as temperature subsides.
> *2.6 Stevens–Johnson Syndrome*. Associated conjunctivitis and often urethritis; lesion in throat may be slight.

Complications
   Note: main importance of haemolytic streptococcal infection lies in frequency and severity of complications.

1. Septic complications
> *1.1 Local.* Acute otitis media in children under 5 years, suppurative cervical adenitis, sinusitis, retropharyngeal abscess, bronchopneumonia.
> *1.2 General.*
> *1.2.1* Septicaemia. May be fulminating condition, death occurring in a few hours in young babies.
> *1.2.2* Febrile convulsions in older infants. Due to associated pyrexia.

2. Allergic manifestations
> *2.1 Acute Rheumatism.* Attack or relapse usually preceded by β-haemolytic streptococcal tonsillitis.
> *2.2 Acute Nephritis*
> *2.3 Henoch–Schönlein Purpura*
> *2.4 Erythema Nodosum (see below).*

Treatment
Take throat swab and give penicillin until results known.

Erythema Nodosum

Definition
A non-specific reaction characterized by painful, raised, red nodules occurring mainly on front of shins.

Aetiology
Many possible causes: e.g. streptococcal infection, tuberculosis, BCG, sarcoidosis, coccidioidomycosis, sulphonamides.

Clinical Features
Character of rash. Tender, erythematous patches, raised in centre, up to 2 cm in diameter; tend to appear in crops. Lesion turns purple, then brown as rash fades.
Duration. Usually last 7–14 days. Occasionally up to 3 weeks.
Site. Extensor surfaces of legs below knees. Bilateral. Rarely extensor surfaces of arm around elbow or on thighs. In streptococcal cases may be preceded by sore throat and transient joint pains.

Investigations
Child should be investigated for:
1. Streptococcal infection by: throat swab; antistreptolysin titre.
2. Tuberculosis by: Mantoux reaction; radiography of chest.

Chapter 28   # MENINGOCOCCAL INFECTIONS

Meningococcal infection occurs sporadically and occasionally in epidemics in impoverished communities.

Aetiology

1. Bacteriology. Causative organism: *Neisseria meningitidis* ('*diplococcus intracellulans meningitides*' of Weichselbaum). Usually called the meningococcus. Grows best in presence of carbon dioxide.

2. Toxic Properties. Mainly due to lipopolysaccharides or endotoxin.

3. Age. Rare under 3 months; 40 % of all cases occur under 5 years.

4. Epidemiology. Disease occurs sporadically and in epidemics. Spread by carriers. Epidemics comparatively rare although carrier rate high. One attack confers immunity. Predisposing causes: Overcrowding and malnutrition.

Manifestations

1. Septicaemia. Fulminating:
        1.1 Mainly septicaemic.
        1.2 Mainly encephalitic.
        1.3 Mainly adrenal.

2. Meningitis. Most important manifestation of meningococcal infection. Occurs in about 90% of cases. Types:
        2.1 Cerebrospinal type (acute).
        2.2 Posterior basic type (rare, chronic).

3. Waterhouse–Friderichsen syndrome is a fulminating infection with sudden onset with high fever, prostration, and either clear mentality (adrenal type) or convulsions and loss of consciousness (encephalitic type). Purpuric rash develops which rapidly becomes massive. Peripheral circulatory failure occurs with cyanosis.

Treatment

  1. Penicillin parenterally in massive dosage.

  2. Adrenal replacement therapy: hydrocortisone 100 mg i.v., if evidence of adrenal insufficiency. Some give massive doses.

  3. Plasma i.v. may be required for shock and to correct dehydration.

  4. Oxygen of value.

  5. Test for disseminated intravascular coagulation and treat accordingly.

  6. Isolate patient for 48 h.

  7. Give prophylaxis to contacts.

Chapter 29   # DIPHTHERIA

Rare disease but may become more frequent because of drop in immunization rate.

Epidemiology

1. Age. Very rare under 6 months. Majority 2–6 years.

2. Incubation period. 2–5 days.

General Considerations

  1. Factors which alter signs, symptoms, severity and prognosis of diphtheria:
        1.1 Strain of Organism. Gravis, intermedius or mitis.
        1.2 Site of Lesion. Sites most commonly involved:

1.2.1 Fauces. (Includes tonsils, pharynx and larynx)—Severe.

1.2.2 Nose and Skin. Including mucous membranes of eyes; wound or sore; vagina. Less severe but can also give rise to complications.

1.3 Age of Patient. More severe in young children.

2. Diphtheria bacillus gives rise to signs and symptoms by following means:

2.1 Immediate generalized toxic effect.

2.2 Local effect.

2.3 Remote generalized toxic effect (*described under* 'Complications').

Clinical Types

1. Faucial diphtheria. Varying grades of severity.

Onset: Gradual with general malaise; loss of appetite; limb pains. Child toxic, may or may not complain of sore throat. Temperature 38·3–39·4°C (101–103°F). Pulse rapid. Tonsils inflamed and a membrane formed; breath smells fetid. 'Tonsillar' lymph nodes enlarge. May be considerable painless oedema around lymph node giving rise to 'bull-neck' appearance.

2. Laryngeal diphtheria

Onset: Usually acute, with loss of voice and stridor leading to respiratory embarrassment.

3. Nasal diphtheria. General malaise slight. Thin bloodstained discharge present with crusting of external nares.

Complications

1. Cardiovascular. Myocarditis may appear about 12th day. If commences before 5th day prognosis poor. May cause sudden death.

2. Peripheral nervous system. Three types of paralysis occur:

2.1 Local

2.2 Specific. Due to absorption of toxin from blood stream.

2.2.1 Site: Ciliary muscles, external rectus or diaphragm, special affinity may be due to fact that these muscles are in constant action.

2.2.2 Time Relationship: 3rd–4th week for ciliary muscle and external rectus palsy. 5th–7th week for diaphragm.

2.2.3 Clinical Manifestation of Ciliary Paralysis: Loss of power to accommodate. Often passes unnoticed unless tested.

2.2.4 Duration of Ciliary Paralysis: about 3 weeks.

2.3 General

Clinical manifestation of late paralysis (up to 7th week) following severe infections. Swallowing and breathing may become difficult. Paralysis of limbs may not be appreciated until child starts to get up. Duration of Peripheral Paralysis: May be 6 months, with eventual complete recovery.

Diagnosis

Rests on following evidence:

1. Clinical. Severe toxaemia with little local features.

Note: Diagnosis should be made on clinical grounds. If any doubt exists diphtheria antitoxin must be given.
2. Culture from swab
3. Contact history

Treatment
1. Immediate antitoxin serum therapy
   Dose. Depends on severity of disease, not age of patient.
   Mild Case (i.e. involving tonsil, larynx or anterior part of nose only). 10 000–20 000 u.
   Moderate Case (i.e. involving pharynx, associated with periadenitis). 20 000–1 000 000 u.
Severe Case (i.e. 'bull-neck' type). 1 000 000–2 000 000 u.
Note: Because of danger of sensitization, give single, adequate, intravenous dose. Test for sensitivity first. Adrenaline should always be available.
2. Penicillin or erythromycin.
3. Corticosteroids for acute laryngeal diphtheria.

Chapter 30   *WHOOPING-COUGH (Pertussis)*

Epidemiology
Age. Disease of infants and young children. May occur even in newborn. No inborn immunity.
Epidemics. Occur about every 4 years.
Transmission. By droplet infection: most commonly.
Incubation. 7–10 days.

Clinical Features
1. Catarrhal phase (first 2 weeks). Insidious onset with short dry nocturnal cough; becomes progressively worse and diurnal. Paroxysmal sneezing or coryza may be present. Sometimes low fever.
2. Spasmodic phase (3rd–5th week). Cough becomes paroxysmal, occasionally spasmodic sneezing.
Character of Cough. Child emits series of short vigorous coughs, 10–20 in number. Breathing suppressed during this time: face becomes blue and congested, veins distended, eyes bulge and tongue protrudes. Sudden inspiration then occurs, with whoop. Process may be immediately repeated. Paroxysm usually ends with expectoration of little thick mucus or with vomiting. During attack urine may be voided. When paroxysm ended child lies back exhausted and distressed.
   In babies under 3 months of age, paroxysm may commence with or end in apnoea. Fatal asphyxia can occur.
Common associated findings
   a. Temperature: Normal, if raised usually indicates bronchopneumonia.
   b. Signs in chest: usually nil initially but after second week scattered rhonchi and coarse crepitations common.

3. Convalescent phase (5th week onward). Child no longer infectious. Paroxysms less frequent and severe but may persist for weeks. Intercurrent coryza months later sometimes induced return of whoop.

4. In vaccinated children. Disease may be very mild with only slight cough and minimal whoop. Whoop usually absent in infants.

Investigations
1. Isolation of organism by per nasal swab.
2. White blood count
   1st week: leucopenia may be present.
   2nd week: lymphocytosis almost invariable. Absolute count of over 10 000 lymphocytes per cmm suggestive. Occasionally very high counts (50 000–80 000 per cmm) seen.
3. Radiological exmination. Nil or patchy areas of segmental collapse common even in apparently mild cases.

Complications
Common.
1. Respiratory system
   1.1 Pulmonary Collapse. Often multiple, usually persists for some weeks. Rarely diagnosed clinically.
   1.2 Bronchopneumonia. Due to secondary invaders, e.g. haemolytic streptococci, pneumococci, staphylococci, etc. Temperature rises, child toxic and has respiratory difficulty.

2. Central nervous system. Convulsions serious. Possible causes:
   2.1 Anoxia. Fits occur at height of paroxysm. Probably due to cerebral hypoxia.
   2.2 Intracranial haemorrhage often seen in cases coming to autopsy. In survivors may lead to paralysis, hemiplegia, etc.
   2.3 Unknown. May be due to encephalopathy.
3. Mechanical damage. From repeated paroxysms. May result in:
   3.1 Haemorrhages: Subconjunctival, Retinal, Cerebral, Purpuric: Spots often occur on head and shoulders.
   3.2 Rupture of Lung Alveoli. Pneumothorax or interstitial emphysema.
   3.3 Oedema of Face. Uncommon, due to congestion of veins.
   3.4 Fraenal Ulcer. If lower incisors present.

Differential Diagnosis
Other causes of paroxysmal cough:
1. Cystic fibrosis. No whoop occurs: paroxysm usually short and child does not go blue in face; does not end in vomit.
2. Asthma. Wheeze present.
3. Obstruction within trachea, e.g. foreign body.
4. Pressure on trachea from without, e.g. enlarged hilar lymph nodes due to tuberculosis, mediastinal tumours.

Prognosis.
Good except in young (less than 3 months) infants.

Prophylaxis
1. Combined prophylaxis. Diphtheria, tetanus and pertussis. *See* p. 520.
   Dangers: Encephalopathy reported following use of whooping-cough vaccine in less than 1 in 100000 children. Occurs few hours after injection. Convulsions, paralysis, death or mental deterioration may result. Vaccination should not be given if infant has had any complication following previous vaccine injection. Epilepsy and perinatal asphyxia are official contraindications.
2. Newborn babies particularly susceptible to whooping-cough; should never be allowed to come into contact with disease.
3. If previously immunized child comes in contact with case, booster immunization can be given to prevent attack.

Treatment
Give cough sedatives. Salbutamol often helpful. Ampicillin or erythromycin may help only if given very early.

Chapter 31   # SYPHILIS

Syphilis may be congenital or acquired.
1. Acquired. In children lesion usually extragenital, e.g. on lip. Primary chancre forms and course of events similar to that seen in adults.
2. Congenital. Infant contracts disease by infection from mother. Condition now very rare in developed countries.

Congenital Syphilis

Transplacental infection by the mobile spirochaete, *Treponema pallidum*.

Clinical Features
Early Manifestations. Constitutional symptoms may be absent, slight or extreme, with failure to thrive, jaundice and anaemia. Purulent, sometimes sanguineous, nasal discharge ('snuffles') may develop, often with associated laryngitis and hoarse cry.
   Skin manifestations include a red or copper-coloured rash on the buttocks, bullous lesions on palms and soles, sores and fissures around lips and anal condylomata. Osteitis with bony tenderness may be present. Organ involvement with hepatosplenomegaly and nephrotic syndrome may occur, as well as neurological signs, such as bulging fontanelle, hydrocephalus and delayed development.
Later Manifestations. Periostitis gives rise to thickening of bone, best seen in tibia (anterior bowing—'sabre tibia'), skull, fingers (dactylitis), hard palate (gumma, leading to perforation), and the nasal bridge collapses to give a characteristic saddle shape.
   Abnormalities of the permanent teeth include notching of central incisors ('Hutchinson's teeth') and tapering molars ('Moon's molars').

Painless effusions into the knee joints are known as 'Clutton's joints'. Interstitial keratitis causes visual impairment, and deafness may also occur. Typical 'adult' forms of neurosyphilis—meningitis, tabes dorsalis or general paralysis—are seen after the age of 10 years.

Diagnosis
1. *Radiology.* Periostitis in infancy is a useful diagnostic sign.
2. *Serological Tests.*
> 2.1 May not necessarily be positive during first few months even in infected case.
>
> 2.2 Positive reaction in child without symptoms within first 3 months of life does not necessarily mean child is infected, although mother almost certainly is.

Prevention
1. Routine test for syphilis should be performed on every pregnant woman.
2. If mother found to be infected immediate treatment should be instituted.

Treatment
Penicillin alone in large doses probably adequate, but wise to give several courses. Tests for syphilis should be repeated from time to time and further courses given if positive.

Chapter 32   # TUBERCULOSIS

Natural History of Tuberculosis in Childhood

Primary Tuberculosis
Primary tuberculous complex: consists of:
1. *Primary Focus.* Local inflammation at site of lodgement of tubercle bacillus.
2. *Involvement of Regional Lymph Nodes*
Sites. Primary tuberculous complex:
1. *Primary Focus in Lung* (Ghon Focus) *and Mediastinal Lymph Nodes.* Tubercle bacilli enter lung by inhalation, usually by direct droplet infection from infected contact, become lodged in alveoli.
2. *Tonsillar Infection and Cervical Lymph Nodes*
3. *Skin Lesion and Lymph Nodes draining the Part.* Finger, eye, etc. From cut, abrasion or injections infected with human or bovine strains. Note especially BCG injections.

Secondary or Postprimary Tuberculosis
Results from either overwhelming new infection, or reactivation of existing dormant lesion (even calcified lesion may contain living bacilli).

Aetiology
Organisms usually acquired from infected adult—rarely from infected milk.

Diagnosis
From contact history, clinical features and skin sensitivity test.
Mantoux reaction. By intradermal injection. Heaf multiple puncture technique or commercially available Tine test.
   Solution used. Fresh solution of PPD (purified protein derivative).
   Result. Site should be observed at 48 and 72h. Positive reaction: Redness; palpable area of induration, one diameter of which should be at least 6mm. If violently positive central vesiculation or even necrosis occurs.
   Uses and Limitation
   1. Measures sensitivity to tuberculin. Sensitivity develops about 6 weeks after individual has been infected by tubercle bacilli. Individual then said to have undergone 'Mantoux conversion'.
   2. Mantoux reversal: Reaction may become negative with time or overwhelming tuberculosis or intercurrent infection, e.g. measles.
   Organisms should be sought by appropriate means, including stomach wash out.

Prevention
BCG useful in developed countries but much less effective elsewhere. Used now for school leavers and contacts.

Intrathoracic Primary Tuberculosis

Definition
Uncomplicated primary complex in lung consists of Ghon focus in lung parenchyma and enlarged lymph nodes in mediastinum.

Clinical Picture
Child usually appears perfectly well, but occasionally vague, non-specific malaise is observed. Mantoux reaction becomes positive in about 6 weeks.

Radiological Appearances
Ghon focus sometimes seen as blurred opacity associated with increased hilar shadows due to enlarged lymph nodes.

Prognosis (Fig. 32.1)
Most commonly condition arrests spontaneously and is only incidentally discovered by positive tuberculin reaction and/or presence of calcified lesion on radiography of lung.

Postprimary Tuberculosis

Tuberculous Pleural Effusion
Now rare. Typical clear, straw-coloured fluid which may form clot on standing and which contains occasional tubercle bacilli. More common in adolescence. Occurs 3–12 months after primary infection.
   Commonly pleural involvement first indication of tuberculous infection.

Diagnosis
By X-ray, pleural aspiration and Mantoux.

Fig. 32.1. Complications of childhood tuberculosis

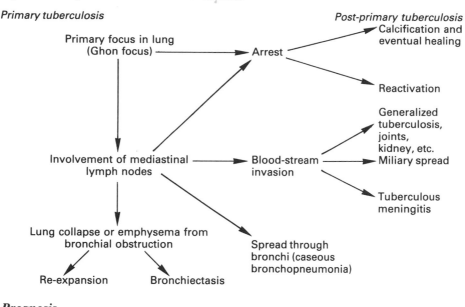

Prognosis
Good.

Treatment
Routine antituberculous therapy. Corticosteroids often helpful.

Miliary Tuberculosis

Definition
Form of tuberculosis due to massive blood-stream invasion (tuberculous septicaemia). Manifested pathologically by appearance of miliary tubercles in lungs or other viscera, including the central nervous system; and clinically by severe toxaemia with or without localizing signs. Occurs most commonly 1–3 months after primary infection.

Clinical Features
Usually presents as acute non-specific illness with general malaise, tachycardia, high swinging temperature. Child may complain of headache or appear drowsy. In later stages child obviously toxic and ill. Wasting marked. On examination spleen may be palpable.

Choroidal tubercles: Can be found in about 60% of cases. Fundi must be examined fully dilated in dark room. Usually multiple. Do not occur in uncomplicated tuberculous meningitis. Of great diagnostic value.

Appearance: (1) About half size of disc, not raised, appear to fade off into choroid, pale yellow, along retinal vessels. (2) Later become smaller, paler and more distinct. (3) Eventually become white, clear cut, heavily pigmented around—stage of scarring.

Clinical features of lung lesion often limited to cough and raised respiratory rate.

Investigations
1. *Chest radiography.* Typical 'snowstorm' appearance—fine mottling of both lungs may be present. Absence does not rule out diagnosis in early stages. Mediastinal lymph nodes often enlarged.
2. *Mantoux reaction* almost always positive; may occasionally be negative in overwhelming infection.
3. *Gastric lavage.* Tubercle bacilli often found, but usually only on culture or guinea-pig inoculation, of little value in diagnosis of acute condition.
4. *Lumbar puncture* should always be performed; fluid examined for tubercle bacilli and cultured. Concurrent meningitis often present.

Prognosis. With treatment almost 100% recovery in uncomplicated miliary tuberculosis.

Tuberculous Meningitis

Aetiology
Age. Commonest 1–4 years. Rare before 6 months.
Time relationship to primary infection. Usually occurs 1–3 months after.

Pathogenesis
Small tuberculoma forms near meninges — the Rich focus. From this organisms are carried into meninges.

Pathology
1. Small tubercles, often best seen on ependymal lining of lateral ventricles, and on cortex and walls of ventricles.
2. Gelatinous exudate fills spaces at base of brain.
3. Hydrocephalus.
4. Areas of brain softening from vascular obstruction.

Clinical Picture
N.B. Importance of early diagnosis: Prognosis of tuberculous meningitis very much worse with late diagnosis.
1. *Premonitory stage.* Symptoms: Vague. Child's mentality appears to alter, cross and irritable, sleeps frequently, restless, unaccountable vomiting, constipation, headache.
2. *Stage of irritation.* Child becomes drowsy, turns away from light. Commencing dehydration. Child tends to pick skin, grind teeth. Pulse slow. Signs of meningeal irritation, neck stiffness, etc., often appear late.
3. *Terminal stage.* Child in coma; squints; facial or other palsies occur. Incontinent; may cry out with peculiar meningeal cry, wasting occurs.

Investigations
1. *Mantoux reaction* usually positive in initial stages. May become negative in late stages.
2. *Lumbar puncture.*
        2.1 Pressure (normal 100–200 mm CSF). Early cases normal. Later raised.
        2.2 Cells (normal below 5 cells/mm^3). Early case:

almost always raised up to 40 or 50. Later: raised to 100–1000. Cells mainly lymphocytes.

2.3 Protein   (normal   below   0·25 g/l)   1·0–10 g/l. Spider-web clot may form in later cases.

2.4 Glucose (normal above 2·5 mmol/l (45 mg%)). Usually below 2·5 mmol/l even in early stages. Often 0·85–1·7 mmol/l (15–30 mg%).

2.5 Organisms. 10 ml of CSF centrifuged; drop from deposit placed on microscope slide and allowed to dry; stained for acid-fast bacilli. Fluid should be cultured.

3. Radiography of chest. Repeat monthly. May show evidence of other tuberculous manifestation, especially primary tuberculous complex with enlarged hilar lymph nodes, pleural effusion or miliary tuberculosis.

4. Gastric lavage for culture of tubercle bacilli.

5. Fundi examination for choroidal tubercles.

Prognosis
Good if treatment commenced early.

Treatment
General.   Usual nursing care for critically ill child required. Particular care must be taken to give psychological support to child during prolonged treatment involving frequent injections and lumbar punctures.

Drugs—used in tuberculosis:

  Drugs which penetrate inflamed meninges: Isoniazid, rifampicin, streptomycin and ethambutol.

  Regimes alter with availability of new drugs.

  Consult textbook on tuberculosis for further information.

Extrathoracic Tuberculosis, Primary and Post-primary

Tuberculous Lymphatic Involvement
  1. Involvement of lymphatic tissue essential part of primary tuberculous complex.

  2. In miliary tuberculosis lymphatic tissue often affected as is any other tissue.

  3. Generalized involvement of lymph nodes, liver and spleen may occur in older children.

  4. Selective lymphatic involvement common, especially cervical lymph nodes.

Tuberculous Cervical Adenitis
(*Scrofula; Tuberculous Glands of Neck*)

Virtually only occurs from infection with bovine tubercle bacilli from infected cow's milk. In countries in which cows are not infected and in which milk is pasteurized, the disease is unknown. But *see* Atypical Mycobateria, p. 108.

Clinical Features
Insidious onset. Lump which gradually increases in size. Constitutional upsets mild. Lymph nodes matted, immobile, only slightly tender; may remain enlarged

for months and eventually calcify. Alternatively, lymph node caseates, bursts through deep cervical fascia, forms typical 'cold abscess'. Obvious swelling occurs which may be quite large and fluctuate, skin appears red or purple, in later stages is stretched and shiny, only slightly tender.

Differential Diagnosis of Enlarged Lymph Nodes in Neck
1. Acute lymphadenitis. Commonest. Due to infection in throat or from lesion on scalp often caused by pediculi. Differentiation usually easy by history, acute onset, constitutional disturbance, considerable pain and tenderness. Occasionally difficulty arises, especially if chemotherapy has been given in inadequate dosage, thus masking symptoms.
2. Atypical mycobacterial infection. Now commoner than true tuberculosis in most western countries.
3. Leukaemia and lymphoma. Other groups of nodes often involved. Spleen palpable, characteristic blood picture, child usually appears ill.
4. Branchial cyst often resembles breaking down lymph node.
5. Cat scratch disease, glandular fever, sarcoidosis and fungal infections.

Abdominal Tuberculosis, Tuberculous Mesenteric Lymphadenitis (*Tabes Mesenterica*)
Very rare manifestation of primary tuberculosis complex but primary focus in intestine rarely discoverable. Regional mesenteric lymph nodes may be caseous or calcified. Usually no symptoms. Rarely general malaise and steatorrhoea.

Tuberculous Peritonitis
Tuberculous mesenteric lymph node may rupture into peritoneal cavity, causing tuberculous peritonitis. Types:
  1. Ascitic type—Gross ascites.
  2. Plastic type—Abdomen distended with matted omentum and gut. Prognosis poor.

Primary Tuberculosis of Skin
Primary lesion occurs infrequently and is often missed. Sequence of events occurs as in primary tuberculous complex anywhere, i.e. primary lesion with involvement of regional lymph nodes.

Predisposing Causes of Primary Lesion
History of preceding injury in about 40% of cases. Wound subsequently becoming contaminated by tubercle bacillus. Theoretically ordinary BCG vaccination can be classified as primary tuberculosis of skin *see* p. 103.

Unclassified Mycobacteria (atypical; anonymous)
Increasing evidence that certain unclassified mycobacteria can be pathological to man.

In many parts of world these organisms can be cultivated from soil, water, animals, etc. Local small epidemics occur.

Clinically two main types:
  1. Lymph-node involvement—especially cervical and submandibular. Resem-

bles classical tuberculosis but more indolent and resistant to antituberculous therapy.

2. Localized deep, undermining skin ulcers—*M. ulcerans*.

Diagnosis
Mantoux test performed as for classical tuberculosis using a battery of PPD-like material including Avian and Battey strains. Some cross-immunity with classical tuberculosis.

Treatment
Resistant to most antituberculous agents. Erythromycin may be of value. Excision of lymph node.

Leprosy
Very rare except in few localities. *See* textbook of medicine.

Chapter 33   ***TETANUS***

Aetiology
Tetanus bacillus introduced into body via infected wound, umbilical stump. Source of entry sometimes unknown. Bacillus multiplies locally in wound, produces powerful exotoxins which spread via peripheral nerves.

Clinical Course
Incubation period—3–10 days. Onset with gradually increasing jaw stiffness until there is difficulty in opening mouth. Progressing to *risus sardonicus*—retraction of angle of mouth. Later: stiffness and rigidity of back and abdominal muscles develop; as back muscles are more powerful, opisthotonos occurs. Limbs involved last.
Note: Rigidity present all the time (differentiates from strychnine poisoning). Spasm occasionally superadded. May be induced by touching patient, sudden light or noise. Excrutiatingly painful, as both prime mover and antagonist muscles contract simultaneously. Patient remains conscious to the end.

Differential Diagnosis
1. Trismus may be presenting sign in following: (*a*) Any painful condition of mouth and jaw such as quinsy, bad teeth, inflamed cervical lymph nodes, etc. These are commonest causes in children. (*b*) Encephalitis especially postvaccinial.

2. Other conditions causing muscular spasm, e.g. tetany, rabies, strychnine poisoning.

Prognosis. Depends on:
1. Amount of exotoxin absorbed.
2. Site of wound—more dangerous near face.
3. Length of incubation period. If short (<10 days) prognosis grave.
4. Interval between first symptom and first major spasm—'period of onset'. If rapid (under 1 week) prognosis grave.

5. Treatment. Availability of skilled nursing care and team to effect assisted ventilation if needed.

Prophylactic Treatment

1. Booster dose of tetanus toxoid to previously immunized wounded children.
2. Human tetanus-immune globulin 250u i.m. to child not previously immunized.
3. I.m. penicillin for 3 days if circumstances suggest tetanus likely.

Management of Case

1. General: (*a*) Nurse in quiet darkened room. For severe cases team of specialists required, anaesthetist being most important. (*b*) Penicillin. (*c*) Human tetanus immune globulin in a single dose of 5000–10 000u i.m. and infiltrated around wound if possible should be given as soon as possible. Does not influence present state of patient, but prevents formation of further toxins. (*d*) Wound should be treated as required.
2. Mild cases. Sedation with diazepam or chlorpromazine.
3. Severe cases: (*a*) Complete paralysis by curarizing drugs. (*b*) Intermittent positive-pressure respiration.
4. Active immunization in convalescence as infection does not confer permanent immunity.

Chapter 34   # MALARIA

Very common infectious disease of tropics and subtropics in many parts of world. Incidence falling following efforts to eradicate mosquitoes. Only features of importance to childhood will be discussed here.

Infection

Caused by four species of protozoa: *Plasmodium falciparum, P. vivax, P. malariae* or *P. ovale*. Transmitted by female anopheline mosquito.

Life Cycle (Fig. 34.1)

Immunity

1. Passive. Infants of malarial mothers acquire transfer of antibodies contained in IgG fraction of serum. For this reason malarial attack rare under 6 months of age.
2. Natural. Non-specific (cellular immunity). Perhaps associated with increased stimulation of reticulo-endothelial system.
3. Acquired (humoral immunity). Produced by active infection with malarial parasite. Associated with circulating IgG antibody.
4. Partial protection by some haemoglobinopathies, e.g. S, and G-6-PD deficiency. Also possibly thalassaemia.

Clinical Features

Incubation period: 9–30 days. Non-immune child with primary attack: fever, listlessness, drowsiness or irritability, vomiting, diarrhoea. Convulsions common.

Fig. 34.1.   Life cycle of *P. falciparum*.

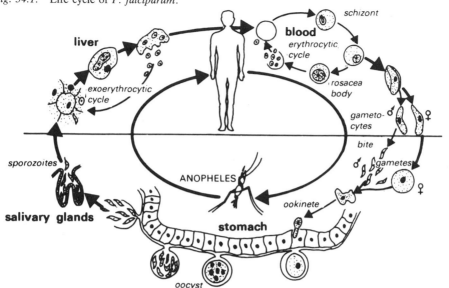

Older children complain of headache, nausea, thirst and abdominal pain. Rigors may occur. May have cough.

On examination. High fever which may be short-lived or continuous at first but later tends to settle to regular 48 h pattern (for *P. vivax*). Enlarged, tender liver and spleen. Anaemia marked.

Course and Prognosis
Cerebral malaria, hyperpyrexia, anaemia, severe diarrhoea and vomiting all common in children. Death may occur. Blackwater fever, an acute haemolytic anaemia with haemoglobinuria, only with poorly controlled *P. falciparum* infection.

Differential Diagnosis
In endemic areas, malaria is *the* great mimic and must be considered in the diagnosis of every ill child. Blood smear must always be examined.

Treatment
1. Of acute attack: Chloroquine or Camoquin (4-amino-quinoline) will cure *P. falciparum* but will not prevent relapse of *P. vivax* or *malariae*. Dosage depends on age and severity.

2. For prophylaxis: Pyrimethamine or chloroquine weekly, or paludrine (Proguanil) daily. Chloroquine-resistant falciparum now widespread in SE Asia and elsewhere. Give Fansidar, or if Fansidar resistant give quinine.

Chapter 35   *TOXOPLASMOSIS*

Toxoplasma gondii is a protozoal parasite which is widespread but very rarely gives rise to disease. Cats are the main carrier but epidemics have followed ingestion of raw meat. The acquired disease resembles that in adults with malaise, muscle pain, weakness, painless lymphadenopathy and skin rashes.

If a mother becomes infected during pregnancy the outcome will depend on the age of the fetus and the size of the infecting dose. It may result in fetal death, or a live birth with stigmata of congenital toxoplasmosis:

Acute: Jaundice, purpura, hepatosplenomegaly, lymph-node enlargement, skin rashes etc.

Chronic: Choroidoretinitis which may be the only manifestation and may not be discovered until school age. Hydrocephalus, microcephaly and other brain lesions occur in infancy, giving rise to mental deficiency or fits. Calcification of brain lesions seen on radiograph of skull, maximal in walls of ventricles causing curvilinear shadows.

Chapter 36   *VISCERAL LEISHMANIASIS (Kala-azar)*

Uncommon disease of tropical and some subtropical countries, characterized by chronic febrile illness with weight loss and marked hepatosplenomegaly.

Aetiology
Causative organism is an intracellular parasite, *Leishmania donovani*. Transmitted by the bite of infected sandflies in which it occurs as a flagellated 'leptomonad'; it is engulfed by skin macrophages, changes to the leishmanial form and multiplies in the reticulo-endothelial system, particularly the liver and spleen, as well as the skin and intestinal mucosa.

Clinical Features
Insidious onset, with irregular fever, weight loss, progressive (often massive) hepatosplenomegaly, anaemia and leucopenia. Secondary infections occur late in the course of the disease, which may be fatal if untreated, after a course varying from a few months to two years.

Laboratory Investigations
1. Blood films show leucopenia, often pancytopenia if there is hypersplenism, but relative mononucleosis.
2. The ESR is high and hypergammaglobulinaemia is present.
3. The diagnosis is confirmed by finding the parasite (Leishman-donovani bodies) in smears of peripheral blood, bone marrow, spleen or liver aspirates, or jejunal biopsies. Repeated biopsies may be needed before kala-azar can be ruled out.
4. Serological tests including immunofluorescent and ELISA tests are positive in more than 80% of cases.

Treatment
Pentavalent antimonial drugs are the first choice, but if there is no improvement after a full course, amphotericin B may be successful.

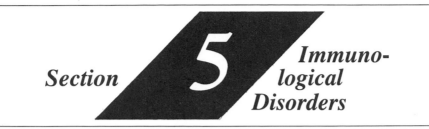

Chapter 37   *NORMAL DEFENSIVE RESPONSE*

Function of immunological system is defence against infective agents, malignant cells and foreign proteins. Mediated by lymphoid cells, immunoglobulins and opsonins. Serious immune deficiencies may account for 2% child deaths. Deficiencies in immunological defences should be suspected when a patient has recurrent or persistent infections or infection by organism not usually considered to be pathogenic. e.g. candida or a saprophyte. Normal response in two phases:

1. *Phagocytosis* by polymorphs or macrophages, followed by destruction of engulfed particles. *Opsonins*, including some immunoglobulins and serum complement system, alter surface of bacteria to enhance phagocytosis. Tuftsin produced by spleen also stimulates ingestion by acting on leucocyte membrane.

2. *Lymphocytic reaction.* Two different cell lines:

(i) T-cells (thymus-dependent cells) responsible for cellular immunity. Exposure of mature T-cells to antigen generates several types of effector cells: (*a*) Helper T-cells, which cooperate with B-cells in induction of antibody responses; (*b*) Suppressor T-cells, which limit the extent of both antibody and cell-mediated immune responses, and (*c*) Cytotoxic T-cells which are particularly important in defence against viral infection, and are sensitized to kill foreign cells bearing appropriate antigens. Subpopulations of helpers and suppressor cells can be distinguished by monoclonal antibodies which recognize different cell surface 'marker' characteristics.

Products of T-cells are known as lymphokines, which act by stimulating lymphocyte multiplication, increasing vascular permeability, cytotoxic effect on antigen-bearing cell, inhibiting migration of macrophages from site of immunological reaction, and transferring characteristics of sensitized cells to other lymphocytes (transfer factor). Tests for lymphokine function include transformation of lymphocytes to lymphoblasts on stimulation with phytohaemagglutinin (PHA) or other antigens. Some T-cells (memory cells) have very long life span and are responsible for prompt response on subsequent contact with antigen.

(ii) *B-cells*, responsible for humoral immunity, i.e. immunoglobulins (antibodies). Lymphocytes in contact with antigen become activated to produce daughter cells, some of which differentiate into plasma cells, characterized by large amounts of cytoplasm and extensive cytoplasmic reticulum. Plasma cells are relatively short-lived, and secrete large amounts of immunoglobulins.

Immunoglobulins are composed of units of 2 long ('heavy') and 2 short ('light') peptide chains. Molecular weight about 150000 except IgM (about 900000) which consists of several basic units linked together. Light chains are identical for all immunoglobulins, but heavy chains are distinct for each class. *Deficiency of immunoglobulins with opsonizing properties increases susceptibility to pyogenic infections.*

The main characteristics of the different immunoglobulins are given in *Table 37.1* and blood levels are indicated in *Table 37.1* and *Fig. 37.1.*

Fig. 37.1. Blood levels of immunoglobulins.

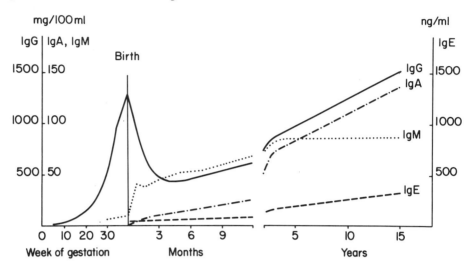

Chapter 38　　　　DISORDERS OF PHAGOCYTIC PHASE

A group of rare disorders, mainly hereditary.

1. *Congenital chronic neutropenia.* Recurrent severe skin infections, septicaemia. Permanent low neutrophil polymorph count.

2. *Cyclic neutropenia.* Periodic (about every 12 days), severe reduction in neutrophils (0–500/mm^3), lasting about 7 days. Fever, stomatitis and risk of severe infection during neutropenic episodes.

3. *Shwachman–Diamond syndrome.* Chronic or cyclical neutropenia, with exocrine pancreatic insufficiency. Autosomal recessive inheritance. Symptoms of cyclic neutropenia combined with malabsorption and absence of pancreatic enzymes (p. 270).

4. *Acquired agranulocytosis.* May be idiosyncratic response to drugs, or follow exposure to volatile chemicals. Acute onset with stomatitis and risk of overwhelming infection. Milder form of neutropenia following splenectomy in young children, also carries risk of septicaemia which may endanger life.

5. *Chronic granulomatous disease.* X-linked recessive disorder, affecting male children of female carriers. Phagocytosed bacteria not destroyed. Clinical features include chronic suppurating lesions in lymph nodes, pulmonary infections, eczema, hepatosplenomegaly. Lymph-node granulomas often due to relatively innocuous bacteria. Defect is inborn error of leucocyte oxidation system, demonstrated by failure to re-oxidize reduced nitroblue tetrazolium to

Table 37.1.　Classification of immunoglobulins

Immunoglobulin	Level	Formed in	Main features	Crosses the placenta	Complement fixation
IgG	High at birth (maternal), falls by 6 months. Adult levels by 4 years 7–14 g/l (700–1400 mg/dl)	Plasma cells	Predominant serum Ig 0·8 g/l (80 %) Gram-positive bacteria. Viruses. Toxins	Yes	Yes
IgM (macroglobulin)	Adult levels by 9 months 0·6–0·7 g/l (60–70 mg/dl). Low at birth unless intra-uterine infection	Lymphocytes	Isohaemagglutinins. Bacteriolysis. Opsonizing properties against Gram-negative bacteria. First antibodies produced in immunological response, brucella, diphtheria, respiratory infections	No	No
IgA	Adult by 5 years 1·5–2·5 g/l (150–250 mg/dl)	Plasma cells	Bactericidal in presence of lysozyme, passes through mucosal surfaces, combines with 'secretory piece' to form secretory IgA which resists proteolysis. Predominant immunoglobulin in all exocrine secretions. Antibody to oral antigens	No	No
IgD	Adult 0·03 g/l (3 mg/dl)	Plasma cells	Uncertain	No	No
IgE	Adult 0·0003 g/l (0·03 mg/dl)	Plasma cells	Mediates atopic reactions, fixes to mast cells, affects histamine and SRS-A release	No	No

blue colour (NBT test). Treatment symptomatic, early radical surgery where indicated; appropriate antibiotics—rifampicin penetrates into leucocytes and often used. Leucocyte transfusion may be life-saving but sensitizes patient to donor cells. Bone marrow transplantation has been successful.

6. *Job's syndrome*. Rare. X-linked or autosomal dominant condition characterized by chronic eczema, recurrent staphylococcal skin infection, eosinophilia, elevated serum IgE and a defect in granulocyte chemotaxis. Treatment is unsatisfactory but clinical improvement with ascorbic acid and transfer factor has been reported.

7. *Chediak–Higashi syndrome*. Recurrent skin infections and partial albinism. Leucocytes contain giant lysosomes. Steroids beneficial.

8. *Myeloperoxidase deficiency*. Metabolic error in phagocytes associated with inability to kill fungi. Candida septicaemia is usual result.

Chapter 39   # DISORDERS OF COMPLEMENT SYSTEM

Complement (C) system consists of a series of serum proteins (C_1–C_9), which work by a chain reaction (complement cascade). Primary selective deficiencies of individual complement fractions are very rare but have been recorded.

Defects may be in chemotaxis, phagocytosis or bacterial lysis, with resulting increased susceptibility to bacterial and fungal infection. Hereditary absence of a specific inhibitor of activated C_1 (C_1 esterase inhibitor) allows complement cascade to proceed spontaneously, resulting in angioneurotic oedema. Low C levels in pre-term infants correlate with decreased opsonizing activity against *E. coli, P. aeruginosa, Serratia marescens* and *S. aureus*. (Neonatal susceptibility to gram-negative infections is also related to low IgM levels.)

Chapter 40   # DISORDERS OF LYMPHOCYTIC PHASE

1. T-cell Deficiency

Defective cell-mediated immunity manifests itself by severe chronic infections appearing during the first 3 months of life. Symptoms include failure to thrive, chronic diarrhoea, chest infections, thrush, skin rashes and fever. Resistance to viral, bacterial and fungal infections are all reduced; there may be severe candida septicaemia, *Pneumocystis carinii* infection or severe illness with generalized infection following smallpox or BCG vaccine. Immunoglobulins normal. Marked lymphopenia. Four distinct syndromes are described:

  a. Thymic dysplasia (*Nezelof syndrome*). Symptoms as above.

  Pathology: Hypoplastic thymus, no Hassall's corpuscles, no T-lymphocytes. B-lymphocytes present in spleen and blood. Basic defect is probably defective colonization of thymus by medullary stem cells.

  Treatment: Maintain child in germ-free environment until bone marrow transplantation.

b. Thymic aplasia with hypoparathyroidism (DiGeorge syndrome). Defect in structures derived from 3rd and 4th branchial arches. May be associated malformations of ear, nose, mouth or great vessels. Severe neonatal hypoparathyroidism with tetany. Subsequently infections develop as above. Chest X-ray indicates absent thymus.

Pathology: Aplastic thymus, absent parathyroids, no T-lymphocytes, low serum calcium, high phosphorus.

Treatment: Maintain in germ-free environment, treat parathyroid deficiency, do fetal thymic transplant.

c. Thymic dysplasia with hypothyroidism (Good syndrome). Extremely rare combination of thymic hypoplasia and hypothyroidism.

d. Mucocutaneous candidiasis. Specific inability of T-cells to respond to *C. albicans*. Causes persistent candida infection of skin, nails, mouth. Treatment with transfer factor from lymphocytes of normal person may cure.

2. B-cell Deficiency

Predominant feature of defective humoral immunity is recurrent, frequent and severe bacterial infection (pharyngitis, otitis media, sinusitis, pneumonia, pyoderma, septicaemia, meningitis). Diminished or absent antibody response to infections or immunizations, but infections respond normally to antibiotics. T-cell function maintains normal response to fungal, mycobacterial and viral infections.

a. Physiological hypogammaglobulinaemia. Age 3–6 months, maternal IgG catabolized and infant's immunoglobulin synthesis still poor. Danger period for repeated infections. Occasionally there is delayed maturation of immunoglobulin synthesis up to 2 years—*transient hypogammaglobulinaemia*—which must be differentiated from true inherited hypogammaglobulinaemia because ultimate prognosis good.

b. Congenital agammaglobulinaemia (Bruton's Disease) X-linked recessive. Incidence 1 in 100000 live male births.

Recurrent pyogenic infections, onset usually toward end of first year of life. Normal clinical response to most viral infections and vaccinations, but no antibodies formed. N.B. Infective hepatitis may be fulminant. Non-infective arthritis of rheumatoid type often occurs, as does malabsorption which may be associated with *Giardia lamblia* infestation. Lymph nodes and tonsils aplastic. A non-sex-linked variety also occurs and carries a very bad prognosis.

Investigations: Radiographs reveal normal thymic shadow, hypoplastic adenoids. Marked hypogammaglobulinaemia affecting IgG, IgM and IgA. Lymphocyte count normal.

Inadequate antibody response to vaccines and regional lymph node after vaccination shows absence of lymphoid follicles and plasma cells. Low titre of isohaemagglutinins.

Treatment: (i) Antibiotics for individual infections according to sensitivities. (ii) Replacement of gammaglobulin by injections sufficient to increase IgG above $2.0 g/l$ (200mg/dl). Usually weekly dose of $0.025 g/kg$ is adequate.

Prognosis: Good during early childhood, with adequate replacement therapy. In later life some patients develop hepatitis or dermatomyositis.

c. Dysgammaglobulinaemia. Selective deficiencies of one or two major immunoglobulin classes. Commonest is *isolated IgA deficiency*, affecting both serum and secretory IgA. Main symptom is recurrent respiratory infection. Also increased incidence of coeliac disease, and giardiasis.

d. Acquired hypogammaglobulinaemia. Two varieties, according to which immunoglobulin predominantly deficient.

Low IgG, normal IgA and IgM: Seen in excessive immunoglobulin loss (nephrotic syndrome, intestinal lymphangiectasia) or catabolism (corticosteroid therapy), or inadequate synthesis (malnutrition, bone-marrow diseases).

Low IgM ± IgA, normal IgG: Seen in malignancy, uraemia, cytotoxic therapy, coeliac disease, diabetes mellitus, and severe infections. Symptoms of susceptibility to infection seen in association with underlying disorder.

3. Combined T- and B-cell Deficiency
Cellular and humoral immunity both affected.

Inheritance: several varieties, may be autosomal or X-linked recessive.

Symptoms: Repeated skin and respiratory infections from second month of life, thrush, chronic diarrhoea, persistent fever. Susceptibility to opportunistic bacteria, fungi and viruses, and infection with live attenuated vaccines may be fatal.

Investigations: Lymphopenia, negative PHA Test indicate defective humoral immunity. No antibody response to vaccines.

Pathology: Rudimentary thymus and lymphoid tissue. Absent Hassall's corpuscles. *Basic defect* in maturation or migration of medullary stem cells.

Severe combined immune deficiency (*SCID*). One identifiable defect is adenosine deaminase (ADA) deficiency in which abnormalities of purine metabolism occur which are toxic to both T and B-lymphocytes. In another disorder, purine nucleoside phosphorylase (PNP) deficiency, the toxic effects of the biochemical error are limited to the T-cells and relatively normal humoral immunity is preserved.

Treatment: Bone-marrow transplant, but danger of graft *v* host reaction. ADA deficiency may improve temporarily after blood transfusion.

Prognosis: Patients usually die during first year if untreated.

4. Atypical Immune Deficiences
a. Wiskott–Aldrich syndrome. Rare, X-linked recessive. Affected males have chronic eczema, thrombocytopenic purpura and recurrent fungal and bacterial infection beginning in first year. Various immunological defects are described, particularly deficiency of IgM. No lymphopenia but defective cellular immunity usually demonstrable. Prognosis poor but administration of transfer factor may be valuable.

b. Ataxia-telangiectasia. Rare, autosomal recessive. Progressive ataxia commencing in early years, with telangiectasia of conjunctivae and exposed skin, often appearing much later. Recurrent respiratory infections but lymphoid tissue not enlarged. Risk of lymphoreticular malignancy developing. Low IgA levels and evidence of cellular immune deficiency. Transfer factor has been beneficial.

Section 6

Diseases of Nutrition

Note:
1. In the developing world, undernutrition is by far the most important factor in childhood mortality and morbidity. By contrast, overnutrition is commonest primary nutritional abnormality in 'affluent' countries.
2. A good diet contains sufficient calories and proper balance between its constituents.
3. Many growth disturbances are result of a pathological process and a secondary effect on nutritional intake.

Chapter 41   ## FAILURE TO THRIVE

Clinical picture of infant under 1 year of age who 'fails to thrive' is common. Following conditions should be considered:

1. Primary 'syndrome' disorders. e.g. Russell–Silver dwarf, chromosome abnormality, etc.

2. Alimentary causes. Starvation; chronic vomiting from any cause; gastroenteritis; coeliac disease; cystic fibrosis; chronic intussusception.

3. Infections. Urinary tract; respiratory; tuberculosis; congenital infections, e.g. rubella, toxoplasmosis, cytomegalovirus.

4. Congenital malformations. Usually obvious, e.g. cleft palate; congenital heart disease; other causes of heart failure.

5. Metabolic. Idiopathic renal acidosis; hypercalcaemia; hypophosphatasia; nephrogenic diabetes insipidus; diabetes mellitus; Fanconi syndrome; uraemia.

6. Central nervous system. Mental retardation resulting in poor food intake; degenerative diseases of the nervous system, diencephalic syndrome.

7. Prematurity

8. Malignant disease e.g. Letterer–Siwe disease, neuroblastoma.

Emotional Deprivation
Part of the spectrum of child abuse and neglect. Usually associated with some degree of undernutrition, i.e. caloric deprivation. Should be suspected in any young child with failure to thrive who has no features suggesting chronic illness or congenital disorder, and in whom parent-child relationship seems abnormal.

Clinical Features of Emotional Deprivation
Child may be apathetic, adopting catatonic postures, or attention-seeking and

over-affectionate. Appetite usually good even in apathetic children, while older, mobile child will eat ravenously and hoard food if possible.

Investigation

In suspected case, good weight gain on admission to hospital suggests that home environment is unsatisfactory. Social service report may confirm medical suspicion. Fall in weight on discharge home followed by a further gain on readmission, if otherwise unexplained, is virtually conclusive and should initiate the procedure for management of non-accidental injury if this has not been invoked previously.

Laboratory investigations usually normal although growth hormone secretion is often reduced, returning to normal during nutritional recovery.

Malnutrition

The distinction between 'marasmus' and 'kwashiorkor' useful on clinical and aetiological grounds. Kwashiorkor, i.e. malnutrition with oedema, is a more acute condition than marasmus. Metabolic adaptation to starvation is therefore more effective in the marasmic child. Kwashiorkor is rare in some countries where malnutrition is common, e.g. some parts of Latin America. Mixed forms (marasmic kwashiorkor) frequently seen in many areas.

Table 41.1. Classification of malnutrition syndromes (Wellcome)

	Weight for age as % of Boston 50th centile	Oedema
Underweight	60–80	–
Marasmus	<60	–
Kwashiorkor	>60	+
Marasmic kwashiorkor	<60	+

In chronic malnutrition, a useful distinction is also made between 'stunting', i.e. failure of longitudinal growth, and 'wasting', i.e. discrepancy between height and weight. Stunting may indicate very chronic malnutrition or lack of a specific nutrient essential for linear growth, e.g. zinc. Wasting is indicative of recent or active malnutrition.

Table 41.2. Classification of malnutrition syndromes (Waterlow). Standards are Boston centiles

Stunting (Height for age)	Wasting (Weight for height)
0 = >95%	0 = >90%
1 = 95–90%	1 = 90–80%
2 = 89–85%	2 = 79–70%
3 = <85%	3 = <70%

$$\text{Weight for height} = \frac{\text{weight of patient}}{\text{weight of normal subject of same height}} \times 100.$$

Metabolic Consequences of Malnutrition

Reduced protein intake causes fall in serum proteins and reduced cell synthesis, particularly affecting tissues with rapid turnover, i.e. skin, gut and blood cells. Immunological defences impaired because synthesis of neutrophils, lymphocytes, complement and imunoglobulins is reduced.

Clinical Complications of Malnutrition
1. Oedema and reduced blood volume secondary to hypoproteinaemia.
2. Hypothermia even in presence of infection.
3. Depression, misery, anorexia and reduced activity.
4. Malabsorption with villous atrophy.
5. Increased susceptibility to infection.
6. Negative Mantoux in presence of active tuberculosis.

Marasmus

Very common in many parts of developing world. Mainly in first year of life.

Aetiology
May follow prematurity or illness in neonate with inadequate lactation as result of poor suckling. Also when breast feeding over-prolonged without supplement. Infections, particularly diarrhoea, often contributory.

Clinical Features
Growth failure, wasting of muscles, slack skin, often dehydration, may be vitamin deficiencies. May be associated with enteritis, malaria, tuberculosis, respiratory infection, etc. In contrast with kwashiorkor *no oedema*, pigmentary and skin changes slight or absent, usually good appetite.

Treatment
(1) Reduce heat loss but do not add warmth. (2) Frequent small feeds with high protein, high calorie content, e.g. dried skimmed milk, sugar and edible oil supplemented by local ingredients. Nasogastric tube feeding may be necessary at first. Give standard daily volume for expected weight. (3) Treat associated diseases if present, e.g. i.v. fluids for enteritis, vitamin A for xerophthalmia, antituberculous therapy, antimalarials, antihelminthics and iron, etc. (4) Educate mother to avoid relapse.

Prevention
(1) Education of parents. (2) Adequate supplies of suitable weaning foods, to be introduced by age 6 months. (3) Early detection by local health personnel, and suitable management of infants underfed at breast. (4) Prevention and control of infectious disease.

Kwashiorkor (*Protein–energy Malnutrition; Protein–calorie Malnutrition*)

Common condition in areas where protein foods not given to growing child because of scarcity, cost or local practice, e.g. many parts Africa, Asia, W. Indies. Child usually aged 1–3 years.

Aetiology
Growing child requires positive protein balance, whereas adults need only maintain protein equilibrium. Protein foods often expensive, may also be withheld from young child because of ignorance or local superstition. Severe protein lack leads to kwashiorkor, often associated with vitamin deficiency, anaemia, intestinal parasite infestation, diarrhoea, malaria and other infections.

Clinical Features
Onset fairly sudden, often follows infection, e.g. measles, pertussis, gastro-enteritis. Child may be abruptly displaced from breast by further pregnancy.

Typically anorexic, miserable child, with oedema. Diarrhoea common. Muscles weak and thin. Skin may show dermatitis ('flaky paint'). Hair sparse, friable, may be depigmented. Liver usually enlarged, with fatty change. Serum albumin low.

Differential Diagnosis
Other causes of oedema, e.g. nephrotic syndrome, cardiac failure.

Treatment
(1) Reduce heat loss but do not warm. (2) Initially correct fluid/electrolyte imbalance, and feed ½ strength milk ad lib up to 90 cal/kg for 1–2 days. Nasogastric tube feeding often necessary. (3) When appetite returns, increase volume and energy content of intake, give protein 2 g/kg, mineral mixture (including Mg, K, Zn, Cu) and multivitamins including folate. Useful mixture is dried skimmed milk, sugar and oil. (4) After 7–10 days reinforce milk with edible oil, feed at least 150 cal/kg. Intake by this time limited only by appetite. Use local food mix, e.g. meat, vegetables, beans. (5) Treat associated infections, malaria, parasitosis, avitaminosis, anaemia. (6) Educate mother to avoid relapse.

Prevention
(1) Education of parents. (2) Adequate supplies of suitable weaning foods with sufficient protein. (3) Prevention and control of infectious disease and parasitic infestation e.g. by immunization. (4) Early detection of poor weight gain by local health personnel.

Chapter 42   # VITAMINS

Vitamin A (Retinol)

Fat-soluble vitamin derived from liver, fish, milk, eggs or from precursor carotenes in plants, and stored in liver. Necessary for synthesis of visual pigments in retina, and for normal development of bones, teeth and epithelium. Daily requirements: 2000–4000 i.u. Dietary deficiency very rare in developed countries but may occur in malabsorption syndromes.

Deficiency Effects
1. Eyes: night blindness, photophobia; later, xerophthalmia followed by greyish plaques on conjunctiva (Bitot's spots) and keratomalacia leading to blindness.

2. Retarded mental and physical development.
3. Skin dry, scaly, may be hyperkeratotic.

Hypervitaminosis A
Gross, prolonged overdosage with vitamin A may lead to tibial thickening similar to cortical hyperostosis. Increased fontanelle tension may occur in young infants.

Vitamin B Complex

Deficiency Syndromes
All very rare in UK. Combination of lesions frequently occurs. May occur in infants given special foods for metabolic diseases if adequate vitamin supplements not given.

Vitamin	Daily requirements Infants	Older children	Deficiency disease	Principal manifestations
Thiamine B₁	0·4 mg	0·6–1·2 mg	Beri-beri	1. Cardiac: tachycardia, heart failure, oedema. 2. Nervous: apathy, ptosis of eyelids
Riboflavin	0·6 mg	1–2 mg	Glossitis, etc.	Angular stomatitis, smooth tongue
Nicotinic acid	3–5 mg	7–12 mg	Pellagra*	1. 'Dermatitis'—erythema and scaling of exposed skin 2. 'Diarrhoea'—gastro-intestinal lesions 3. 'Delirium'—mental symptoms
Pyridoxine (B6)	0·3–0·5 mg	0·5–1·5 mg	Anaemia, Convulsions, etc.	1. Microcytic anaemia 2. Neonatal fits 3. Peripheral neuropathy
Folic/folinic acid	20 μg	50 μg	Megaloblastic anaemia (secondary to malabsorption or dietary deficiency, e.g. goat's milk)	Megaloblastic anaemia

*See Hartnup Disease, p. 155.

Pyridoxine Dependence
Very rare condition of early infancy, manifested by myoclonic seizures or generalized fits, accompanied by a hypsarrhythmic EEG pattern. IV, injection of 100 mg stops fit and restores normal EEG pattern. Daily maintenance dose necessary.

Vitamin B12 (*Cyanocobalamin*)
Present in green vegetables, liver. Complex with gastric intrinsic factor necessary for absorption, which takes place in terminal ileum. Malabsorption of B12 may

occur in juvenile pernicious anaemia due to congenital absence of intrinsic factor, or specific absorption defect in ileum (both extremely rare), Crohn's disease or surgical resection of terminal ileum. Deficiency produces megaloblastic anaemia.

Vitamin C

Infantile Scurvy (*Avitaminosis C*)

Definition
Now rare disease in most countries. Caused by lack of vitamin C (ascorbic acid) in diet. Manifested by haemorrhages mainly under periosteum of bone and to lesser extent in the gums.

Sources of Vitamin C
Green vegetables, fresh fruit particularly citrus fruits, blackcurrants, rose hips. More plentiful in human milk than cow's milk.

Requirements
25–50 mg ascorbic acid per day for infant, overdosage virtually impossible.

Aetiology of Scurvy
Inadequate intake of vitamin C may occur in occasional infants fed unmodified cow's milk or weaned late on to diet with inadequate fruit and vegetables.

Clinical Features
Irritability, bony tenderness from subperiosteal haemorrhages, spongy purple swelling of gums and gingival haemorrhage if teeth have erupted.
   Ascorbic acid level reduced in leucocytes, nil in urine. X-rays show thin long bone cortex and perhaps subperiosteal haemorrhages.

Treatment
Ascorbic acid by mouth, 500–1000 mg daily. Symptomatic improvement is prompt.

Vitamin D

Rickets (*Avitaminosis D*)

Definition
   1. Metabolic disorder of growing bone with impaired deposition of minerals in bony matrix. Usually due to primary deficiency of vitamin D or its active metabolites but may be complication of other conditions.
   2. Vitamin D-resistant rickets produces a similar clinical picture but results from an inherited metabolic disorder (p. 127).
   3. Higher incidence in dark-skinned races results from combination of dietary inadequacy and lack of exposure to sunlight (*see below*).

Sources of Vitamin D
   1. Dietary. Vitamin D_3 (fat soluble) found in some dietary fats, including milk, fish, eggs. Rich sources include fish liver oils. Some foods such as oatmeal contain

phytic acid, which forms insoluble calcium complexes and inhibits calcium absorption.

Physiology: Vitamin D_3 (cholecalciferol) absorbed in small intestine, bile salts necessary for its absorption, and there is an enterohepatic circulation of D_3. Conversion to active metabolite 25-hydroxycholecalciferol (25OHCC) occurs in liver, and an even more active substance 1,25-dihydroxycholecalciferol is further synthesized from 25-HCC in the kidneys. 1,25-DHCC acts on small bowel mucosa to enhance calcium absorption in combination with binding protein, and on bone to stimulate calcium mobilization. Synthesis of 1,25-DHCC controlled by parathormone (PTH). Fall in serum calcium causes increased PTH secretion, which promotes synthesis of 1,25-DHCC and thus increases calcium absorption (*Fig. 42.1*).

2. *Synthesis* in skin by action of ultraviolet light on 7-dehydrocholesterol.

Incidence
Difficult to assess. Rare in developed countries except in some immigrant communities. May occur in very small pre-term infants not receiving sufficient vitamin D. Common in countries where mother and babies kept out of sunlight.

Radiological Appearances
Best seen in anteroposterior view of lower end of radius and ulna.
1. *Early active rickets*
    1.1 Fraying of epiphysial plate. Often first noticed at lower end of ulna.
    1.2 Cupping and broadening of epiphysis.
    1.3 Rarefaction of shaft of bones.
2. *Advanced active rickets*
    1.1 Lengthening of distance between shaft and epiphysial centre of ossification (owing to development of rachitic metaphysis).
    1.2 Appearance of early condition, as above, but in greater degree.
    1.3 'Periostitis' appearance due to subperiosteal osteoid deposits.
    1.4 Bony deformities.
    1.5 Greenstick fractures.

Pathological Biochemistry
1. Usual biochemical findings in rickets:
    1.1 Serum calcium usually normal. (Normal = 2·25 – 2·65 mmol/l.)
    1.2 Serum phosphorus low 0·64–1·1 mmol/l. (Normal = 1·1–1·6 mmol/l.)
    1.3 Serum alkaline phosphatase raised (over 100 SI units).
    1.4 Low 25-OH cholecalciferol. (Normal up to about 1 ng/ml.)
    1.5 Elevated parathormone levels. (Normal up to about 1 ng/ml.)
2. Theory of pathogenesis. Lack of vitamin D leads to calcium malabsorption in gut with tendency to hypocalcaemia. This is corrected by secondary

Fig. 42.1. Vitamin D metabolism. 25-OHCC, 25-hydroxycholecalciferol; 1,25/DHCC, 1,25-dihydroxycholecalciferol.

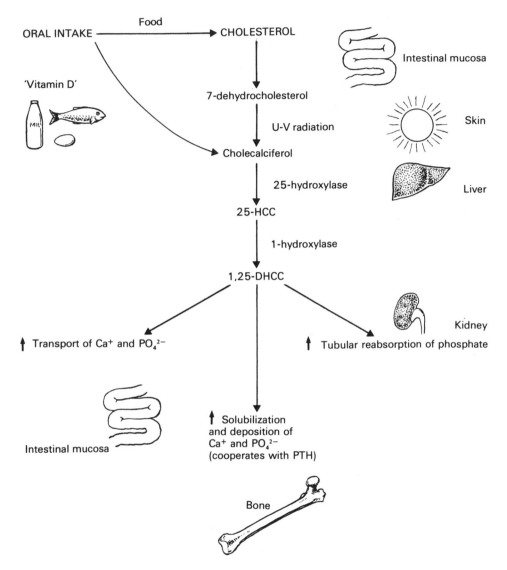

hyperparathyroidism resulting in low serum phosphorus, which gives rise to rickets with low phosphorus and normal calcium (usual type).

3. Urine often contains excess amino acids.

Clinical Features of Moderate Rickets (Low-phosphorus Type)
    1. Bony deformities. Severe case.
           1.1 Head
           1.1.1 Frontal bossing
           1.1.2 Late closing of fontanelle

1.2 Thorax. 'Rickety rosary'.
1.3 Arms and Legs. Epiphysial enlargement common. Best felt at wrists. Bowing of long bones.
   Note: Physiological bowing of legs very common. May be due:
   1.3.1 To position of fat and muscle, but radiograph demonstrates straight bones.
   1.3.2 Bones are bowed. If an isolated occurrence with no other evidence of rickets, prognosis good as spontaneous regression of bowing occurs.
2. *Ligaments and muscles*. Hypotonia often marked.
3. Following deformities classically described but no longer regarded as evidence of rickets:
   3.1 Pigeon Chest. Often genetically determined.
   3.2 Harrison's Sulcus
   3.3 Funnel Sternum. Often congenital.
   3.4 Craniotabes. Skull soft, can be indented like table tennis ball. Usually most prominent over occiput near sutures. Often found in normal newborn babies or in low birth weight infants.

Prophylaxis
Pre-term infants: 400–800 iu vitamin D per day from 1st week. Full term infants receive adequate supplies from proprietary milk or weaning foods which are fortified with vitamin D.

Treatment.
1500 iu vitamin D per day.

'Late Rickets'

Classification
1. Vitamin-D resistant rickets
   1.1 Now commonest type of rickets in many parts of the world. Signs, symptoms, radiological and pathological appearance resemble infantile rickets except that picture modified by older age of bones. Serum calcium usually lowered. If untreated, active rickets continues throughout years of growth.
   1.2 Genetically inherited disease. Inherited as X-linked dominant. Actual enzyme defect uncertain but 25-hydroxylation of D_3 is known to be normal in some patients, abnormal in others.
   1.3 Treatment. 1,25-dihydroxyvitamin D_3 or 1α-hydroxyvitamin D or huge doses of vitamin D (20 000–25 000 iu) daily required to control activity. Meticulous clinical, radiological and biochemical control required as toxic level and therapeutic level may be almost the same. 25-HCC much more effective if obtainable. Aim to keep serum calcium below 2·5 mmol/l with slight elevation of alkaline phosphatase. Hypercalcaemia will produce nephrocalcinosis.

2. *Rickets due to defective absorption of vitamin D*. As in:

> *2.1 Coeliac Disease. Note*: rickets only occurs during active growth. Will therefore only appear during recovery from coeliac disease. Villous atrophy impairs calcium absorption by 1,25-DHCC/calcium-binding protein system. Large doses of D_3 may be rquired.
>
> *2.2 Chronic Obstructive Jaundice*. Bile acids necessary for micelle formation and D_3 absorption in jejunum.

3. *Rickets due to renal defect*

> *3.1 Chronic Renal Failure*. Failure of 1,25-HCC synthesis by kidneys.
>
> *3.2 Tubular Insufficiency*. (i) Fanconi syndrome, *see* p. 154. (ii) Idiopathic renal acidosis. (iii) Familial hypophosphataemic rickets. Defective reabsorption of phosphorus in renal tubule. Usually X-linked, can be autosomal recessive.

4. Anticonvulsant rickets. Consequence of hepatic enzyme induction leading to increased breakdown of D_3 to inactive metabolites. Low plasma levels of 25-HCC.

Hypervitaminosis D
Excess vitamin D produces toxic symptoms: hypertension, vomiting, as well as calcification in soft tissues. Renal calcification may lead to permanent renal damage.

Hypophosphatasia
Very rare autosomal recessive condition.

Clinical Features
1. Newborn. Severe skeletal deformities with absence of bone formation, especially of skull.
2. Infants. At about 6 months of age develop vomiting, constipation, fits, failure to thrive, fever and hypotonia. Cranial sutures wide at 1 year but craniostenosis by 2 years.
3. Young children. Dwarfism, poor gait, premature loss of deciduous teeth.

Investigations
Most cases show markedly low serum alkaline phosphatase, and inconstant hypercalcaemia. Urine contains phosphoethanolamine. These changes may also be found in asymptomatic heterozygotes.

Radiology
Changes similar to rickets.

Course
Vitamin D does not help. Steroids said to benefit some patients. Severe cases die in infancy.

Vitamin E (α-*tocopherol*)

Fat-soluble vitamin derived from green leaf vegetables, nuts and seed oils. Requirements vary with fatty acid intake. Deficiency occurs occasionally in preterm infants and in severe malabsorption states, particularly cholestatic liver disease. Prevents oxidation of unsaturated fatty acids.

Deficiency Effects
Haemolytic anaemia, thrombocytosis, muscle weakness. Long-standing deficiency (as in abetalipoproteinaemia) may lead to degenerative changes in the central nervous system, particularly the spinocerebellar tracts.

Vitamin K

Fat-soluble vitamin present in liver and some vegetables but mainly synthesized by intestinal bacteria. Necessary for prothrombin synthesis in the liver. Prothrombin deficiency manifested as a haemorrhagic disorder may occur in malabsorption states such as cystic fibrosis, suppression of intestinal flora by antibiotics, in the newborn (haemorrhagic disease, p. 422) and in liver disease.

Chapter 43   **FLUOROSIS**

Alteration of calcification of teeth due to ingestion of fluorides.

Aetiology
Excess fluoride in drinking water in some areas. Also follows industrial contamination, especially aluminium manufacture. Teeth affected only during stage of development.

Degrees
1. Mild (Drinking water containing fluoride $0.05–0.1$ parts/10^6). Enamel shows white opaque areas. Results in better teeth, with less dental caries.
2. Moderate (Little more than 0.1 part/10^6). Whole enamel opaque. May be brown mottling. Resistance to dental caries.
3. Severe (Considerably more than 0.1 part/10^6). Extensive brown mottling and pitting occur. Spinal deformity may develop in later life. Even if absorption extreme bone changes rarely manifested for considerable time.

Chapter 44   **OBESITY**

No clear line of demarcation can be drawn between 'normally' fat children and those 'pathologically' obese. Fatness should be regarded as excessive if it interferes with child's activities or makes him cause for comment. Arbitrary definition is weight more than 20 per cent above appropriate weight for height centile.

Causes
1. Early onset. Early introduction of cereals and overfeeding with carbohydrate

important cause of obesity in first year. Early-onset obesity may be associated with permanent increase in total number of body fat cells.

2. Overeating. Commonest cause, and an associated cause even in true endocrine obesity. Overeating sets up vicious circle of obesity, leading to lack of physical exercise which results in greater obesity.

3. Constitutional. Certain races or families tend to be fatter than others.

4. Emotional. Child may be unhappy and seek consolation in overeating.

5. Nervous. Rarely follows cerebral disease, e.g. chorea encephalitis or chronic (e.g. tuberculous) meningitis.

6. Endocrine

> *6.1 Pituitary*
> 6.1.1 Cushing's Disease
> 6.1.2 Fröhlich's Syndrome (dystrophia adiposogenitalis). (*See* p. 467.)
> 6.1.3 Prader–Willi Syndrome. Usually males with low birth weight, hypotonia, mental retardation, compulsive eating, early obesity, small genitalia; girls hypoplasia labia minora; sometimes diabetes in early adult life. Aetiology unknown, probably hypothalamic disorder.
> *6.2 Adrenal.* Cushing's Syndrome. Very rare in children, except where secondary to corticosteroid therapy.
> *6.3 Sexual.* After castration.

Complications
1. Strong likelihood of childhood obesity persisting into adult life.
2. Mortality in adults increases 13% for each 10% overweight.
3. Obese adults more liable to coronary artery disease, hypertension, diabetes, osteoarthritis, cholecystitis.
4. Fat infants more prone to chest infections.
5. Fat children often object of teasing. Loss of self-esteem leads to depression, may seek consolation in further excessive eating.
6. Fat children prone to flat feet, knock knees, effort dyspnoea, limb pains and psychosomatic symptoms.

Clinical Features of Overeating Type
1. Distribution of fat. Mainly over breasts, hips and abdomen.
2. General build. Child tends to be taller than average.
3. Genitalia. Normal size, although may be lost in fat.

Treatment
1. Motivation. Treatment never succeeds without active cooperation of parents and child. Sometimes parents unconcerned, and morbidity of obesity may need to be stressed. Group therapy often helpful, e.g. summer camps for obese adolescents, or joining organization such as 'Weight Watchers'.
2. Diet. Diet should contain 600–800 cal per day initially, more later. Adequate protein and vitamins must be taken. Initial 'crash' diet in hospital may be valuable in selected cases.
3. Exercise. Increasing activity often helpful but must be without increasing diet.

Chapter 45	***ANOREXIA NERVOSA***

A behavioural disorder, mainly affecting adolescents, 90% female. Complex psychological background in which ambivalence or fear of the sexual changes of puberty is often present, combined with a need to control the body's configuration and hence its function. Frequently begins with simple attempt by an obese teenager to lose weight, but affected individuals unable to stop when appropriate weight is attained. Although thin, patients often perceive themselves as fat.

Clinical Features
Progressive weight loss as patient eats very little leading to emaciation. In girls, menses cease. Lanugo hair often present on body and face. Limbs become stick-like, cheeks sunken, but activity continues as usual. Sometimes patients will eat adequate meals but then induce vomiting. Deception common, with surreptitious disposal of food claimed to have been eaten.

Treatment
In severe cases, admission to hospital and withdrawal of privileges may be necessary. Tube feeding is sometimes needed. Patient may be confined to bed in a single room and gradually allowed up, or allowed visitors, as a reward for compliance with prescribed feeding regime. Skilled psychological help should be enlisted to complement nutritional management. About 40% are probably cured eventually, others run varying steady or relapsing courses from chronic state of emaciation but ability to live an otherwise normal life over many years, to rapid deterioration and death in a few months. Death may be sudden, due to acute cardiac failure. Suicide not uncommon.

Chapter 46

**FLUID, ELECTROLYTES AND
ACID–BASE BALANCE**

General Considerations

1. Body water distribution is regulated by osmotic pressures across cell walls. Sodium (Na^+) is main determinant of extracellular fluid (ECF) osmolality, potassium (K^+) mainly in intracellular fluid (ICF). Oncotic pressure of plasma proteins important for maintenance of intravascular volume.

2. Total body water as percentage of weight decreases during fetal life and more slowly after birth, mainly due to contraction of ECF compartment.

3. Fluid balance is deranged more easily and severely in inverse proportion to age of child because of : (*a*) different distribution of body water (*Table 46.1*); (*b*) relatively large surface area of infant; (*c*) higher metabolic rate of infant; (*d*) poor capacity of infant kidney to concentrate urine and thus regulate plasma osmolality.

Table 46.1. Approximate distribution of body water at different ages, as percentage of body weight

	Premature infant	Term neonate	1–24 months	Child	Adult
ICF	30	35	35	36	40
ECF	50	40–45	30–40	30	20
Total body water	80–85	75–80	65–75	65	60

4. Blood volume approximately 8% of body weight.

5. Insensible water loss approximately $300\,ml/m^2/24h$ in child in temperate climate, higher ($\times 3$) in neonate.

6. Obligatory urine output approximately $200\,ml/m^2/24h$ in child, higher in neonate. Actual urine output in healthy child reflects intake, stool and insensible losses, approx. range $1–5/m^2/24h$.

Maintenance Fluid Requirements

Note:

1. Maintenance requirements derived from sum of obligatory urine and stool losses, insensible losses and growth requirements if renal concentrating power is normal.

2. Obligatory renal losses increased in newborn, fever, starvation and renal tubular defect.

3. May be calculated according to age, weight, surface area or calories of basal energy expended (*Table 46.2*).

Table 46.2.   Chart for determining approximate fluid requirements whether based on age, surface area, weight or basal energy expenditure

Age (years)	Birth	2/12	1	3	6	9	12	14	16
Surface area (m²)	0·15	0·25	0·45	0·6	0·8	1·05	1·3	1·5	1·65
Weight (kg)	2	5	10	15	20	30	40	50	60
ml/kg/24 h	132	132	132	110	99	88	77	77	77
Cal/kg†	48	70	63	51	45	38	33	33	31

†Cal/kg × 150 = ml/24 h

Disturbances of Fluid and Electrolyte Balance

Most frequent derangement of fluid balance is dehydration (*below*). Special disturbances occur in pyloric stenosis (alkalosis, p. 141); adrenocortical failure (hyperkalaemia and hyponatraemia, *below*) renal failure (hyperkalaemia and acidosis), diabetes mellitus (acidosis and hypokalaemia, p. 484) and other conditions which are dealt with in appropriate sections.

Dehydration

Water loss usually accompanied by variable deficit of electrolytes. Extracellular fluid may be hypotonic, isotonic or hypertonic, with corresponding shift of fluid from or into cells to maintain osmotic equilibrium.

Hypotonic or Isotonic Dehydration

Commonest form. Usually produced by excessive losses from gut (vomiting or diarrhoea) occasionally from excessive renal loss (diabetes mellitus).

Biochemical Features

1. Absolute deficit of electrolytes—particularly Na^+ and Cl^-. If hypotonic, relative deficit of electrolytes compared with water.

2. Hypotonicity of ECF leads to: (*a*) Shift of water into ICF—intracellular oedema. (*b*) Shift of K^+ into ECF, renal loss of K^+ and overall deficit of K^+ which may not be reflected in serum electrolytes but is important factor in replacement therapy.

3. Hb and PCV elevated from water loss.

4. Blood urea elevated and bicarbonate reduced from impaired glomerular filtration rate.

Clinical Features

1. Mild. Thirst, dry tongue and mouth, irritability, dry warm skin, reduced urinary output (except in diabetes).

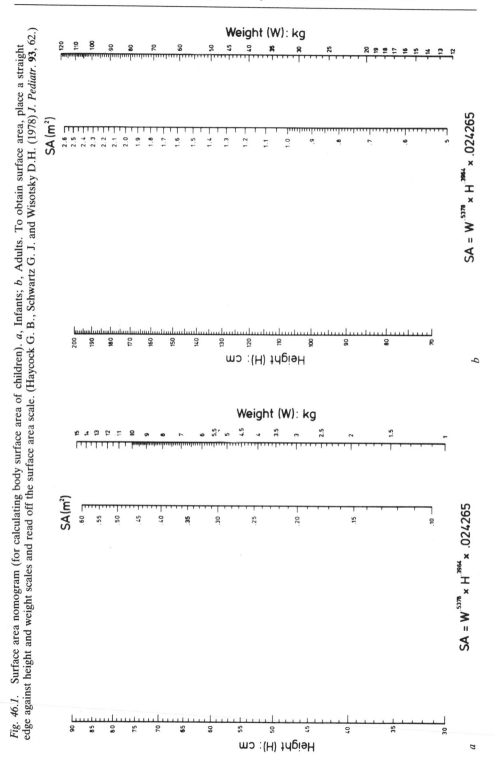

Fig. 46.1. Surface area nomogram (for calculating body surface area of children). *a*, Infants; *b*, Adults. To obtain surface area, place a straight edge against height and weight scales and read off the surface area scale. (Haycock G. B., Schwartz G. J. and Wisotsky D.H. (1978) *J. Pediatr.* **93**, 62.)

$$SA = W^{.5378} \times H^{.3964} \times .024265$$

Corresponds to about 5% loss in body weight in infants.

2. Moderate. Severe thirst, anxiety, restlessness, sunken eyes and fontanelle, dry mouth, skin elasticity lost, tachycardia.

About 7% loss in body weight in infants.

3. Severe. Above features with stupor, hypotonia, inability to suck, signs of shock—rectal temperature elevated but skin cold, pulse weak and rapid, or impalpable.

About 10% loss in body weight in infants.

Assessment

1. History will indicate route and hence nature of fluid losses.
2. Clinical examination will give approximate degree of dehydration.
3. Serum electrolytes and urea will provide best monitor of therapy (combined with clinical reassessment).

Treatment

Correction of fluid loss and electrolyte imbalance. *Route*:

1. Oral. Route of choice. Can be given by intragastric tube if infant unable to drink.

2. Intravenous. Resort to intravenous therapy only when dehydration severe (10%) or electrolyte imbalance, or when mother or nurse unable to cope with oral rehydration. In infants, best intravenous route is scalp vein—difficult over age 6 months when veins not easily visible.

3. Intraperitoneal. Can be used in emergency treatment of severely dehydrated infants in developing countries, when veins collapsed or unavailable from previous use. Needle inserted in midline, midway between xiphisternum and umbilicus, hypotonic fluid (e.g. ½ strength Darrow's solution), fluid run in over 10 min to required volume or until abdominal distension begins.

Amount

Aims:

1. (*a*) Calculate deficit from history and clinical signs as above. (*b*) Severely dehydrated infant will have lost about 10% body weight, i.e. 100 ml water per kg. For older children give about 30% less (i.e. 70 ml/kg) because of relatively smaller ECF compartment.

2. Give daily maintenance requirements.

3. Add excess current losses. Electrolyte losses can be roughly estimated from knowledge of type of fluid lost. *See Table 46.3.* Approximate composition (mmol/l):

Table 46.3.   Approximate electrolyte composition of lost fluids in mmol/l

	Na^+	K^+	Cl^-	HCO_3^-
Blood	135–145	3·5–5·5	100–105	22–36
Gastric juice	30–90	5–20	50–120	—
Small intestine	70–120	5–15	70–120	30

Diarrhoeal fluid approximates to small intestine, i.e. high in Na^+ and HCO_3^-. Serum electrolytes are also useful guide but can mislead in isotonic dehydration, i.e. loss of isotonic fluid. Serial electrolyte measurements offer best guide to adequacy of therapy.

Type of Fluid
1. Oral

1.1 The standard WHO/UNICEF oral rehydration regime is suitable for developing countries and the constituents are available in packets (oral rehydration salts, ORS) to be dissolved in 1 litre of clean water. They contain

Glucose 20 g
Sodium chloride 3·5 g
Sodium bicarbonate 2·5 g   } providing {   Glucose 111 mmol
Potassium chloride 1·5 g Na^+ 90 mmol
                                                                          HCO_3^- 30 mmol
                                                                          K^+ 20 mmol

Volume: ad libitum by month or 20 ml/kg/hour by intragastric tube. *Mother should be told that diarrhoea may continue and the object of treatment is to keep pace with the fluid loss as well as restoring deficit.*
Method. Give small amounts (2·5–5 ml) every minute by spoon. Large boluses often provoke vomiting/diarrhoea. Nasogastric tube feeding is sometimes useful if repeated vomiting is a problem. Reintroduce small tolerated feeds as soon as appetite restored (6–24h), but beware of transient intolerance to lactose or cow's milk protein. Breast milk often well tolerated, also casein hydrolysate formulae without lactose, or rice-water.

1.2 In developed countries where diarrhoea is generally milder, dehydration uncommon and acidosis rare; a solution containing less sodium is preferable to the risk of hypernatraemia, and bicarbonate is usually unnecessary. Suitable commercial preparations (e.g. 'Dioralyte') exist. Our current practice is to use a simple solution (solution A) containing Na 34 mmol/l, K 20 mmol/l, Cl 54 mmol/l and glucose 183 mmol/l.

A domestic substitute is ½ teasponful of salt and 1 tablespoonful of sugar to a litre (or quart) of water.

2. Intravenous (Rehydration)

2.1 When very shocked, plasma or whole blood may be used for initial expansion of intravascular compartment, 20 ml/kg.

2.2 Subsequent fluid can be given by calculation of requirements and giving polyelectrolyte solution such as Ringer-lactate, or physiological saline with added potassium chloride.

2.3 Potassium chloride should be added to intravenous solution to total concentration not exceeding 20 mmol/l as soon as infant passes urine. Ampoules of 7·45% KCl give 1 mmol/ml, *never use undiluted* as this will produce cardiac arrest.

2.4 Aim to rehydrate within 24h; may be reduced to 3–4h without complications in severe diarrhoea syndrome.

3. Intravenous (Maintenance).

3.1 By oral glucose—electrolyte mixture ad libitum or via gastric tube 10–15 ml/kg/h, or

3.2 By intravenous ½-strength Darrow's solution (made up with 5% dextrose) replace continuing stool loss, 10–15 ml/kg/h until infant strong enough to drink, or

3.3 Intravenous ½-strength physiological saline with potassium added to concentration not exceeding 20 mmol/l.

Table 46.4.   Composition of i.v. fluids in mmol/l

	Na^+	Cl^-	K^+	HCO_3^-
Ringer-lactate (Hartmann's) solution	130	109	4	28
Darrow's solution	122	104	35	53

Hypertonic Dehydration

Relatively uncommon. *Causes*:

1. Loss of hypotonic fluid, e.g. in diarrhoea, diabetes insipidus. Diarrhoea usually profuse, and sudden.

2. Excessive administration of sodium salts for treatment of diarrhoea, or extremely concentrated feeds of cow's milk formulae.

Biochemical Features

Water loss disproportionate to electrolyte loss, resulting in:

1. Elevated serum electrolytes (particularly Na^+).

2. Hypertonicity of ECF leading to fluid shift from ICF—intracellular dehydration. *Mild*—serum sodium 150–155 mmol/l. *Moderate*—serum sodium 150–160 mmol/l. *Severe*—serum sodium over 160 mmol/l.

3. Elevated Hb, PCV, blood urea, decreased plasma bicarbonate.

Clinical Features

Mild to moderate—Restlessness, thirst, dry tongue and mouth, reduced urine output. Skin turgor often maintained or increased. *Severe*—Thirst, irritability, fontanelle full, pyrexia, poor pulse volume, sclerematous skin changes, increased reflexes, convulsions. Complications include widespread cerebral haemorrhage and/or thrombosis, subdural effusions and renal tubular damage. Cerebral palsy may be permanent sequel.

Treatment

Slow intravenous rehydration, over 24–48 h is essential, using polyelectrolyte solution of ½-strength isotonic saline (made up with 5% glucose). Potassium chloride should be added.

Note: Rapid administration causes sudden shift of water back into cells, with resultant cerebral oedema, twitching, convulsions and even death.

If serum electrolytes unavailable and clinical doubt exists treat as for hypertonic dehydration, i.e. with ½-strength saline or solution with similar sodium content, because of risk of further increasing hypernatraemia.

Acid–base Balance

General Considerations

1. Blood pH maintained within narrow range in health (7·35–7·45) but system misleading in that small changes in pH reflect very large changes in hydrogen ion (H^+) concentration, and confusing in that fall in pH indicates rise in H^+ concentration, and vice versa.

2. Control maintained by three mechanisms: (*a*) Buffers, i.e. mixtures of weak acids and their salts with strong base. Most important buffer systems in body are: (i) Carbonic acid/bicarbonate, in ECF (H_2CO_3/$NaHCO_3$), normal ratio 1 : 20. (ii) Haemoglobin, proteins and phosphoric acid/phosphate in blood and ICF. (iii) Phosphoric acid/phosphate in ICF. (*b*) Lungs, which remove CO_2 from body. Increased ventilation thus alters equilibrium of carbonic acid and plasma CO_2 ($H_2CO_3 \rightleftharpoons CO_2 + H_2O$) in direction of CO_2 and water, thereby reducing ratio of carbonic acid to bicarbonate in buffer system. Hypoventilation has opposite effect, increasing carbonic acid and thus lowering pH. (*c*) Renal tubules which respond more slowly to pH changes and govern excretion of bicarbonate and H^+ ions. H^+ ions excreted: (i) To neutralize filtered bicarbonate. (ii) As ammonium (NH_4) ions synthesized from ammonia ions in kidneys, and (iii) As titratable acid.

3. Astrup system, using 'arterialized' capillary blood sample, gives following information: (*a*) 'Standard' bicarbonate, i.e. concentration of plasma bicarbonate in mM/l in 'standard' laboratory conditions—whole blood equilibrated at P_{CO_2} 40 mmHg, fully saturated with oxygen at 37°C. (*b*) Base excess, i.e. mM/l of strong acid compared with arbitrary neutrality. In practice base deficit (negative base excess) more frequently encountered, indicates metabolic acidosis. (*c*) pH. (*d*) P_{CO_2}, i.e. partial pressure of dissolved CO_2 in blood, which is in equilibrium with alveolar P_{CO_2}.

Disturbances of Acid–base Balance

A. Metabolic Acidosis

Definition
Blood H^+ ion concentration elevated.

Causes
1. Accumulation of acids (other than carbonic)
        1.1 Renal failure—phosphoric and sulphuric acids.
        1.2 Starvation—ketones and organic acids.
        1.3 Diabetes mellitus—ketones and organic acids.
        1.4 Anaerobic metabolism in hypoxia—lactic acid.
2. Loss of bicarbonate
        2.1 Diarrhoea.
        2.2 Loss of small intestinal fluid (intestinal obstruction or fistula).
        2.3 Renal tubular acidosis.

Clinical Features
1. Those of underlying condition.

2. Hyperventilation (deep, laboured respirations—Küssmaul breathing).

Biochemical Features

See Table 46.5.

Table 46.5.   The 'Astrup' acid–base pattern in simple (unmixed) disturbances

	pH	*Std HCO₃*	*P*CO₂	*Base Excess*
Metabolic acidosis	decreased	Decreased	decreased*	negative value
Metabolic alkalosis	increased	Increased	increased*	positive value
Respiratory acidosis	decreased	increased*	Increased	positive value
Respiratory alkalosis	increased	decreased*	Decreased	negative value

*Partial compensation.
Std HCO₃ and *P*CO₂—capital letter indicates primary disturbance.

Management
1. Correction of underlying condition, and of dehydration.
2. Acidosis will then usually correct itself: renal tubules play major role, by excreting H^- and retaining HCO_3^+ ions.
3. In severe cases, immediate treatment with sodium bicarbonate is indicated (e.g. severe diabetic ketosis, p. 484).

Dosage varies according to base deficit and age of child (for infants, calculate body water as 50% body weight, for older children 33%) using formula:
   (Infants) Base deficit × weight (kg) × 0·5 = mM $NaHCO_3$
   (Children) Base deficit × weight (kg) × 0·3 = mM $NaHCO_3$
$NaHCO_3$ 8% solution gives 1mM/ml. Alternatively, use 1/6M sodium lactate. *Note*: 6·0ml of 1/6M lactate gives equivalent of 1mM bicarbonate. Half volume given immediately, remainder in drip over 2–4h.

B. Respiratory Acidosis

Definition
Accumulation of CO_2 (hence carbonic acid) in blood from inadequate alveolar ventilation.

Causes
1. Acute airways obstruction (e.g. status asthmaticus, croup).
2. Chronic lung disease (e.g. cystic fibrosis).
3. Depression of respiratory centre (e.g. narcotic poisoning, head injury, sleep apnoea hypothalamic disorder—Pickwickian syndrome).
4. Respiratory distress syndrome of newborn (RDS)—usually mixed respiratory and metabolic acidosis.
5. Inadequate mechanical ventilation.

Clinical Features
Those of underlying condition.
   Note: If respiratory disease also causes hypoxia, metabolic (lactic) acidosis is usually superimposed.

Management
1. That of underlying cause of CO_2 retention. *Beware of reducing respiratory drive by overuse of oxygen (CO_2 narcosis).*
2. Metabolic acidosis, if present, revealed by base deficit and may require treatment, e.g. in RDS.

C. Metabolic Alkalosis

Definition
Blood H^+ ion decreased.

Causes
1. Loss of H^+ from ECF by vomiting (e.g. pyloric stenosis, p. 215) or gastric aspiration.
2. Intracellular shift of H^+ in course of K^+ depletion (e.g. pyloric stenosis).
3. Excessive intake of alkalis.

Clinical Features
1. Those of underlying condition.
2. Hypoventilation (rarely detected clinically).
3. Tetany may occur—lowered plasma H^+ ion depresses ionized calcium level, total plasma calcium may be unchanged.
4. Urine alkaline unless associated sodium and potassium deficiency.
Note: K^+ excretion very closely linked with alkalosis and alkalosis with lowered K^+ can only be corrected by giving adequate potassium salts as well as sodium chloride.

Management
1. That of underlying condition.
2. Correction of dehydration and potassium depletion.

D. Respiratory Alkalosis

Definition
CO_2 depletion from alveolar hyperventilation.

Causes
1. Early stages of salicylate poisoning (p. 499).
2. Encephalitis or hypothalamic disturbance causing hyperventilation.
3. Hysterical hyperventilation.
4. Overenthusiastic mechanical ventilation.

Clinical Features
1. Those of underlying condition.
2. Tetany.

Management
1. That of underlying condition.

2. Hysterical hyperventilation can be treated by making patient re-breathe exhaled CO_2, e.g. by breathing into and from a paper bag.

Chapter 47	INTRAVENOUS NUTRITION

Note: The nutritional state can be maintained or improved by total i.v. feeding when the oral route is unavailable, but formidable technical problems and complications make transfer of infant or child to special centre advisable if prolonged i.v. nutrition is indicated. Short-term pre- or postoperative use or i.v. supplementation of oral feeds is practicable for more widespread use.

Indications
Oral feeding must be impracticable or unsuccessful. Following conditions have been successfully managed by i.v. feeding:

1. Following extensive gut resection, particularly in neonate. Objective is to allow time for hypertrophy of villi to occur with improvement in absorption in remaining gut. *Note*: (*a*) Small frequent oral feeds, using elemental diet, will achieve this objective faster, if tolerated. (*b*) Objective may be unattainable in extreme cases, child then kept alive only by i.v. feeding and eventually dies either from complications or lack of suitable veins.

2. Protracted diarrhoea unresponsive to dietary treatment.

3. Severe and uncontrolled inflammatory bowel disease (ulcerative colitis/ Crohn's).

4. Extreme prematurity. *Note*: Although faster growth rate can be achieved, risk of complications may be considerable. May reduce incidence of necrotizing enterocolitis (NEC).

5. Renal failure.

6. Coma, e.g. following head injury.

7. Swallowing disorders, e.g. infectious polyneuritis, poliomyelitis.

8. Burns. *Note*: high protein intake can be achieved and may be valuable in early management of extensive burns.

Fluids
Must contain source of calories, adequate water, amino acids, minerals including trace elements, electrolytes, vitamins and, if treatment prolonged, essential fatty acids. Many available commercial preparations have high osmolality or other drawbacks making them unsuitable for paediatric use.

1. Amino acids. May be from synthetic mixtures (D- and L-forms) or hydrolysates of animal protein such as casein (L-forms only). Should be good balance with adequate essential amino acids. *Note*: 8 'essential' amino acids but histidine, proline, alanine, taurine and cysteine also regarded as 'essential' for young infants because of rapid growth demands.

2. Carbohydrates. May be given as glucose, fructose or sorbitol. Glucose or glucose + fructose best for infants, fructose alone may cause acidosis or osmotic diuresis.

3. Fats. Commercial preparation ('Intralipid') derived from soya bean oil. Fat mainly present as triglycerides. Eight-five per cent fatty acids unsaturated, high proportion (54%) of linoleic acid (c.f. human milk 50%).

4. *Vitamins*. Multivitamin preparation should be added to infusion fluid.

5. *Minerals*. Iron best given by i.m. injection at intervals of 2 weeks. Requirement 1 mg/kg/day.

Trace elements can be given by a weekly infusion of plasma, 10 ml/kg. Daily requirements of sodium, potassium, magnesium, calcium and phosphorus given as i.v. fluids.

Technique

1. Strictest possible asepsis at all times.
2. Intensive nursing by trained staff essential.
3. Excellent biochemical facilities with full use of microtechniques essential for frequent monitoring of electrolytes, acid–base status, etc.
4. Dehydration, electrolyte depletion or deranged acid–base status should be corrected before nutrition commenced.
5. Drip sets should be changed daily. A continuous infusion pump very useful.
6. Use peripheral veins first, for as long as possible. Ultimately an indwelling catheter in vena cava may be required, and should be inserted by surgeon in operating theatre.
7. Monitor electrolytes, pH and acid–base status, blood sugar *daily*; calcium, phosphorus, magnesium, aspartate transaminase, haemoglobin, WBC and platelets *twice weekly*.
8. Discontinue *slowly*: danger of hypoglycaemia with abrupt termination.

Complications

Following have been reported, more or less frequently:

1. Septicaemia: *Strep. faecalis, Staph. aureus, Candida albicans*, etc.
2. Metabolic acidosis, electrolyte imbalance.
3. Phlebitis and venous occlusion, including superior vena cava.
4. Catheter dislodgement with extravasation of fluid sometimes into pleural cavity.
5. Cardiac failure.
6. Hypoglycaemia.

Schedule

Following schedule used in many centres, but many alternatives available which follow similar principles. Quantities used are for newborn infants, per kg per 24h, except where stated.

1. Amino acid/glucose mixture, e.g. 'Vamin-glucose'   30 ml
2. Fat emulsion, e.g. 'Intralipid'   20 ml
3. Glucose 10–15%   150 ml
4. Sodium chloride   4–5 mmol
5. Potassium chloride   3–4 mmol
6. Calcium gluconate   0·5 mmol
7. Phosphorus, as sodium phosphate   0·45 mmol
8. Magnesium, as magnesium chloride   0·15 mmol
9. Vitamins, e.g. 'Multibionta'   2 ml/l of fluid
10. Total fluid intake   200 ml
11. Vitamin K 1 mg/week i.m.
12. Vitamin B_{12} 50 µg i.m. or i.v. every 2 weeks
13. Folic acid 1 mg every 2 weeks i.m.
14. I.m. iron, e.g. 'Imferon' 0·5 ml every 2 weeks

Definition
Symptom-complex with many different causes characterized clinically by increased irritability of muscles and biochemically by low ionized serum calcium.

Causes
1. Due to low ionized calcium

1.1 Tetany of Newborn. Much commoner in babies fed with unmodified cow's milk. Associated with high phosphate content of milk and deficient fat absorption. Limited to first 2 weeks of life. Low magnesium may also be present, and requires correction before calcium levels can be elevated.

1.2 Rickets. Calcium level is usually normal in this disease, but occasionally it is due to lack of calcium as well as vitamin D in diet. Tetany then results.

1.3 Renal Failure resulting in low serum calcium and retention of phosphates.

1.4 Hypoparathyroidism from any cause—rare in children.

1.5 Exchange Transfusion. Due to removal of calcium and chelating effect of anticoagulant (sodium citrate).

2. Due to alkalosis

2.1 Excessive vomiting with loss of hydrochloric acid, e.g. pyloric stenosis.

2.2 Excessive ingestion of alkalis, e.g. sodium bicarbonate.

2.3 Hyperventilation due to hysteria or encephalitis lethargica.

Clinical Features
Major convulsions occur in young infants. Increased irritability of muscle may occur, with carpopedal spasm, at all ages.

Treatment
Administration of calcium. Neonatal tetany: Calcium gluconate 5–10 ml of 10% solution slowly i.v. for acute symptoms, maintain with oral calcium chloride 1·0 g daily for up to 10 days. *Note*: Danger of cardiac arrest during intravenous treatment. Give slowly.

Idiopathic Hypercalcaemia of Infancy

Very rare disease, symptomatically similar to idiopathic renal acidosis, in which principal biochemical finding is raised serum calcium. In severe form

(Williams' syndrome) bone changes, hypertension, supravalvular aortic stenosis, characteristic facies and mental retardation occur. These features may also occur in combination without hypercalcaemia.

Chapter 49   *INBORN ERRORS OF METABOLISM*

General Considerations
  1. Name 'inborn errors of metabolism' coined by Garrod in 1908 referring to group of rare genetically inherited diseases (albinism, alcaptonuria, cystinuria and pentosuria). Since then many more conditions have been described.
  2. Metabolic errors are due to absence of a specific enzyme, and inherited as single gene defects. Most are autosomal recessive. Many conditions dealt with elsewhere are due to known inborn metabolic errors (e.g. adrenal hyperplasia) or other enzyme deficiencies as yet unidentified (e.g. cystic fibrosis).
  3. Some may not be manifest until later life (e.g. Wilson's disease).
  4. If enzyme is absent one or more of the following may occur:
     4.1 End product is not formed; if vital for life, child will not survive.
     4.2 Precursor substances will accumulate; this may not matter, but if toxic then particular disease symptoms will develop.
     4.3 Alternative pathways may be developed. Normal metabolites may accumulate or be excreted in abnormally large amounts.
  5. If missing enzyme can be identified and offending metabolic pathway traced, it may be possible to institute treatment by elimination (e.g. in phenylketonuria) or by other means (*see below*).
  6. For purposes of classification only big groups of well-recognized conditions will be included.

Prenatal Diagnosis
Some conditions can be diagnosed prenatally by examination of fetal cells or liquor amnii obtained at amniocentesis for enzyme activity or metabolic products. These include: Tay–Sachs disease, certain mucopolysaccharidoses, homocystinuria, galactosaemia and glycogen storage disease Type II.

Principles of Management
The following therapeutic possibilities may be employed where appropriate:
1. Dietary
     1.1 Restriction of intake of toxic substrate, e.g. phenyl-ketonuria.
     1.2 Provision of essential end product, e.g. corticosteroids in adrenal hyperplasia, Factor VIII in haemophilia.
     1.3 Large doses of coenzymes (vitamins), e.g. homocysti-nuria.
2. Biochemical
     2.1 Induction of enzyme synthesis, e.g. phenobarbitone in Dubin–Johnson or Crigler–Najjar disease.
     2.2 Removal of stored substances, e.g. penicillamine in Wilson's disease.

2.3 Inhibition of enzymes, e.g. allopurinol in gout.

3. Enzyme replacement

3.1 Plasma infusion, e.g. experimental use in mucopoylsaccharidoses.

3.2 Purified protein fractions or pure enzyme. Experimental.

3.3 Organ transplant, e.g. renal transplant in cystinosis.

4. Genetic engineering. Viral transduction, e.g. experimental trial in arginosuccinic aciduria.

5. Genetic counselling. For prevention of recurrence if justified.

6. Prenatal screening. For prevention of recurrence with abortion if parents willing, legally possible and ethically justified.

Classification

1. Errors in amino acid metabolism

1.1 Errors in phenylalanine metabolism.

1.2 Errors in tyrosine metabolism.

1.3 Errors in methionine metabolism, e.g. homocystinuria.

1.4 Errors in urea cycle, e.g. arginosuccinic aciduria.

1.5 Errors in branched-chain amino acid metabolism, e.g. maple-syrup urine disease.

1.6 Errors in propionate metabolism, e.g. methylmalonic acidaemia.

1.7 Errors in histidine metabolism, e.g. histidinaemia.

1.8 Errors in imino acid metabolism, e.g. hyperprolinaemia.

1.9 Error in amino acid transport, e.g. Hartnup disease.

2. Errors in protein metabolism

2.1 Haematological (see Chapters 131, 135).

2.1.1 In clotting mechanisms.

2.1.2 In erythrocyte metabolism.

2.1.3 Haemoglobinopathies.

2.2 In Plasma Protein, e.g. disorders of immunoglobulins (p. 117); Wilson's disease; hypophosphatasia (p. 128).

2.3 In Muscle Protein, e.g. muscular dystrophy (p. 447).

3. Errors in carbohydrate metabolism

3.1 Defects in Carbohydrate Absorption, e.g. lactose, sucrose/isomaltose, glucose/galactose.

3.2 Defects in Mucopolysaccharide Metabolism, mucopolysaccharidoses.

3.3 Defects in Monosaccharide Metabolism, e.g. galactosaemia, hereditary fructose intolerance.

3.4 Disorders of Glycogen Metabolism, glycogen storage diseases.

4. Errors in lipid metabolism

4.1 Hyperlipidaemias, e.g. hypercholesterolaemia, skin xanthomatosis.

4.2 Hypolipoproteinaemias

4.3 Lipid Storage Diseases, e.g. Gaucher's disease, Niemann–Pick disease, Tay–Sachs disease.

4.4 Defects in Steroid Metabolism, e.g. adrenal hyperplasia (p. 468).

5. *Errors in pigment metabolism*
      5.1 The Porphyrias
      5.2 Methaemoglobinaemia
      5.3 Defects in Glucuronide Conjugation, e.g. Crigler–Najjar disease.
6. *Errors in purine metabolism*
      6.1 Gout
      6.2 Hyperuricaemia (Lesch–Nyhan syndrome).
7. *Errors in mineral metabolism*
      7.1 Iron, e.g. sideroblastic anaemia, haemochromatosis.
      7.2 Copper, e.g. Kinky-hair syndrome (Menkes), Wilson's disease.
      7.3 Zinc, e.g. Acrodermatitis enteropathica.

Chapter 50   # ERRORS IN AMINO ACID METABOLISM

Errors in Phenylalanine Metabolism

Phenylketonuria (PKU)

Definition
Commonest inborn error of amino acid metabolism, manifested biochemically by absence of phenylalanine hydroxylase and elevated plasma phenylalanine, clinically by severe mental retardation, hyperactivity, skin lesions, fair hair and blue eyes, eczema.

Inheritance
Autosomal recessive.

Incidence
In classic form, 1 : 10000 to 1 : 20000 live births in Caucasian populations.

Biochemistry
Absence of phenylalanine hydroxylase in liver leads to accumulation of phenylalanine in plasma and CSF. Phenylalanine and metabolites (phenylpyruvic and phenyl-lactic acid) appear in urine when blood levels exceed 0·6–1·2 μmol/ml (10–20mg/dl). Elevated phenylalanine levels damage brain, cortical atrophy may occur.

Screening
In most developed countries, newborns screened for phenylketonuria. Infant must be fed adequate dietary protein for phenylalanine to rise. Tests are:
    1. Blood (Guthrie test). Test made after at least 48h. Blood spot collected on filter paper, placed on culture plate inoculated with *Bacillus subtilis*. Organism

requires phenylalanine for growth, colonies flourish if blood levels elevated. Detects levels above 0·25 μmol/ml (4 mg/dl).

2. Blood amino acid chromatography. Advantage is detection of other inborn errors as well as PKU, can use eluted blood spots from filter paper, or capillary specimens.

3. Urine chromatography. Less sensitive than (2) but samples (filter paper) easier to obtain.

4. Urine ferric chloride test. Green colour with phenylalanine metabolites. Unreliable because adequate accumulation may take several weeks after birth.

5. Heterozygotes detectable by raised blood phenylalanine levels after oral phenylalanine load (100 mg/kg).

Clinical Features
Severe mental deficiency if untreated. Child characteristically blond with blue eyes due to competititve inhibition of tyrosinase by phenylalanine. Hyperactive, distractable. Vomiting common in early infancy. Convulsions, marked EEG dysrhythmia. Skin dry, tendency to eczema. Peculiar 'mousey' smell often noted. Occasionally normal or near-normal intelligence despite lack of treatment.

Treatment
Dietary restriction of phenylalanine as soon as diagnosis made. Aim to maintain plasma phenylalanine between 0·15 and 0·45 μmol/ml (2·7–7·5 mg/dl). Extremely low levels lead to phenylalanine deficiency—failure to thrive, vomiting, diarrhoea, eczema and brain damage. Treatment must be started in early infancy to avoid mental retardation, useless in older untreated patients, but can usually be relaxed after age 7 years in child treated from birth without causing serious fall in IQ (but *see* maternal hyperphenylalaninaemia, *below*).
*Diet.** Low-protein, milk substitutes (e.g. Lofenelac, Minafen, Albumin XP, PK-adc) given, plus a known phenylalanine intake (e.g. from milk) about 30–60 mg/kg/day to maintain satisfactory plasma level.

Hyperphenylalaninaemia
Milder variant of PKU, usually with normal intelligence. Plasma phenylalanine between 0·2 and 1·3 μmol/ml (3–20 mg/dl). *Transient* hyperphenylalaninaemia, usually with hypertyrosinaemia, occurs in some newborns due to late maturation of liver enzymes, and causes confusion in screening tests.

Maternal Hyperphenylalaninaemia
Women with PKU need dietary treatment during pregnancy because high plasma levels may damage brain of developing fetus even though mother asymptomatic.

Errors in Tyrosine Metabolism

Tyrosinaemia
Very rare metabolic error, caused by deficiency of *p*-hydroxyphenylpyruvic acid oxidase. Manifested clinically by failure to thrive, cirrhosis, hypoglycaemia, vitamin D-resistant rickets, renal tubular defect. Severe form causes death in

---

*For details, *see* Francis, Dorothy E. M. (1982) *Diets for Sick Children*, 4th ed. Oxford, Blackwell.

infancy from liver failure, milder form similar to Fanconi's syndrome. *Treatment*: low tyrosine diet.

Neonatal Hypertyrosinaemia
Elevated blood levels of tyrosine, with increased urinary tyrosine metabolites (tyrosyluria) occur transiently in 10% of pre-term infants and some neonates. Caused by immaturity of liver enzymes. Probably benign, but can be cured by reducing protein intake and giving vitamin C (coenzyme). Elevated blood levels of other amino acids may also occur.

Symptomatic Hypertyrosinaemia
May occur in liver disease, scurvy and malabsorption.

Albinism
Metabolic error seen in all races and in animals, due to defect in tyrosinase and resulting in failure of melanin synthesis. Two forms:
1. Generalized. Autosomal recessive inheritance. Skin pale, hair white, irides very pale blue, nystagmus, photophobia, pale retinae. Sunburn and later skin cancer is major hazard.
2. Ocular. X-linked inheritance. Limited to ocular features.

Alkaptonuria
Rare metabolic error in conversion of homogentisic acid to aceto-acetic acid in tyrosine pathway. Manifested biochemically by excretion of homogentisic acid (a reducing substance) in urine, which turns brown on standing; clinically in adult life by pigmentation of ears, nose and sclerae (ochronosis), and by degenerative arthritis. *Treatment*: none available.

Goitrous Cretinism
Tyrosine is thyroxine precursor.

Errors in Methionine Metabolism

Homocystinuria

Definition
Uncommon metabolic error involving sulphur-containing amino acid pathway, which normally proceeds from methionine via homocysteine and cystathionine to cysteine. Two forms;
   1. Defect in cystathionine synthetase. This blocks synthesis of cystathionine from homocysteine, which then uses alternate pathway via homocystine.
   2. Defect in folate metabolism. Pyridoxine is coenzyme.

Clinical Features
Body build resembling Marfan's syndrome with long limbs and arachnodactyly. Chest deformity, pes cavus and dislocation of lens common. Mental retardation in 50%. Risk of thrombosis. Medial necrosis of aorta leads to dissecting aneurysm.

Investigations
   1. Urine contains homocystine and methionine.

2. Blood levels of methionine elevated but no homocystine present.
3. Liver biopsy and fibroblast culture confirm defect of cystathionine synthetase.

Treatment
1. Low methionine diet—soya milk substituted for cow's milk. Cystine and serine supplements necessary.
2. Oral pyridoxine (100–500 mg/day) corrects biochemical defect in some patients.

Errors in Urea Cycle

Urea cycle converts ammonia to urea, mainly in liver (*Fig. 50.1*). Defects in cycle have high blood ammonia (normal 17–35 μmol/l, 30–60 μg/dl) as common feature, sometimes only seen after protein load test. Hyperammonaemia also seen in liver failure and Reye's syndrome. Defects at all enzyme sites in cycle have been described.

Fig. 50.1. The urea cycle. 1, Carbamyl phosphate synthetase; 2, Ornithine transcarbamylase; 3, Arginosuccinic synthetase; 4, Arginosuccinase; 5, Arginase.

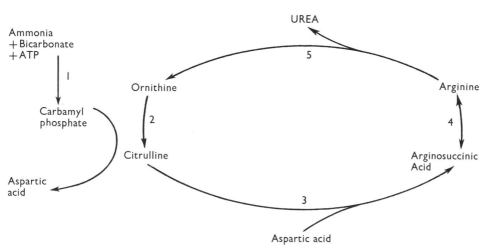

Clinical Features
Neonatal period: Progressive lethargy, tremors, convulsions, progressing to coma. Marked hypotonia. Respirations become shallow, eventual apnoea. Septicaemia may coexist.
Differential diagnosis in neonatal period: Transient hyperammonaemia of the newborn.
Older children: Mental retardation, episodic lethargy and ataxia, trichorrhexis nodosa (fragile hair) in arginosuccinic aciduria. Sodium valproate may precipitate severe/fatal symptoms.

Investigations
1. Blood ammonia elevated.

2. Blood urea usually normal.
3. Plasma amino acids may be abnormal, depending on site of enzyme block. Glutamine elevated. Arginosuccinic acid unstable in analysis and specimen needs special preparation.
4. Urinary amino acids may be abnormal, e.g. arginosuccinic acid.
5. Enzyme assay — defect demonstrable in liver or red cells.

Treatment
Reduced protein intake, minimum daily requirements of essential amino acids. In acute crises, dialysis, sterilization of gut and anabolic steroids may be required.

Transient Hyperammonaemia of the Newborn
More common than urea cycle defects, this condition presents in the first 48 h with severe hyperammonaemia, lethargy, apnoea and eventual coma. If treated energetically with exchange transfusion and/or peritoneal dialysis, infant may survive unscathed and the metabolic abnormality corrects itself in a few days. Exact cause unknown.

Errors in Branched-chain Amino Acid Metabolism

Maple Syrup Urine Disease

Definition
Disorder of leucine, isoleucine and valine metabolism, resulting in elevated levels of these branched-chain amino acids in blood, urine and CSF. Manifested clinically by neonatal convulsions, coma and early death if untreated.

Inheritance
Autosomal recessive.

Clinical Features
Several forms exist:
Severe form. Neonatal vomiting, convulsions, spasticity, hypoglycaemia and keto acidosis. Coma follows and death in a few weeks. Peculiar malt-like smell to urine.
Mild form. Later onset of above symptoms, precipitated by infection or high protein intake. Variants occur associated with mental retardation and recurrent hypoglycaemic attacks.

Investigations
Urine. Positive ferric chloride test. Elevated branched-chain amino acids.
Blood. Elevated plasma branched-chain amino acids, especially leucine.
Fibroblasts and leucocytes. Enzyme deficiency demonstrable.

Treatment. Diet low in natural protein, which is replaced by synthetic amino acid mixtures omitting offending substances. Crises treated by high-carbohydrate, protein-free diet, and perhaps anabolic steroids, for a few days until blood levels of branched-chain amino acids fall. Peritoneal dialysis sometimes necessary.

Errors in Propionate Metabolism
(*Organic Acidurias*)

Propionic Acidaemia

Definition
Intolerance to multiple amino acids: isoleucine, valine, threonine and methionine due to deficiency of propionyl coenzyme A carboxylase. Autosomal recessive.

Clinical Features
Presents as overwhelming illness in first 3 months, preceded by frequent vomiting and failure to thrive. Later, episodes of severe acidosis, ketonuria, hypoglycaemia, vomiting and dehydration, lethargy, flaccidity, progressing to coma. These episodes may be precipitated by infection and are reversible by treatment with i.v. fluids and bicarbonate. Frequently accompanied by haematological problems: neutropenia, anaemia, thrombocytopenia. Candidiasis common.

Investigations
Blood and urine. Elevated levels of propionic acid, glycine.

Treatment
May require nasogastric feeding. Limited intake of offending amino acids to essential requirements. Monitor by blood levels of propionic acid and glycine (elevated in uncontrolled cases). Some patients respond to treatment with biotin.

Methylmalonic Acidaemia
Clinically indistinguishable from propionic acidaemia but metabolic defect is in methylmalonyl CoA mutase and blood and urine contain both propionic and methylmalonic acids. Hepatomegaly present. Autosomal recessive.

Treatment
Diet as for propionic acidaemia. Close biochemical monitoring is essential, best by urinary level of methylmalonic acid. If successfully treated, prognosis for life and intelligence is good. Some patients respond to large doses of the cofactor, vitamin B_{12} (1 mg daily).

Multiple Carboxylase Deficiency
Clinical features of propionic acidaemia with bright red, scaly, weeping skin eruptions and patchy alopecia. Skin lesions resemble biotin deficiency and fundamental defect may be in activation of biotin to produce active carboxylases. Urine contains increased organic acids.

Treatment
Biotin 10 mg once or twice daily controls all clinical manifestations.

Errors in Histidine Metabolism

Histidinaemia
Rare metabolic error due to histidase deficiency. May produce no symptoms, but

can also be associated with speech defects and/or mental retardation. Blood and urine histidine elevated. Defect present in liver and skin cells.

Treatment
Low-histidine diet. Controversial—may not be necessary.

Errors in Imino Acid Metabolism

Hyperprolinaemia
Rare inborn error due to defective proline metabolism. Plasma and urinary proline levels elevated, also urinary glycine and hydroxyproline. Patients have familial nephritis, deafness (cf. Alport's syndrome, p. 380) and EEG abnormalities. No specific treatment.

Disorders of Amino Acid Transport

Note: Generalized amino aciduria occurs normally in first 3 months of life, more marked in pre-term infants. Also occurs in liver disease and renal tubular damage from any cause.

Cystinuria

Definition
Autosomal recessive disorder of transport of cystine, lysine, arginine and ornithine across wall of gut and renal tubule. Manifested clinically by renal calculi.

Clinical Features
Recurrent cystine stones in urine may lead to renal failure. Normal intelligence.

Investigations
Urine contains excess cystine and basic amino acids. Blood amino acids normal.

Differential Diagnosis
Other causes of cystinuria, e.g. Fanconi's syndrome.

Treatment
D-Penicillamine 20 mg/kg/day increases solubility of cystine in urine. Side-effects include fever, skin rashes, leucopenia, thrombocytopenia.

Cystinosis

Definition
Rare generalized metabolic disorder, characterized biochemically by increased synthesis of cystine from cysteine and clinically by deposition of cystine crystals throughout body. Manifested clinically by blond hair, photophobia, renal disease (Fanconi's syndrome) and vitamin D-resistant rickets.

Clinical Features
May present in early childhood. Progressive renal tubular failure usually produces death in a few years. Photophobia due to corneal involvement, hair becomes

blond due to inhibition of melanin synthesis. Vitamin D-resistant rickets and renal tubular acidosis.

Investigations
Urine. Generalized amino aciduria, cystine not particularly excessive. Glycosuria.
Blood. Hypokalaemia, hyperchloraemia, low bicarbonate.

Treatment
Renal transplantation may be effective as transplanted kidneys not affected by cystinosis. Vitamin D and alkalis orally.

Hartnup Disease

Definition
Rare metabolic error affecting transport of 13 amino acids in gut and kidney. Characterized by aminoaciduria and increased gut loss of amino acids. Tryptophan deficiency causes symptoms. Clinically mimics pellagra.

Clinical Features
Ataxia, photosensitivity, psychiatric disturbances. May lead to progressive mental impairment but often improves with age and may be manifest only at times of stress.

Treatment
(1) High-protein diet. (2) Nicotinic acid 25 mg/day

Blue Diaper Syndrome
Very rare defect in tryptophan transport across gut. Unabsorbed tryptophan degraded by bacteria to indoles, which are then absorbed.

Clinical Features
Blue colour in napkins from interaction of bleach and urinary indican. Calcium in gut chelated by indoles and absorbed causing mental retardation, hypercalcaemia and nephrocalcinosis.

Differential Diagnosis
Other causes of blue stain in napkins—*Ps. pyocyanea*, contact with brass, methylene blue.

Lowe Syndrome
Very rare X-linked condition manifested clinically by buphthalmos, cataracts, hypotonia, mental retardation and cryptorchidism. Renal tubular defect causes proteinuria, amino aciduria, organic aciduria and acidosis.

Bibliography

Urea cycle symposium (1981) *Pediatrics* **68**, 273.

Chapter 51	# ERRORS IN CARBOHYDRATE METABOLISM

The Mucopolysaccharidoses

Group of inherited diseases characterized by progressive abnormal deposition of acid mucopolysaccharides (glycosaminoglycans) in tissues and/or their excretion in urine. Several distinct types exist, Type II commonest. (*Table 51.1.*) Antenatal diagnosis in Type II possible from amniocentesis and fibroblast culture. Basic defect is abnormality of a lysosomal enzyme. Replacement of missing enzyme theoretically possible.

Mucopolysaccharidosis Type IH (Hurler)

Definition
Rare autosomal recessive disease characterized clinically by progressive chondro-osteodystrophy, hepatosplenomegaly, corneal opacities and mental retardation; pathologically by abnormal deposits of heparan and dermatan sulphates in reticulo-endothelial system and other organs.

Pathology
Abnormal intracellular storage of glycosaminoglycans in most tissues of body, notably brain, heart, liver, spleen and bones.

Clinical Features
Insidious onset, but symptoms usually apparent by age 2 years. Moderate growth failure. Frequent chest infections. Cardiac valve involvement ultimate cause of death in most cases.
Appearance of fully developed case
1. *Skull*. May be scaphocephalic, brachycephalic or hydrocephalic.
2. *Face*. Becomes very ugly, with large lips and tongue, and gingival hypertrophy. Features coarsen owing to thick skin. Ears low-set. Hypertelorism, depressed nasal bridge. Nasal discharge present.
3. *Eyes*. Corneal opacities develop. In early cases only visible with slit-lamp, later vision becomes impaired.
4. *Spine*. Kyphosis, with thoracic or lumbar gibbus.
5. *Abdomen*. Big, owing to enlargement of liver and spleen. Umbilical and inguinal hernias present.
6. *Joints*. Cannot be fully extended, especially fingers, thus giving rise to claw-hand.
7. *Mental Defect*. Usual but not invariable.
8. *Deafness* frequent.
Formes frustes. Any of above features may be absent. Corneal opacity probably only constant feature, but may not appear till age 7–9 years.

Investigations

1. *Radiological appearance*
        1.1 Skull. Large. Sella turcica elongated.

Table 51.1.   The mucopolysaccharidoses

Type	Genetics	Skeletal changes	Corneal opacity	Aortic disease	Hepato-megaly	Spleno-megaly	Mental retardation	Short stature	Urine
IH(Hurler)	Autosomal recessive	+ (characteristic)	Usual (82%)	Often (45%)	Usual (75%)	Often (45%)	Marked	+	HS + DS 1:3
Is (Scheie)	Autosomal recessive	+	Usual	Often	Usual	Often	Often (? 50%)	+	HS + DS 1:3
II (Hunter)	Sex-linked recessive	+	Unusual (25%)	–	Usual (83%)	Often (58%)	Usual but less severe than Hurler	+	HS + DS 1:1
III (Sanfilippo)	Autosomal recessive	Usual	–	–	Often (67%)	Unusual (25%)	Severe	+	HS
IV (Morquio)	Autosomal recessive	+ (characteristic)	Usual	?	Usual	Usual	Usually normal	+	KS
VI (Maroteaux–Lamy)	Autosomal recessive	+	–	Usual (75%)	+	Usual (75%)	Normal	+	DS only
VII β-glucuronidase deficiency	Autosomal recessive	+	±	–	Usual	Usual	Severe	+	DS + HS + CS

CS = chondroitin 4,6 sulphate, DS = dermatan sulphate, HS = heparan sulphate, KS = keratan sulphate.

1.2 Vertebral Bodies. Small, wedge-shaped. First or second lumbar displaced backwards with upward-pointing hook.
1.3 Long Bones. Thickened. Irregularity of epiphyses.
1.4. Metacarpals. Short and broad. Distal phalanges pointed.
2. *Urine*. Contains dermatan sulphate and heparan sulphate.
3. *Fibroblast culture*. Dermatan sulphate present. Decreased β-galactosidase activity.

Prognosis
Death usually occurs before age 10 years.

Treatment
Bone marrow transplants to young children are giving promising results.

Muycopolysaccharidosis Type Is (Scheie)
Rare, autosomal recessive. Manifested clinically by stiff joints, coarse facies, cloudy corneas, aortic regurgitation and normal or slightly impaired intelligence. Urine contains dermatan sulphate. Biochemically resembles Type I$_H$.

Mucopolysaccharidosis Type II (Hunter)

Definition
Rare, X-linked recessive disease characterized clinically by retarded growth and changes similar to those of Type I. Pathologically by abnormal deposition of dermatan and heparan sulphates in tissues and their excretion in urine.

Clinical Features
Less severe than Type I, mental retardation less marked but behaviour problems frequent. No corneal clouding. Joints stiff. Life expectancy 30 years or more. May be cardiac involvement.

Mucopolysaccharidosis Type III (Sanfilippo)

Definition
Rare, autosomal recessive disease characterized clinically by severe mental retardation with mild skeletal changes; pathologically by urinary excretion of heparan sulphate and deposition of dermatan sulphate in tissues.

Clinical Features
Mild coarse facies, some joint stiffness, clear corneas. Hyperkinetic. Progressive mental retardation, eventually severe. Long survival.

Mucopolysaccharidosis Type IV (Morquio)

Definition
Rare, autosomal recessive disease, characterized clinically by dwarfism, skeletal deformity, mild corneal clouding and generally normal intellect; pathologically by urinary excretion of keratan sulphate.

Clinical Features
Bony changes increasingly evident from late infancy with prominent sternum,

marked lumbodorsal kyphosis and short trunk. Corneal clouding varies from obvious to minimal. Intelligence normal or slightly reduced. Aortic incompetence sometimes develops later. Odontoid hypoplasia may produce death or neurological abnormalities from cervical dislocation. Joints may be enlarged.

Investigations
(1) Radiographs show flattened vertebrae with irregular shapes and uneven surfaces. First lumbar vertebra particularly affected, displaced backwards, giving rise to kyphosis. Epiphyses of long bones normal at first, but become disorganized in severe cases. (2) Urine contains keratan sulphate.

Prognosis
Deformities become progressive, dwarfism more severe, but intelligence usually spared.

Mucopolysaccharidosis Type VI (Maroteaux–Lamy)
Autosomal recessive, similar to Type I but milder, without mental retardation. Dermatan sulphate in urine.

Mucopolysaccharidosis Type VII (β-Glucuronidase Deficiency)
Autosomal recessive. Coarse features, mental retardation, hepatosplenomegaly. Urine contains chondroitin sulphate.

Defects in Monosaccharide Metabolism

Galactosaemia (*Galactose Diabetes*)

Definition
Rare familial disorder characterized clinically by jaundice in newborn period, failure to gain weight, enlargement of liver, mental deficiency and often lamellar cataracts; pathologically by excretion of sugar in urine identifiable as galactose.

Aetiology
Autosomal recessive.

Pathogenesis
Lactose present in human milk or cow's milk formula is digested to glucose and galactose in jejunum. Absorbed galactose is normally converted to glucose-1-phosphate (*Fig. 51.1*).

1. Primary defect is deficiency of the specific enzyme galactose-1-phosphate uridyl transferase. This enzyme is present in erythrocytes where its absence can be detected, probably also in other cells.

2. Lack of specific enzyme results in accumulation of galactose-1-phosphate which may: (*a*) be toxic itself (*b*) interfere with glucose utilization.

3. With increasing age, symptoms and galactose-tolerance test improve, suggesting that alternative metabolic pathway has developed.

Clinical Features
Jaundice and fever often presenting feature in neonatal period. Child gains weight slowly and may have enlargement of liver but not spleen. Later hepatic and often

Fig. 51.1. Disease caused by enzyme defect: (1) Type I glycogenosis. (2) Type II. (3) Type III. (4) Type IV. (5) Type V. (6) Type VI. (7) Type VII. (8) Type VIII. (9) Types IX, X. (10) Galactosaemia. (11) Galactokinase deficiency.

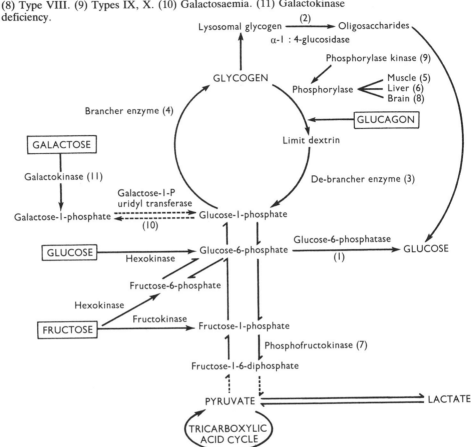

renal insufficiency occurs. Fairly severe mental defect. Lamellar cataract usually develops.

Laboratory Investigations

1. Urine. (*a*) Found to contain reducing substance—usually at first assumed to be glucose. May be present as trace only or in large amounts. (*b*) Also contains abnormal amino acids.

2. Erythrocyte galactose-1-phosphate test should be performed on cord blood of babies whose siblings have galactosaemia. Can be performed on venous blood of older babies.

3. Galactose-tolerance curve: blood sugar remains high as long as 5h after ingestion of sugar. *Dangerous test* as dose of galactose will harm child.

Differential Diagnosis

1. Glycogen storage disease. Liver enlargement found, but no sugar excreted in urine. Ketosis usually present. Low blood sugar.

2. Gaucher's disease. Liver moderately enlarged; spleen very large.

Treatment
Synthetic milk must be substituted for breast and cow's milk. Completely milk-free diet required.

Prognosis
With elimination of galactose from diet from birth it is possible for child to grow up normal mentally and physically. *Early diagnosis essential.* In later years tolerance to galactose may develop and normal diet can be given.

Errors in Fructose Metabolism

Adult fructose intake 50–100 g/day (mostly in sucrose). Metabolized in liver, kidney and small bowel mucosa. Absorbed unchanged, as fructose. Can be phosphorylated and converted to glucose in small gut mucosa.

Essential Fructosuria
Very rare; harmless; autosomal, recessive; 99% Jewish. Fructokinase lacking. Very high blood levels of fructose, 10–20% appears in urine.

Hereditary Fructose Intolerance
Deficiency of fructose-1-phosphate aldolase, which mobilizes fructose-1-phosphate to enter metabolic pathway.

Acute Syndrome
Clinical features. Oral fructose produces sweating, nausea, vomiting, convulsions, disturbance of consciousness, fructosuria, amino aciduria, hyperbilirubinaemia, elevated SGOT.

Chronic Syndrome
(Most often observed when sucrose added to diet at weaning).
Clinical features. Child fails to thrive, has hepatomegaly leading to cirrhosis, jaundice, bouts of vomiting and dehydration, oedema, ascites, convulsions. Symptoms worse the younger the age of weaning on to sucrose.

Investigations
Frutosuria and fructosaemia present. Amino acidaemia and amino aciduria may develop. Liver cell damage leads to abnormal liver function tests.

Prognosis

If initial severe illness is survived, aversion to sweets leads to protection and child may develop normally—physically and mentally. Marked lack of dental caries due to low sugar intake.

Disorders of Glycogen Metabolism

Glycogen Storage Diseases
Group of diseases in which excessive glycogen accumulates in tissues, producing functional impairment of affected organs associated with biochemical derange-

ment of carbohydrate metabolism. Specific enzyme defects can be identified (*see Fig. 51.1*). Major clinical features listed in *Table 51.2*.

Inheritance
Types I–VII autosomal recessive; Type VIII X-linked.

Type I (*Glucose-6-phosphatase Deficiency; Von Gierke's Disease; Hepatic Glycogenosis*)

Commonest of the glycogenoses, manifested clinically by hepatomegaly and ketosis. Enzyme deficiency demonstrable in liver and kidney.

Pathology
Liver may be huge, sometimes kidneys enlarged. Deposits of normal glycogen present.

Clinical Features
Considerable variation in severity of disease:
1. *Mild*. Condition may not be recognized until 2 years of age when size of abdomen and dwarfing are noticed. Skin xanthomas may occur.
2. *Severe*. Symptoms of hypoglycaemia may be presenting feature: vomiting, drowsiness, twitching or convulsions.
On examination. General condition often good. Child small for age. Abdomen large. Liver very big but spleen not palpable.

Investigations
1. *Urine* contains acetone in morning and often throughout 24h. Rarely contains sugar and amino acids.
2. *Blood glucose*. Fasting hypoglycaemia. Hyperlipaemia common.
3. *Carbohydrate challenge tests* (*see Table 52.3*).
4. *Very low glucose-6-phosphatase* in liver, intestinal biopsy and platelets.

Prognosis
Patients often live for many years.

Treatment
Symptomatic treatment of hypoglycaemia: frequent meals, if necessary at night. High-protein diet (25–30% total calories given as protein) helps to raise blood sugar. Glucagon of value in some cases. Nocturnal feeds via nasogastric tube and slow pump prevent hypoglycaemia and promote growth.

Type II (*Lysosomal-Glucosidase* (*acid maltase*) *Deficiency; Pompe's Disease; Cardiac Glycogenosis*)

Very rare disease; glycogen stores in heart, liver, skeletal muscle.

Clinical Features
Onset within first month of life. Failure to thrive, muscular hypotonia, cyanosis, cardiac failure, often systolic murmur. May be macroglossia.

Table 51.2. Classification of major glycogen storage diseases (adapted from Mahler*)

Type	Enzyme defect	Tissue affected	Clinical features
I (von Gierke's disease)	Glucose-6-phosphatase	Liver, kidney, gut	Hepatomegaly, hypoglycaemia, ketosis, acidosis
II (Pompe's disease)	Acid maltase (lysosomal α-1,4 glucosidase)	Generalized, particularly heart, tongue, brain, WBC	Cardiomegaly, heart failure, enlarged tongue, muscle weakness, death in infancy
III (Limit dextrinosis)	'Debrancher' amylo-1,6 glucosidase	Liver, heart, muscle, RBC. WBC	Hepatomegaly, moderate fasting hypoglycaemia, muscle weakness, and wasting
IV (Amylopectinosis)	'Brancher'	Liver, spleen, heart, muscle, RBC, WBC	Cirrhosis, hepatic failure
V (McArdle's syndrome)	Muscle phosphorylase	Skeletal muscle only	Pain, stiffness, weakness on exercise only; occasionally myoglobinuria
VI (Hers' disease)	Liver phosphorylase	Liver, WBC	Hepatomegaly, moderate fasting, hypoglycaemia
VII	Phosphofructokinase	Skeletal muscle only	Similar to V
VIII	Brain phosphorylase	Brain	CNS degeneration, death in infancy
IX	Liver phosphorylase kinase	Liver, WBC	Similar to VI. Mildest of glycogenoses
X	Liver and muscle phosphorylase kinase	Liver, muscle	Hepatomegaly

*Mahler R.F. (1977) Disorders of glycogen metabolism. In *Clinics in Endocrinology and Metabolism*, 5. London, Saunders, pp. 579–598.

Investigations
1. Radiographs show enlarged globular heart; ECG abnormal.
2. Muscle biopsy may show excess glycogen, also occasionally seen in WBCs.
3. Blood biochemistry normal
4. Carbohydrate challenge tests normal (*Table 51.3*).
5. Absence of lysosomal α-1,4-glucosidase in liver and leucocytes.

Table 51.3.   Summary of clinical and functional differentiation between the ten major types of glycogen storage disease

Tissue affected	Response to diagnostic test	Type of glycogen storage disease
Liver and kidney only		I, VI, IX
Muscle only		V, VII
Many tissues		II, III, IV
	Fasting	
	Severe hypoglycaemia	I
	Moderate hypoglycaemia	III, IV, VI, IX
	No hypoglycaemia	II, V, VII, VIII, IX, X
	Glucagon	
	No increase in blood glucose } Fasting	I, III, IV, VI
	Normal increase in blood glucose	II, V, VII, VIII, IX, X
	No increase in blood glucose } Post-prandial	I, VI, IX, X
	Normal increase in blood glucose }	II, III, IV
	No increase in blood lactate	VI IX
	Normal increase in blood lactate	II, III, IV, V, VII
	Gross increase in blood lactate	I
	Intravenous galactose or fructose	
	No increase in blood glucose	I
	Normal increase in blood glucose	II, III, IV, VI, VII, IX
	Abnormal increase in blood lactate	I
	Ischaemic forearm exercise	
	No increase in blood lactate	III, IV, V, VII
	Normal increase in blood lactate	I, II, VI, IX

Type III (*'Debrancher' Enzyme Deficiency; Limit Dextrinosis*)

Very rare, partially degraded glycogen ('limit dextrin') stored in most body tissues. Fasting hypoglycaemia usually mild, other features resemble mild Type I. Glycogen present in biopsies has simple structure, enzyme deficiency can be demonstrated in RBCs and WBCs. Treatment as for Type I.

Type IV (*'Brancher' Enzyme Deficiency; Amylopectinosis*)

Extremely rare, produces cirrhosis, portal hypertension and hepatic failure in childhood. Stored 'glycogen' is abnormal, starch-like amylopectin.

Type V (*Muscle Phosphorylase Deficiency; McArdle's Disease*)

Very rare. Muscle pain, stiffness and weakness after exercise, occasional myoglobinuria. Normal glycogen stored in muscle. No hypoglycaemia.

Type VI (*Hepatic Phosphorylase Deficiency; Hers' Disease*)

Very rare. Mild fasting hypoglycaemia, hepatomegaly.

Type VII (*Muscle Phosphofructokinase Deficiency*)

Clinically similar to Type V. Metabolic pathway blocked by absence of phosphofructokinase in muscles. No liver disease.

Type VIII (*Hepatic Glycogen Storage with Progressive Degeneration of CNS*)

Very rare, fatal form in which CNS changes predominate. Low brain phosphorylase activity due to incomplete activation of adenyl cyclase system. Causes spasticity, decerebration, death in infancy. Urinary catecholamines elevated.

Type IX (*Hepatic Phosphorylase Kinase Deficiency*)

Almost identical to Type VI. May be autosomal (Type IXa) or X-linked recessive (Type IXb).

Type X (*Hepatic and Muscle Phosphorylase Kinase Deficiency*)

Only 1 case described, girl with asymptomatic hepatomegaly. Phosphorylase present in liver and muscles inactive because of kinase deficiency.

Bibliography

Hobbs J. R. (1981) Bone marrow transplantation for inborn errors. *Lancet* 2, 735.

Chapter 52   # ERRORS IN LIPID METABOLISM

A. Hyperlipidaemias

Lipids (cholesterol and triglycerides) exist in plasma as complexes with proteins. Disorders classified according to electrophoretic characteristics of lipoproteins (Fredrickson). Appearances of serum on standing may suggest diagnosis. Five main types described (*Table 52.1*).

Type I (*Familial Hyperchylomicronaemia*)

Rare autosomal recessive disorder.

Clinical Features

Table 52.1.   Types of hyperlipidaemia

Type	Chylomicrons	Cholesterol	Triglycerides	LDL (beta-lipoprotein)
I	↑+++	↑++	↑+++	N
II	N	↑+++	↑+	↑++
III	N	↑++	↑++	↑++
IV	N	N or ↑	↑+++	↑++
V	↑++	↑++	↑+++	↑++

May present in childhood with recurrent abdominal pain, or frank pancreatitis. Xanthomas occur in crops, mainly in limbs and buttocks. Hepatosplenomegaly.

Investigations
1. Chylomicrons increased, due to low activity of lipoprotein lipase enzyme. Creamy supernatant on standing serum. Retinal blood vessels appear whitish.
2. Marked elevation of plasma triglycerides.
3. Moderate elevation of cholesterol.

Treatment
Low fat diet. MCT supplements can be used. Avoid high carbohydrate intake as this increases endogenous triglyceride production.

Prognosis
Attacks of pain and xanthomas recur if untreated. No increase in atherosclerosis.

Type II (*Familial Essential Hypercholesterolaemia*)

Fairly common autosomal dominant. Onset of symptoms before age 20 only in homozygote.

Clinical Features
Xanthomas, arcus senilis and premature atherosclerosis.

Investigations
1. Hypercholesterolaemia.
2. Triglycerides normal or slightly elevated.
3. Increased beta-lipoprotein.

Treatment
1. Low animal-fat diet.
2. Cholestyramine increases bile salt excretion and this depletes body cholesterol.

Prognosis
Ischaemic heart disease in early adult life almost inevitable unless preventive measures taken. Efficacy of treatment doubtful.

Type III (*Broad Beta Disease*)

Rare. Genetics uncertain. Manifested as xanthomas and atherosclerosis in young adults.

Type IV (*Familial Hyperprebeta-lipoproteinaemia*)

Common disorder, genetics not clear. Manifested clinically in adults as xanthomas, premature atherosclerosis, obesity and tendency to diabetes. Children may have abdominal pain. Hypertriglyceridaemia increased by carbohydrate in diet. Low calorie diet is principal treatment.

Type V (*Mixed Lipaemia*)

May be a variant of Type IV. Symptoms rare in childhood, include xanthomas, diabetes, obesity and abdominal pain.

B. Hypolipoproteinaemias

Absence of Alpha-lipoprotein (*Tangier Disease*)
Extremely rare. Manifested as peculiar orange enlargement of tonsils, with hepatosplenomegaly, peripheral neuropathy and lipid deposits in cornea. Plasma cholesterol low but triglyceride may be raised, electrophoresis shows absence of alpha-lipoproteins.

A-Beta-Lipoproteinaemia (*Acanthocytosis; Bassen–Kornzweig Syndrome*) *see* p. 271.

C. Lipid Storage (*Lipidoses*) (*See* p. 330).

Bibliography

Beaumont J. L. et al. (1970) Classification of hyperlipidaemias and hyperlipoprotinaemias. *Bull. WHO* **43**, 891–915.

Chapter 53   # ERRORS IN PIGMENT METABOLISM

The Porphyrias

A group of rare metabolic disorders with excessive production of porphyrins or their precursors.

Acute Intermittent Porphyria
Very rarely present in childhood. Autosomal dominant.

Clinical Features
Bouts of acute abdominal pain, vomiting, constipation, paresis, other CNS

symptoms, hypertension and psychiatric disturbance. Often provoked by drugs or infection. Urine contains porphobilinogen. Treatment: symptomatic.

Cutaneous Hepatic Porphyria
Autosomal dominant.

Clinical Features
Bullous lesions of skin on exposure to sunlight, heal with severe scarring. Liver disease frequent. Precipitated by drugs. Urinary porphyrins elevated during attack. Liver function tests abnormal.

Porphyria Variegata
Almost confined to South Africa. Autosomal dominant. Manifestations very rare in childhood. Combines features of acute intermittent and cutaneous hepatic porphyrias.

Congenital Erythropoietic Porphyria
Extremely rare autosomal recessive. Severe solar photosensitivity from early childhood, with extensive bullous eruption followed by scarring, hyperpigmentation and deformity. Eyes may be damaged. Teeth coloured brownish-pink from porphyrins. May be anaemic with shortened RBC survival. *Prognosis*: Poor.

Congenital Erythropoietic Protoporphyria
Rare, autosomal recessive, manifested from infancy by irritant urticarial rash on exposure to sunlight. No anaemia. May be liver disease but prognosis otherwise better than in erythropoietic porphyria.

Chapter 55   *ERRORS IN PURINE METABOLISM*

Primary gout rarely occurs in childhood. Signs, symptoms and treatment as for adults. Secondary hyperuricaemia occurs in leukaemia and chronic renal disease, may cause gout.

Lesch–Nyhan Syndrome

Definition
Very rare X-linked recessive disorder characterized clinically by mental retardation, spasticity, choreoathetosis and self-mutilation, biochemically by hyperuricaemia and absence of hypoxanthine guanine phosphoribosyl transferase in cells.

Clinical Features
Severe mental retardation. Self-destructive biting of tongue, lips and fingers, and neurological features involving pyramidal and extrapyramidal tracts. Gouty tophi develop in older patients.

Treatment
Allopurinol may control gouty manifstations but has no effect on intellectual or nervous defects.

For Further Reading

Stanbury J. B., Wyngaarden J. B and Fredrickson D.S. (ed.) (1983) *The Metabolic Basis of Inherited Disease*, 5th ed. New York, McGraw-Hill.

9

INTRODUCTION

Disorders of the respiratory system, principally upper and lower respiratory tract infections, asthma and cystic fibrosis, constitute a large part of paediatric practice. Upper respiratory tract infections (URTI), mainly viral in origin, are common in all communities in the winter months. But URTI proceeding to pneumonia are particularly common in young children, especially when poor nutrition and unhygienic surroundings combine. Under-privileged children are at special risk because of the increased likelihood of cross-infection, the immunological overload for parasitic and gastrointestinal infections and the absence or abuse of antibiotic therapy.

The pattern of respiratory diseases in children differs from that found in adults for the following reasons:

1. Anatomical and Pathological

1.1 The small larynx and trachea of the child easily become blocked by inflammatory oedema or exudate so that stridor is common.

1.2 Plugs of mucus in the small lower air passages may cause segmental collapse and/or consolidation.

1.3 The short distance between the upper and lower respiratory tract means that infection can readily contaminate the whole respiratory system.

1.4 The chest wall of the infant is soft as the ribs are incompletely calcified; in-sucking of the chest may be marked.

1.5 The infant's mediastinum is very mobile so that considerable shift may occur.

1.6 The lymphatic system is well developed, hence hilar lymph nodes enlarge readily.

2. Physiological

1.1 Respiration rates are labile and are easily influenced by external surroundings and disease.

1.2 Normal rate
Birth about 40/min
1 year about 30/min
3 years about 25/min

3. Clinical

Respiratory infections. Children encounter about six new respiratory viral infections each year, usually from other children. For this reason the first child in a family tends to suffer from few infections until he goes to school, but during the first year at school he succumbs to many. His younger siblings, however, catch infections from him in the first 5 years of life and do not have so many on entering school.

Sputum. Rarely obtainable from a child under about 8 years as it is swallowed. Cystic fibrosis (CF) children with their copious sputum expectorate earlier.

Foreign bodies. Inhalation of food, vomit, etc. is common in infants owing to poor respiratory coordination; 1–3 year age group maximal for inhalation of foreign bodies, such as peanuts.

4. Examination of the Child

Gentleness, warm hands and stethoscope chest piece, are essential. Signs in the chest can be misleading. Examination should proceed as for adult, but the following points are of special importance:

Percussion. Should be light, as chest wall thin. As much can be deduced by feeling with pleximeter finger as by listening.

Auscultation. Breath sounds are puerile in type (louder than in adult and more bronchial in character). May even be heard through thin layer of fluid. Voice sounds may also be heard through fluid.

5. Radiology

Of particular importance owing to the difficulty in clinical examination (but note danger of excessive radiation). Films in children are hard to interpret because:

5.1 Difficult to position accurately an ill or restless child.

5.2 Child may move, exposures must be very short.

5.3 Films vary greatly with phase of respiration: in full inspiration, heart long, diaphragm low and lung fields appear translucent; in full expiration, heart transverse, mediastinum appears broad, diaphragm high and lung fields more opaque.

5.4 Crying may alter appearance of film considerably, especially in infants. Hilum often appears abnormally broad.

5.5 Thymus may be large. Often appears as sail-shaped shadow in upper zone.

Chapter 56	# ACUTE INFECTIONS OF THE UPPER RESPIRATORY TRACT

The clinical picture differs in the child and adult for the following reasons:

Response to Infective Agents varies with Age

Infants, children and adults may react differently to same agent, even if transmitted from one to another.

Overlap of Clinical Syndromes
Almost identical signs and symptoms may be produced by different aetiological
agents: viral, bacterial and other (e.g. *Mycoplasma pneumoniae,* rickettsiae etc.).

The Short Respiratory Tract
In the child makes the distinction between upper and lower respiratory tract
infections even less meaningful than in adults.
    Infection may trigger off an attack of asthma which modifies the clinical picture.

Acute Rhinitis

Classification
The common cold; coryza; upper respiratory tract infection (URTI).
Specific infective rhinitis, e.g. prodromal signs of measles; pertussis.
Allergic rhinitis, e.g. 'hay fever'.

The Common Cold
The clinical features of URTI are too well known to require description.
However, note that the small nasal passages of babies are easily blocked by
secretions, resulting in dyspnoea and difficulty in sucking from breast or bottle.
Normally the baby breathes through his nose while feeding. If the nose is blocked
the baby has to remove his mouth from the nipple or teat frequently to take gulps
of air. This leads to restless feeding, air swallowing and vomiting.
    Infection easily spreads to the sinuses, ears, and larynx.
    The common cold, although mild in adults, can lead to dangerous pneumonia in
a child. Contact between an infected adult or older child and a baby should
therefore be avoided as far as possible. This is particularly important in the
hospital situation when the baby is already sick.

Acute Pharyngitis

(Including Influenza; Febrile Sore Throat; Feverish Colds; Adenopharyngoconjunctival Fever; APC Syndrome)
    Acute pharyngitis is an epidemic disease with a mixed picture depending on the
type of virus, age, and the general health of the child. If the systemic symptoms are
marked, is often described as influenza. Symptoms include headache, malaise and
fever of sudden onset. Later, sore throat, shivering, blocked nose and often aches
and pains in the muscles, vomiting and abdominal pain. Signs of pharyngitis,
laryngitis and cervical lymph node involvement common. In some epidemics
conjunctivitis (bilateral or unilateral) is prominent feature, in some it is absent.
    In infants, pharyngitis may present as pyrexia of unknown origin; diarrhoea and
vomiting; or febrile convulsions.
    In older children may present with abdominal pains. Differential diagnosis
from appendicitis may then be difficult.

Antibiotic Therapy in Upper Respiratory Infections
The abuse of antibiotics in respiratory infections is becoming a major problem.
The free use of antibiotics in paediatrics is contributing to the high incidence and
severity of allergies in later life. It is often stated, in favour of giving antibiotics to
URTI, that the practice has diminished the incidence of acute rheumatic fever and

Table 56.1. Viruses causing respiratory illnesses (shading indicates relative frequency)

	Common cold	Feverish colds Influenza	Pharyngitis Laryngitis Tracheitis	Bronchiolitis	Pneumonia	Herpangina
Influenza A, B	▨	▨	▨	▨	▨	
Para-influenza	▨	▨	▨		▨	
Respiratory syncytial	▨			▨	▨	
Adenovirus	▨		▨		▨	
Enterovirus	▨		▨		▨	
Rhinovirus	▨	▨	▨	▨	▨	
Coronavirus	▨	▨				
Coxsackie						▨

septic complications such as otitis media and pneumonia. This may be true but against this must be set the increased incidence of allergies, diarrhoea, the indoctrination of the public to expect a medicine at every visit to the doctor and the financial cost to the community.

Viruses do not respond to antibiotics, the important bacterium is the β-haemolytic streptococcus with its major complication, rheumatic fever. Unfortunately, it is difficult to distinguish streptococcal from virus infections, but the following are some guides:

In viral infections the constitutional signs are often mild and the temperature is low (this may also be so in subacute streptococcal sore throat). With viruses there are always coryzal signs by the 2nd or 3rd day; adult members of the family may have obvious colds. The appearance of the throat gives little guidance although exudate is uncommon with virus infections. *Antibiotics should only be given if the probability of a streptococcal infection is high, or if there has been previous rheumatic fever.*

Herpangina

An uncommon respiratory infection caused by Coxsackie viruses Group A. It mainly affects infants and young children. The clinical features are sore throat; high fever; tiny vesicles with red areola found on pillars of fauces which burst to form little ulcers.

Acute Epiglottitis

Uncommon disease almost invariably due to *Haemophilus influenzae*, type B.

Peak incidence 3–5 years. May occur in small epidemics. Can be fatal.

Sudden onset with sore throat; dyspnoea and fever. May be considerable bacteraemic shock, severe pain in throat, dysphagia and stridor.

Examination should be performed with great caution and a means of establishing an airway under anaesthetic should be available. The epiglottis is seen to be very swollen and fiery red. Looks like red cherry obstructing the pharynx. Antibiotics and steroid therapy should be given urgently.

Acute Laryngitis ('Croup')

Croup is due to a combination of an infection—usually viral but occasionally *H. influenzae*—with a narrowing of the larynx. This may be an anatomical lesion (mild or severe) or due to an allergic diathesis. Children with croup often develop asthma later. Therefore, as would be expected, croup is often recurrent.

Laryngitis develops gradually, often a few days after the onset of coryza or tonsillitis, or it may develop suddenly with considerable stridor in the early hours of the morning.

There is hoarseness or loss of voice, a harsh barking cough which is often painful. Condition may resolve rapidly or slowly. The child should be nursed in a moist atmosphere.

For differential diagnosis *see Table* 56.2.

Acute Obstructive Laryngotracheitis and Laryngotracheobronchitis

This is an uncommon disease which presents as a severe form of laryngitis and spreads to involve the trachea and bronchi. It is probably caused by a more virulent organism. Clinically there is a sudden onset of stridor a day or so after an URTI. Respiratory distress and prostration may be severe from a combination of hypoxia and toxaemia. The larynx and trachea are acutely inflamed and may contain a purulent membrane. For further details *see* ENT textbooks.

For differential diagnosis *see Table* 56.2.

| Chapter 57 | CHRONIC INFECTIONS OF THE UPPER RESPIRATORY TRACT |

Perennial Allergic Rhinitis

A disorder affecting atopic children, characterized by persistent clean nasal discharge, sneezing and blocked nose. The nasal mucosa is swollen and pale. Children have characteristic rubbing of the nose — 'Bowen's allergic salute'.

Hay Fever (Allergic Rhinitis)

Part of the allergic diathesis. The child has frequent intermittent attacks of watery nasal discharge with sneezing and rubs the nose because it itches ('Bowen's allergic salute'). Mucosa is pale, swollen, with clear mucus overlying it. Often

Table 56.2.   Differential diagnosis of stridor ('croup')

	Common age range	Principal features
Onset before 3 months Congenital laryngeal stridor syndrome: Inspiratory laryngeal collapse.	0–18 months	No cyanosis. Child well.
Cysts, web, etc.	Birth onwards	Often cyanosis. Progressive
Onset after 3 months Acute laryngitis	4 months onwards	Mild to severe hoarseness. Other members of family may have respiratory infection
Acute laryngotracheo-bronchitis	4 months to 6 years	Child very ill. Marked respiratory distress with stridor
Diphtheria (Very rare)	6 months to 12 years	Child ill. Membrane usually visible. If in doubt treat
Foreign body	4 months onwards	Abrupt onset. History often obtained. X-ray
Onset after 6 months Laryngeal papillomas or haemangioma	1–3 years	Insidious onset. Hoarse voice. Progressive condition
Angioneurotic oedema	1 year onwards	Usually associated widespread urticaria
Inhaled steam	1–5 years	History of accident. Scalds on lips and tongue
Onset after 2 years Asthma	2 years onwards	Often inspiratory and expiratory, wheezing prominent

associated with conjunctivitis, chronic rhinitis, sinobronchitis or asthma. Seasonal, related to release of grass, plant or tree pollens into the atmosphere.

Therapy for rhinitis: Cromoglycate (Rynacrom) or steroid insufflators (Beconase).

Therapy for conjunctivitis: Cromoglycate eye drops (Opticrom).

Disease of Nasal Sinuses

The maxillary antra and ethmoidal sinuses are present from birth. The sphenoidal and frontal sinuses develop from about 3 years. The latter are present radiologically from 7 years. Sinusitis is rare in young children but is common in older ones. For details *see* ENT textbook.

Recurrent Infection of Tonsils and Adenoids

The tonsils and adenoids are thought to act as a 'filter', preventing organisms in pharynx reaching general circulation. If frequently infected, tonsils may become nidus of infection. With repeated infection lymphoid tissue either hypertrophies or becomes small and fibrotic. Tonsils in older child may therefore be large or small.

With repeated attacks of tonsillitis, the tonsillar lymph nodes often enlarge. Rarely, the tonsillar enlargement is sufficient to cause obstruction to the breathing, particularly at night. Apnoeic attacks then occur which can be quite prolonged. Enlargement of the adenoids also occurs. When this happens the airway is diminished and the child becomes a mouth breather. Also, because the Eustachian tube becomes obstructed, otitis media or 'glue ear' may result, causing deafness.

Indications for Tonsillectomy

1. Recurrent (more than 3 per year) attacks of tonsillitis in a child over 3 years old which fail to respond to adequate courses of continuous prophylactic oral penicillin. Adenoids should also be removed.
2. Very large tonsils giving rise to sleep apnoea or obstruction.

Cases for which Tonsillectomy should not be advised

1. The appearance of asymptomatic 'big tonsils', 'infected-looking tonsils', etc.
2. As possible focus of infection in acute rheumatism, nephritis, etc.
3. Before 3 years old.

Note: If tonsillectomy performed a small number of children are undoubtedly improved, small number made worse, most unaffected. Local custom varies widely.

Indications for Adenoidectomy

Any case in which the adenoids are enlarged and causing symptoms, especially 'glue ear'.

Chapter 58   # DISEASE OF THE NOSE, EAR AND LARYNX

Congenital Choanal Atresia

A rare genetically inherited condition in which there is congenital obstruction of the air passages in nose. Obstruction may be membranous or bony, unilateral or bilateral. Very important condition as failure to recognize it may result in death during first few hours of life.

Clinical Features

Normal babies only breathe through their nose, but baby with choanal atresia can only breathe when his mouth is open. This art may not be learnt for several days.

The infant is usually a good colour when crying but goes blue when he is quiet and mouth shut.

Emergency treatment consists in maintaining an airway through the mouth until surgical intervention can be performed.

Foreign Bodies in Nose

Children quite commonly push beads, bits of paper, pebbles, etc. into the nostril.

This should be suspected if there is a unilateral nasal discharge, which may be purulent or bloodstained.

Epistaxis (*Nose-bleed*)

Common condition. Blood usually comes from rupture of a dilated vein on the septum just inside the external nares. This may occur spontaneously, from a blow or in association with a general disease such as purpura or leukaemia.

Hereditary Haemorrhagic Telangiectasis (*Rendu–Osler–Weber Disease*)

Usually commences as recurrent epistaxes in childhood; later bleeding occurs from vagina, urethra, stomach, etc. Telangiectases may not appear until 20–30 years of age. May present as pulmonary arteriovenous aneurysm.

Diseases of the Ear

Note: For detailed description consult ENT textbooks. Only problems particularly related to medical paediatrics will be considered.

Pre-auricular sinus is not uncommon. Tiny dimple is visible usually just beside the tragus. The sinus may track forward. This gives rise to no trouble unless the track becomes infected. If this occurs a pre-auricular abscess develops 1 cm or so away from the origin of the sinus. This will keep recurring unless the sinus track is found and laid open.

Acute Otitis Media

A very common and important condition which is responsible for much pain and unexplained fever in childhood, particularly in young babies. If the disease becomes chronic there is a risk of eventual deafness. Some factors which may contribute to the frequency of otitis media in children are:

1. Short, relatively wide Eustachian tube. Probably reason for prevalence of condition in babies. Infection can easily travel from nasopharynx to middle ear.
2. If baby fed lying down infected material may flow up tube into ear.
3. Enlarged adenoids. Pad of adenoids may block Eustachian tube which then cannot drain middle ear.
4. Poor environment. Often a feature in the triad: malnutrition, chronic infection, worm infestation—seen in children in developing countries.
For further details *see* ENT textbooks.

Serous Otitis Media (*'Glue-ear'*)

A condition where the middle ear is full of an amber or greyish exudate which may be thin or thick and viscid. Glue ear is a very important cause of partial deafness, up to 50 dB loss; bone conduction is normal. On otoscopy the drum appears to lack lustre and to be a grey colour. It may bulge or be indrawn perhaps because a blockage of the Eustachian tube results in negative pressure in the inner ear. This gives rise to a compensatory exudate. The treatment is surgical, usually with the insertion of grommets.

Congenital Laryngeal Stridor Syndrome

This not uncommon condition may be familial. The onset is within the first few days of life or may be delayed up to a month or two. The majority of cases are due to weakness or deformity of the epiglottis. The infant's larynx normally has loose aryepiglottic folds; these may collapse on inspiration causing crowing (inspiratory laryngeal collapse syndrome, ILC).

A small minority of cases are due to cysts, haemangiomas, cleft larynx, web or other causes. Also occurs in hypoplasia of mandible—Pierre Robin syndrome.

With inspiratory laryngeal collapse there is inspiratory crowing, expiration is normal. The crow is more obvious when the baby is crying or excited, or when there is a superadded respiratory infection. It may become less marked or even disappear during sleep. Respiratory distress is absent. Sucking does not cause difficulty. The condition becomes less noticeable as the child grows. Has often disappeared by about 12–18 months. May recur during crying for longer periods.

Laryngoscopy should always be performed, a removable cause may be found. Radiograph with opaque substance in the larynx or xerography may be of value.

For differential diagnosis *see Table* 56.2.

Chapter 59   **THE NON-COMMUNICATING CHILD**

Differential Diagnosis
The non-talking child is common. Following conditions must be considered.
1. Delayed maturation. Most normal children say two or meaningful words by 15 months. Those who do not should be examined by a doctor. Many are perfectly normal but speech is late in maturing. This condition is commoner in boys than girls: may be genetically inherited. Child may not talk even up to 4 years and yet be normal. When speech starts he makes up for lost time rapidly. *Note*: Delayed speech is also common following prematurity as part of generalized delay in milestones.
2. Deafness. This is the most important cause of speech delay. Early recognition of deafness is vital so that treatment can be started.
3. Mental retardation. Perhaps commonest cause of speech delay. Reasons:
    3.1 The Intellectual Factor. Level of mental ability of subnormal child usually correlates well with level of language development.
    3.2 Physical Factors. Subnormal child may also have brain damage; heavy sedation for fits, cleft palate, etc.
    3.3 Psychological Factors. Lack of motivation to speak; subnormal child may be given all he wants without asking for it; over-protection.
    3.4 Social Factors. Parents may not realize the need to communicate with the child. May not meet other people. The speech standards at home may be poor.
    3.5 Emotional Factors. Behaviour problems common.
4. Neurological problems
    4.1 Inability to think: Amentia; dementia, e.g. cerebral sclerosis, lipidosis.
    4.2 Inability to translate thought into word symbols: Motor dysphasia, e.g. brain injury, infection, vascular lesions, etc.

4.3 Inability to understand the spoken word: Receptive aphasia, e.g. constitutional.
4.4 Inability to transmit motor impulses (central loss): Dysarthria, e.g. cerebral palsy, chorea, tumours of posterior fossa, etc.
4.5 Inability to transmit motor impulses (peripheral loss): Dysarthria, e.g. peripheral neuropathy.

5. *Infantile autism, see* p. 355.
6. *Emotional deprivation.* The child deprived of love and affection tends to withdraw into himself and frequently will not talk. This especially happens if the child has been ill-treated.

Deafness

Normal development of Hearing and Speech
At the age of 2–3 months a new sound will momentarily arrest the child's attention; he gives evidence of delight at meaningful sounds such as voice or footsteps.

At the age of about 5 months the child turns his head toward sound; vocalizes in response; babbles when alone.

At the age of 10–12 months the child recognizes his name and may say a few words.

At the age of 15 months the child should say at least two or more meaningful words.

Importance of Normal Hearing
Hearing is a social attribute, for instance:

The sound of a voice indicates the presence of an adult to comfort and help; or, the sound of key in a lock indicates Daddy coming home, etc. Later, child makes similar noises himself, which gives him a sense of power.

Delay in hearing until 2½ years means speech impairment can never be fully overcome.

Delay till 5 years means total speech impairment.

Young deaf child may mistakenly be thought to be mentally retarded.

With high tone deafness child may have delayed and poor speech, but responds to sounds. Diagnosis then missed unless audiometry done.

The completely deaf child lives in a world of silence. Incomplete deafness is more common. Either a whole range of sounds may be diminished or, more commonly, islands of deafness are present. Here the child may respond to bangs or ringing bells but not to a voice. If the deafness is due to, say, serous otitis media, the quality of sound heard varies from day to day. Thus the same word is heard differently by him on different occasions. Even partial deafness therefore carries a grave educational disadvantge.

Incidence of Deafness
About 5% of schoolchildren are partially or completely deaf. The figure may rise to 40% in some disadvantaged communities with high incidence of glue ear.

Grades of Deafness in Schoolchildren

Grade I
Child who has defective hearing but who, without any special help, can benefit from ordinary school.

Grade II
Child with defective hearing who requires special arrangements. These can vary from favourable position in class to special lip-reading instruction.

Grade III
Child with hearing so defective that methods used for totally deaf have to be employed.
   N.B. This classification takes in intelligence also.

Deafness in Infants and Young Children

Causes of Deafness
The development of the ear occurs mainly during the third and fourth months of fetal life. Causes of deafness include:
1. *Genetic*

    1.1 Isolated deafness—autosomal recessive.

    1.2 Waardenburg–Klein syndrome—white forelock, lateral displacement of inner canthi, broad root of nose, confluence of eyebrows, heterochromia iridis, and uni- or bilateral deafness. Autosomal dominant.

    1.3 Pendred's syndrome—goitre and deafness. Autosomal recessive.

    1.4 Treacher Collins syndrome—micrognathia, sunken cheek bones, antimongoloid slant to eyes, coloboma lower lid, fistula on line between angle of mouth and ear, deformed pinna, deafness. Dominant.

    1.5 Alport's syndrome—deafness and progressive glomerulonephritis; worse in boys. Dominant.

    1.6 Refsum's syndrome—icthyosis, progressive deafness, ataxia, retinitis pigmentosa, myosis, polyneuritis and mental retardation. CSF protein raised. Autosomal recessive.

    1.7 Jervell–Lange-Nielsen syndrome—deafness, prolonged Q–T interval on ECG, syncopal attacks. Possibility of sudden death. Autosomal recessive.

    1.8 Usher's syndrome—deafness and retinitis pigmentosa. Autosomal recessive.

2. *Acquired*

    2.1 Hypoxia and birth injury.

    2.2 Rubella embryopathy.

    2.3 Aminoglycoside e.g. gentamicin therapy.

    2.4 Rhesus incompatibility.

3. Postnatal

The most important postnatal causes are otitis media and recurrent glue-ear, and the three M's—measles, mumps, meningitis. However, in about 40% of cases no cause is ever discovered.

Concept of the 'Child at Risk'

A child coming into any of the above categories should be regarded as being 'at risk' for deafness. Hearing should be tested at 6 months of age and frequently thereafter until state of hearing is known for certain. Screening for deafness should be routine in all infants at 6–7 months.

Any child who does not say two or more meaningful words by 16 months should have hearing tested.

Manifestations of Deafness in Infants

No obvious symptoms arise until about 6 months of age. From then on following may be observed:

Hearing response: baby responds to noise more than to voices. May not respond to either. Some apparent response to noise may be due to vibration.

Sound production: voice monotonous; less experimental sound production than normal infant; may yell or screech.

Visual responsiveness abnormally acute. Child very attentive; comprehends and uses gestures. Lip reads from 1 year onwards.

Emotional behaviour: temper tantrums frequent, due to annoyance at not being understood, or from irritation because he does not understand others.

Social behaviour: interested in things rather than persons; occasional incomprehensible behaviour.

Testing hearing in young or mentally defective children is a task requiring special techniques and expertise. It is unfortunately not difficult to be misled into thinking a child's hearing is normal when it is not.

Principles of Treatment

If doubt exists the child should be treated as if he is deaf.

If he is deaf to the voice, treat even if he responds normally to other noises. The main object is to reach the child by every alternative means of communication in order to bring him up as a normal child. A secondary object is to teach the child to speak. Treatment should be commenced as soon as the diagnosis has been made, before 6 months old if possible. Inability to speak can be due in part to lack of proper training. No deaf child should be dumb. At first training should be mainly at home. Later the child will require special schooling.

Some principles:

The child should be fitted with a hearing aid before six months if possible.

Teach the parents to talk to the child making him watch their lips.

The child should be encouraged to use his voice and to be made to realize that other people regard it as a means of communication.

Use must be made of pantomime and gesture. Sign language or cued speech are sometimes necessary in the severely deaf. Unfortunately, these are not yet standardized. Consult books for details.

Lip-reading. Child should be talked to and taught to speak in same way as normal child.

Help required from expert adviser from early days.

| Chapter 60 | *LUNG INFECTIONS* |

Introduction

In young children the clinical features of bronchitis, bronchiolitis, broncho-pneumonia and bacterial pneumonia merge into each other. Accurate differentiation between them is often not possible. The child's response to infection will depend on such factors as: the nature and virulence of the infecting organism, the physical condition of the child, the presence of any allergic predisposition and the child's environment, e.g. poor housing circumstances, parental smoking, etc.

Acute Bronchitis

Acute bronchitis is common at any age. The clinical picture starts with an upper respiratory tract infection, mainly due to rhinoviruses, which 'goes to his chest', with increasing cough. The respiratory rate is increased with mild dyspnoea, but not so marked as in bronchopneumonia. The child is not shocked. Breath sounds may be rather harsh. Adventitious sounds occur as high and low pitched rhonchi throughout the lung fields.

Acute bronchitis is usually mild and lasts only a few days.

X-ray may show some increase in bronchovascular markings with thickening of the bronchial walls, but often nothing abnormal can be seen.

The presence or absence of an allergic background is important both for treatment and prognosis. Some indicators of an asthmatic background include: associated eczema; family history of allergy; well-marked wheezing, particularly if it persists after the child has apparently recovered; if wheezing occurs without preceding infection; if repeated attacks of 'bronchitis' occur in the absence of parental smoking.

The Wheezy Baby

This condition is sometimes known as 'the fat, happy, wheezy baby syndrome'. It is not uncommon in the age group 3–12 months. It often commences with a virus infection but persists after the coryza. Viruses incriminated are: respiratory syncytial virus (RSV); parainfluenza 1 and 2; adenovirus. RSV is commonest in infants. If similar non-specific wheezing occurs in schoolchild it may be due to RSV or *Mycoplasma pneumoniae*. There is little dyspnoea and cough, but rhonchi are heard all over the chest.

Differential Diagnosis See Table 60.1, p. 184.

Treatment

Treatment is rarely required but the feeding needs care as the child may aspirate.

Antispasmodics and steroids make little difference to course of disease unless more than 3 attacks in which case likely to be early asthma. Antibiotics of value for mycoplasma infection.

If wheezing commences under 1 years of age, is not associated with other

Table 60.1.   Differential diagnosis of acute bronchitis, bronchiolitis and bronchopneumonia

	Acute bronchitis	*Bronchiolitis*	*Bronchopneumonia*
Clinical	Constitutional symptoms mild	Severe dyspnoea full chest	Toxaemia may be severe
Auscultation	Rhonchi	Crepitations or nil abnormal	Rhonchi and/or crepitations
Radiograph of chest	Thickening of bronchial walls	Air trapping	Patchy collapse/consolidation
Causative agent	Rhinovirus	RSV	Mixed viruses, bacterial and other agents

allergic phenomena, e.g. atopic eczema or family history, then it does not portend asthma in later life. If the wheeze commences at age 1–3 years approximately 25% develop asthma. If wheeze present at age 3 years approximately 50% develop asthma.

Sinobronchitis

The combination of sinusitis and bronchitis is very common. Probably due to an allergic background with secondary infection superimposed. The chest condition is perpetuated by a flow of pus into the lungs from the infected sinuses. This may result in segmental or lobar collapse of the lung. The combination of sinus and lung infection is also seen in cystic fibrosis and α_1-antitrypsin deficiency.

Bronchiolitis

This is a common condition mainly occurring in epidemics in the age range 3–18 months. Most cases are due to the respiratory syncytial virus (RSV). Less commonly influenza and parainfluenza viruses.

Clinical
The child presents with an URTI followed by cough and increasing dyspnoea. The signs are similar to those of bronchopneumonia but dyspnoea and emphysema are more marked. The chest is markedly full and 'blown'. Widespread crepitations may be heard or the chest may be silent with poor air entry. As the condition progresses cough becomes feeble and cyanosis and collapse more marked. Dehydration may develop from hyperventilation. Bronchiolitis is usually a self-limiting disease which lasts 5–10 days.

Radiograph shows marked emphysema with evidence of air trapping, little or no collapse or consolidation.

Rapid diagnosis of RSV is possible by indirect immunofluorescence technique on nasopharyngeal aspirate.

Treatment is supportive only, no specific therapy is available.

Bronchopneumonia

Bronchopneumonia is common under the age of 3 years. It may be primary— being caused by any severe virus or bacteria which cause respiratory infection, or secondary—being associated with such disorders as measles or whooping cough; aspiration of infected material, especially milk; any severe illness or surgical operation, especially in debilitated child; burns with fire.

The onset is often acute with sudden high fever and prostration. Sometimes commences with convulsions. Cough may or may not be prominent.

Clinical Examination

Baby obviously ill, may be cyanosed or ashen-grey colour. Tachycardia marked. Respiration rate rapid, often up to 80/min. Usually expiratory grunt. Accessory muscles of respiration in action. Sucking-in of sternal notch, supraclavicular fossa and lower intercostal spaces. Crepitations heard over affected lung fields, may be masked by rattling mucopus in throat. The outlook is good in the majority of cases, but when it is secondary or occurs in a debilitated child the condition may be fatal.

Radiograph shows patches of consolidation and collapse.

Treatment

Treatment of all respiratory infections should be considered under the following headings:

Does the child require:

1. Mechanical aid to clear and maintain the airway?

2. Oxygen? Restlessness and crying are important signs of dyspnoea in an infant.

3. Antibiotics by oral or intravenous route? Amoxycillin or co-trimoxazole useful until organism known.

4. Intravenous infusion or nasogastric tube to maintain fluids, electrolytes and nutrition?

Lobar Pneumonia (Bacterial Pneumonia)

Classic lobar pneumonia as described in adult textbooks is rarely seen in children of any age and virtually never in the young. The usual picture is of a child with a severe lower respiratory tract infection in which signs of consolidation are discovered on chest examination and confirmed by radiography.

A febrile convulsion may occur at the onset in the younger child: herpes febrilis is common on the lips and, uncommonly, meningism is found. If undoubted neck stiffness exists, a lumbar puncture should always be performed. Disease usually due to pneumococcus and illness responds to penicillin G, ampicillin or erythromycin. Intravenous fluids and antibiotics useful initially.

Differential Diagnosis

Other disorders can be mistaken for pneumonia, particularly an acute abdominal emergency, e.g. acute appendicitis. Pain may be abdominal at onset, probably due to involvement of pleura covering diaphragm. Chest signs may be absent or easily missed, e.g. few crepitations heard in one axilla only. The following points indicate an abdominal cause for the pain:

Low fever—usually not above about 38·3 °C (101 °F) occurs in appendicitis.

Vomiting is almost invariable at onset of appendicitis, less common in pneumonia.

Furred tongue and abdominal pain and guarding in the right iliac fossa. May be difficult to persuade a crying child to indicate the point of maximum tenderness, but careful palpation will usually distinguish it.

The diagnosis can almost always be established by radiograph of the chest, but if real doubt exists, less harm is probably done to a child by unnecessary laparotomy as appendicitis and pneumonia may sometimes coexist.

Staphylococcal Pneumonia

This is not an uncommon disease under the age of 2 years. Many cases of cystic fibrosis (CF) are complicated by staphylococcal infection at some time. The condition also occurs apart from CF when it may be clinically severe or surprisingly mild despite considerable radiological change. The condition may follow staphylococcal septicaemia, or arise without apparent cause. Clinically, it is usually thought that the child has an attack of ordinary bronchopneumonia until radiology reveals lung cysts. The child may be toxic or the condition may remain good despite gross radiological findings. Dyspnoea may occur from mechanical pressure of cysts.

Staphylococcal pneumonia must be considered as dynamic, constantly changing. For this reason a constant clinical and radiological watch must be kept on the child for a sudden increase in dyspnoea or toxaemia.

Radiologically there is a mottled or homogeneous consolidation in early stages of disease. Then the consolidated areas become liquefied in the centre forming abscesses. These may be large or small. They are usually multiple. They may be full of pus (opaque), empty (translucent) or half-full (with a fluid level). The pus-filled cysts may communicate with a bronchus. Air may be able to get in but be prevented from leaving by a valve-like mechanism. Air cysts (pneumatocoeles) then develop. These may become very large within a few hours, occupying the whole hemithorax, displacing the mediastinum and compressing the lung on both sides of the chest. Radiological appearances are easily mistaken for a pyo-pneumothorax.

Later, the cyst may rupture into the pleural cavity giving rise to empyema, pyopneumothorax, pneumothorax, or tension pneumothorax. Toxaemia becomes worse if the cyst ruptures.

Radiological skeletal survey should be undertaken if there is any possibility of septicaemia. Concomitant osteomyelitis is common, it may follow lung infection or be the original source of the infection. Surprisingly, it can be almost asymptomatic and must therefore be sought for.

Bacteriology
Bacterial confirmation is often difficult because it may be impossible to obtain a specimen of sputum from a young child. Recovery of staphylococci from the nose and throat swab are of little diagnostic value; cough swab is of more value, especially if a pure growth of coagulase-positive *Staphylococcus aureus* is obtained. Lung puncture is sometimes advocated but is not without risk. Direct aspiration of the trachea by bronchoscopy is the only certain way to obtain a specimen, but this is rarely justifiable.

Prognosis
The great danger is from mechanical obstruction and toxaemia. With good treatment the child usually makes a complete recovery. Permanent lung damage

with bronchiectasis is surprisingly rare. Staphylococcal infection may develop elsewhere, especially in bone.

Differential Diagnosis

Diaphragmatic hernia or eventration of the diaphragm may give comparable radiological pictures, but the child is not toxic. Gurgling sounds may be heard in the chest and the barium meal is diagnostic. Treatment is by adequate antibiotic therapy sufficiently prolonged to eradicate any possible bone lesions. The acute management of the case revolves around the danger of mechanical obstruction of the airways. If acute dyspnoea develops with mediastinal shift, urgent needling of the hyperresonant side with underwater drainage is required.

Empyema

Rare; most commonly found as a complication of staphyloccocal pneumonia. Signs are those of pleural effusion. Treat by aspiration and antibiotics.

Bronchiectasis

Bronchiectasis was at one time common in childhood, but it is now rare apart from cystic fibrosis in which it constitutes a part of the disease profile. Clinical features as for adults.

Chapter 61   # FOREIGN BODIES IN RESPIRATORY TRACT

Foreign bodies (FB) can be divided into three main categories:
   1. Those which give rise to symptoms for mechanical reasons, owing to their large size, e.g. a coin, or to their awkward shape, e.g. a sharp toy or pin.
   2. Those which give rise to symptoms because of their irritative properties, e.g. vegetable matter, especially nuts and peas.
   3. Those which do not give rise to symptoms for a long time, e.g. some small, smooth, metallic or plastic objects.

FB in Larynx or Trachea

Where the FB lodges depends mainly on its size. For example a coin or marble might not pass through the larynx or bifurcation of the trachea. Inhalation of a FB occurs most commonly between the ages of 1 and 3 years.

Symptoms

The higher in the respiratory tract lodgement occurs, the more dramatic are the symptoms—violent cough, stridor, dyspnoea, and cyanosis.

FB in Lung

FBs damage the lung in the following ways:

1. Mechanical blockage resulting in collapse of segment of the lung, the size of which depends on the diameter of the bronchus occluded, or by obstructive emphysema of lobe or segment, caused by FB producing a valve-like action.

2. Irritation of bronchial mucosa from chemical properties of foreign body produces an inflammatory reaction which later may give rise to secondary infection.

The end result of an untreated case depends on the type and size of the foreign body:

1. It may be coughed up, even months after inhalation.

2. If small and comparatively non-irritant the foreign body may be walled off by fibrous tissue and even eventually absorbed.

3. Bronchiectasis sometimes develops owing to combination of obstruction, collapse and infection.

4. The condition may progress to chronic inflammatory reaction or lung abscess.

Clinical Features
Resemble those previously described for larynx and trachea, except that stridor is not common. If the significance of the initial coughing episode is not appreciated, the child presents with vague respiratory illness: dyspnoea, spasmodic cough, slight fever, general malaise. History of sudden bout of choking or coughing few days or weeks previously can sometimes be obtained from parent on careful inquiry.

Clinical Examination
Signs vary greatly: may be absent; may be mainly those of collapse or obstructive emphysema; mainly those of inflammatory reaction; or a combination of these.

Diagnosis should be suspected clinically and confirmed by radiography of the chest. Occasionally radio-opaque foreign body seen. More commonly area of collapse of obstructive emphysema is the only evidence observed. The chest should be screened if the presence of a foreign body is suspected. If obstructive emphysema is present the obstructed lung will not 'light up' on inspiration or become relatively opaque on expiration as does a normal lung. Mediastinum may swing from side to side with respiration.

Bronchoscopy
Must be performed if ever a FB is suspected.

Aspiration Pneumonia

Milk is the most commonly aspirated material. Less commonly other foodstuff or vomitus. Some common causes are:

Babies who vomit frequently from any cause.

Gastro-oesophageal reflux.

Babies with oesophageal atresia fed at birth.

H-type tracheo-oesophageal fistula.

Death only occurs in premature, weakly, or seriously ill babies. Lentil pneumonitis from inhalation of peas and beans is an incidental finding in babies dying from debilitating conditions, e.g. spina bifida. It may also follow inhalation of vomit in an otherwise well child. Diagnosis can be made in life by the appearance of benign miliary mottling on the X-ray of the chest. It can be confirmed by lung biopsy which reveals starch granules with foreign body giant cell reaction.

Chapter 62

LUNG COLLAPSE

Lung collapse due to airway obstruction is common in children. Collapse may be segmental or lobar depending on the site of the obstruction, which can occur anywhere from the main bronchus to the bronchiole. When obstruction occurs, air trapped in alveoli is gradually absorbed. Alveoli then collapse, thus occupying less space than previously. Following compensatory mechanisms fill this space:
Compensatory emphysema, i.e. surrounding healthy lung expands to contain more air.
Diaphragm rises.
Mediastinum shifts to affected side. Interlobar fissure may distort.

Causes of Small, Multiple, Segmental Collapse
(Including right middle lobe collapse). Collapse of this type is most commonly associated with viscid mucus due to asthma, cystic fibrosis, or pertussis. *Note*: because of the stickiness of the mucus which is difficult to shift, these 3 conditions can all give rise to a paroxysmal cough (*see* inspissated mucus plug syndrome in asthma, p. 193).
Less commonly segmental collapse may be due to infected material or blood from the upper respiratory tract.

Causes of Large Segmental and Lobar Collapse
Pneumothorax, pleural effusion, diaphragmatic hernia, or lymph node pressure from TB, leukaemia or other benign or malignant mass.
Lung collapse is not a disease entity, it is a symptom of some underlying disorder. Of itself, it gives rise to little trouble, but may become infected or, if very large, give rise to problems because of mediastinal shift.
Collapse is often clinically unsuspected and is discovered on radiographs of the chest.

Therapy
Collapse may take weeks to resolve. Re-aeration can be assisted by bronchodilators, or planned physiotherapy. Bronchoscopy, performed for diagnosis may also be therapeutic.

Chapter 63

INTRATHORACIC SPACE-OCCUPYING LESIONS

Intrathoracic space-occupying lesions give rise to symptoms and signs mainly because of pressure on surrounding structures, irrespective of nature of lesion.

Some tumours are highly malignant and give rise to metastases. All solid tumours should be regarded as malignant until proved otherwise.

Classification
Lesions in chest
1. Neoplasms

1.1 Benign: Chondroma, haemangioma, bronchial adenoma.
1.2 Malignant
1.2.1 Primary: Neuroblastoma, bronchial carcinoma.
1.2.2 Secondary: Wilms's tumour, neuroblastoma or osteogenic sarcoma.

2. Cysts

2.1 Containing air: Pneumatocele.
2.2 Containing fluid or solid matter. Hydatid, bronchial, diaphragmatic hernia.

Lesions in mediastinum
1. Benign. Ganglioneuroma; lymphangioma; haemangioma, lipoma, enterogenous cyst; dermoid cysts; enlarged thymus; tuberculous lymph nodes; abscess following injury to oesophagus or from tuberculous caries of spine.

2. Malignant. Sympathetic nerve tumours; lymphosarcoma; lymphadenoma, thymic tumours.

Clinical Features of Space-occupying Lesions
Symptoms and signs are caused by pressure on surrounding structures. Thus small masses may give rise to gross symptoms while large tumours can be silent, depending on position. Pressure may be:
1. Generalized. Resulting in distortion of chest wall; pushing down diaphragm.
2. On bronchus. Causing collapse of lobe or of whole lung.
3. On blood vessels. Veins most frequently affected, especially superior vena cava or subclavian. Give rise to venous engorgement.
4. On nerves: (*a*) Recurrent largyngeal; (*b*) Sympathetic chain; (*c*) Phrenic nerve.
5. On oesophagus. Rarely causes obstruction, but may cause displacement which can be revealed by barium swallow.
6. On bone: Giving rise to erosion of rib or vertebrae.
7. On thoracic duct. Resulting in chylothorax.

Radiological Diagnosis
Following points must be noted:
1. Size, shape and position of tumour, especially whether it lies anterior or posterior, in peripheral lung fields, or in mediastinum.
2. What structures are compressed.
3. Whether erosion of bone has occurred.

Diagnosis
Following investigations may give additional information:
1. Tuberculin reaction.
2. Casoni intradermal reaction and hydatid complement fixation test for hydatid disease.

3. Tomography and/or CT scan.
4. Screening chest with barium swallow.
5. Radiography of spine for enlargement of intervertebral foramen or tuberculous caries.
6. Angiography.
7. Bronchoscopy.
8. Thoracotomy.

Chapter 64   # ASTHMA

Asthma is a very common respiratory disorder in childhood One-third of all cases in all age groups commence before the age of 10 years, one-quarter of cases in childhood commence before the age of 1 year, 2–5% of schoolchildren have asthma. The incidence shows a steady fall (to approx. 1%) as age advances towards 16 years. Two males are affected for every 1 female.
Relationship to infantile eczema. Fifty per cent of children with infantile eczema develop asthma; 25% of asthmatic children have had infantile eczema. When coexistent with asthma it is often found that skin lesions become worse as asthma improves and vice versa. Reason unknown.

Aetiology
The asthma threshold. Asthma is a multifactorial disease in which factors summate. When the sum reaches a certain threshold, asthma occurs. Lowering the summation by treating one factor may relieve asthma but best results are obtained by treating all factors concerned.
   1. Constitutional Factors. Some people have a constitutional predisposition to develop asthma. All patients with asthma have this abnormal constitution and perhaps also some people who in fact never develop asthma. Two entities are probably involved:

> 1.1 A liability to develop reagins to certain substances.
> 1.2 A hyper-reactivity of the bronchi manifested by marked bronchoconstriction in response to a variety of substances, some of which are specific, e.g. pollens, and some non-specific, e.g. dusts or cold air.

   2. Hereditary Predisposition. In about 70% of children with asthma there is a family history of: (*a*) respiratory allergic disease (asthma, wheezy bronchitis, hay fever) or (*b*) neurodermatitis (infantile eczema, urticaria). The mode of hereditary transmission is uncertain, probably dominant with variable expression.
   3. Allergic Factors. Allergens causing asthma are almost always inhaled, very rarely from foods.
   Allergic Processes: Commoner type is immediate (Type I) reaction: antigen combines with reaginic antibody (IgE or occasionally IgG) on surface of mast cell in bronchi leading to release of 'spasmogens', e.g. histamine, bradykinins; 5-hydroxytryptamine and slow reacting substance of anaphylaxis (SRS-A). The spasmogens cause bronchoconstriction, increased mucus secretion, oedema of bronchial wall. Obstruction develops within minutes of exposure. In Type III reaction there is a delay of 6–12h between exposure and development of airways

obstruction. This reaction is associated with circulating antibodies, e.g. to aspergillus, house dust, mite, detergents. Patients with asthma often have raised IgE levels in blood, together with positive skin tests and family history. Antigens are pollens, mould spores, fungi (e.g. aspergillus), dander and house dust mite (*Dermatophagoides pteronyssinus*). Foods are more likely to cause urticaria than asthma.

4. Infective Factors. The original attack of asthma sometimes develops 3–6 weeks after a respiratory infection with persisting cough and sputum. Many children (especially young children) develop a wheezy attack with every acute upper respiratory infection, which settles down as the infection subsides. Asthma may fail to settle after acute stage of infection and becomes non-responsive to drug therapy.

Results of Infection
1. Mechanical effect from destruction of ciliated epithelium.
2. Inflammatory oedema with increased production and retention of mucus.
3. Possibly an immunological reaction to bacteria. Persistence of infection causes progressive tissue damage. Treatment does not 'cure' but only restores status quo.

5. Psychological Factors
5.1 Personality: Asthmatic children are usually considered to be overactive and 'highly strung' with intelligence above average. Some doubt has been thrown on this by careful studies. Asthmatic children tend to be more conscientious and try harder.
5.2 Precipitating causes
5.2.1 Acute Emotional Stress or Anxiety: Many asthmatics develop an acute attack during, or more frequently after, acute emotional stress or anxiety (e.g. birthday parties, examinations, etc.). Reason unknown. Possibly due to fall in catecholamine reserves.
5.2.2 Chronic Emotional Stress or Anxiety: In some asthmatics the disease is influenced by emotional factors in their personal environment, usually the home, less often school. May result from restrictions imposed by the disease, e.g. an inability to run.
Note: Psychological factors may cause asthmatic attacks to be more frequent, persistent or severe. Tend to improve in adolescence.

6. Non-specific Factors. In continuous asthma, or during episodes of intermittent asthma, non-specific factors may cause a fall in pulmonary ventilation, producing increased wheezing or even a severe attack, without the child having been in contact with any known specific allergen. The mechanisms involved are obscure.

Examples: Mechanical—exercise, panic and hyperventilation, laughter, heavy meal.

Note: Strenuous exercise sometimes produces lowered ventilation and wheezing without other evidence of asthma especially in children with a family history of asthma.

Physical—cold, change of weather, strong wind.

Chemical—sprays, paint, fumes or tobacco smoke.

Endocrine—menstruation.

Reflex—from nose due to congestion of mucosa.

Fatal cases are usually due to an acute exacerbation of intractable asthma. The findings in the respiratory system are similar irrespective of the aetiology and whether or not steroids have been given:

1. Lumen of small bronchi and bronchioles narrowed by oedema and infolding of mucosa. Occluded by mucus plugs containing fibrin, eosinophils, epithelial cells and lymphocytes.

2. Epithelium. Metaplasia of ciliated epithelium to goblet (mucus) cells or non-ciliated stratified epithelium.

3. Basement Membrane. Much thickened (reason unknown).

4. Submucosa. Oedematous and infiltrated with lymphocytes, plasma cells and eosinophils.

5. Mucus Glands. Marked hypertrophy.

6. Bronchial Muscle. Some hypertrophy usual.

7. Parenchyma. In the absence of chronic infection surprisingly little irreversible change in alveoli and interstitial tissues. Obstructive emphysema is rarely seen in young people even in long-standing continuous asthma.

Summary. Pathological findings indicate that in continuous asthma there is an ongoing production of mucus with deficient removal from the lungs due to damaged ciliated epithelium and narrowed airways. This results in progressive plugging of the bronchial lumen leading to cumulative bronchial obstruction and asphyxia which forms the basis of status asthmaticus.

Pathophysiology

Mechanisms of production and resolution of acute asthma attacks is ill-understood.

1. Asthmatic lungs are hypersensitive to histamine and acetylcholine, aerosols of which readily produce airways obstruction. *Note*: one theory of aetiology is that there is an abnormality in structure or function of β-adrenergic receptor-adenyl cyclase complex.

2. In acute attacks, airways obstruction is produced by:

     2.1 Increased tone and contraction of bronchial muscle.

     2.2 Oedema of mucosa;

     2.3 Increased production of mucus from goblet cells and glands.

3. In attacks the following changes occur in lung physiology:

     3.1 Vasoconstriction of pulmonary circulation to the unventilated areas of lung producing overall hypoxia.

     3.2 Increase in airways resistance (R) and a corresponding fall in lung compliance (C).

     3.3 Distension of the lungs with great increase in total lung capacity (TLC) and residual volume (RV), RV may be increased above the normal vital capacity (VC).

     3.4 Decrease in peak expiratory flow rate (PEF), forced vital capacity (FVC), and forced expiratory volume in 1 s (FEV$_1$). In children, FEV$_1$ should be over 80% cent of FVC, but falls to

50% or less during an attack and may remain low between attacks.

3.5 When pulmonary ventilation (e.g. FEV_1) is low, arterial oxygen saturation may fall. P_{CO_2} is often low because of hyperventilation. A rise is very serious, as it means that resting ventilation is maximal; further reduction from increased airway obstruction, exhaustion or use of depressant drugs may be rapidly fatal.

3.6 As attack subsides all parameters return towards normal, the fall in R preceding by some time the fall in TLC and rise in FEV_1. Symptoms disappear when the FEV_1 reaches more than 50% of expected value. Pa_{O_2} may not reach normal between attacks. In continuous asthma a deficiency of pulmonary ventilation is usually present except when patients given steroids.

Use of Pulmonary Function Tests in Asthma

1. *Estimation of PEF, FEV_1 and FVC* give adequate information. Portable apparatus available, but since tests require good cooperation, they cannot be used in children under about 4 years. PEF useful for assessing progress but too sensitive for use in severe asthma.

2. *Normal range varies greatly.* Relates to patient's height, therefore best to obtain base line for patient when relatively well and compare results later in attacks and during treatment.

3. *Reversibility of airway obstruction* should be established by making initial observations and repeating after use of bronchodilator. Results observed in FVC and FEV_1:

3.1 In normals or in intermittent asthmatics during intermissions: little or no increase following bronchodilatation occurs.

3.2 In acute attack, increase occurs.

3.3 In continuous asthma during intermissions, except sometimes in the presence of chronic infection due to the irreversibility of accumulated mucus and infective inflammatory oedema; increase occurs.

4. *Response of acute attacks* to therapy as judged by FEV_1 measurements:

4.1 The greatest response to treatment is early in an attack, probably due to less oedema and mucus accumulation.

4.2 The lower the initial FEV_1, the less the response to aerosol, salbutamol or isoprenaline.

Note: It follows that asthmatic attacks respond best to early and adequate treatment.

5. *Summary.* The main uses of pulmonary function tests are in:

5.1 Differential diagnosis from other forms of dyspnoea and hyperventilation.

5.2 Assessing the severity of asthma.

5.3 Assessing response to treatment.

Clinical Types

General considerations

1. Asthma should be regarded as continuous spectrum from mild recurrent

rhinitis with wheezing through to severe incapacitating disease or status asthmaticus.

2. If rhinitis, sinusitis and postnasal discharge are dominant features, the condition is sometimes called sinobronchitis.

3. In some children, paroxysmal nocturnal coughing bouts may be only sign of asthma.

Cyclic attacks of childhood. Tend to recur at fairly regular intervals especially during the winter. Often associated with respiratory infections. Typically heralded by lassitude or irritability for 1 day followed by rhinitis and cough developing into wheezing and dyspnoea (which may be severe) in further 12–24h. The attack starts to remit after further 24–48h, whole episode lasting 5–7 days. Abdominal pain may precede or accompany wheezing and dyspnoea. The child is completely well between episodes. This type of asthma is common in young children. The prognosis is good.

Intermittent asthma ('Adult Type'). Not cyclic or preceded by irritability, but may be related to specific aetiology. Often commences about 3 a.m. The duration and course are variable. The attack remits within a few hours or days, child becomes symptomless and pulmonary ventilation returns to normal. Prognosis very good, but many asthmatics who are thought on clinical grounds to be intermittent cases are found to be mild continuous cases by pulmonary function tests.

Continuous asthma (without clinical bronchitis). After an initial attack, pulmonary ventilation improves, but fails to return to normal during intermissions. Presumably persisting mucosal changes. Some dyspnoea, coughing or wheezing is usually present especially after exercise. Acute attacks are exacerbations of continuous state. Prognosis only fair.

Continuous asthma with bronchitis. Irreversible airway obstruction with persisting cough and mucoid sputum. Marked mucosal changes. Pulmonary ventilation usually markedly deficient. This group contains most of the intractable asthmatics who are liable to severe chest deformity, infection and death.

The Asthma Attack

Onset of an asthmatic attack may be insidious with rhinitis, gradually increasing cough and dyspnoea over a few days. It often commences in the evening getting worse over the next few days. This is particularly the picture in young children.

Or the attack may start abruptly with rapidly increasing dyspnoea and distress, often at night.

As the attack proceeds the child becomes obviously distressed. Severe cases may be cyanosed, grey, in shock, alae nasi in action. Some anxiety is commonly present but restlessness, irritability and mental confusion are evidence of cerebral hypoxia.

The breathing is characterized by much noise and effort, but little movement. Dyspnoea can become extreme with greatly overdistended lungs and marked difficulty in expiration. Accessory respiratory muscles in action with no pause between expiration and inspiration.

The percussion note is resonant with obliteration of the normal area of cardiac dullness. Wheezing is often loud with high pitched and low pitched rhonchi heard throughout the lungs, and often crepitations in the young child.

Danger Signs. A 'quiet lung' on auscultation (rhonchi disappear with extreme airflow obstruction), increasing dyspnoea, restlessness, and a shocked appearance are signs of widespread obstruction of small airways by mucus plugs. Other danger features are disturbed consciousness, marked pulsus paradoxus, elevation of P_{CO_2}, very low FEV_1, exhaustion, pneumothorax and pneumomediastinum.

Other features in long-standing cases. In continuous asthma increased lung volumes and airway obstruction produce barrel-shaped (or in younger children match-box shaped) chests with increased anteroposterior diameter, high shoulders and later, dorsal kyphosis. When obstruction is severe, kyphosis is marked and pigeon-chest deformity (retraction of lower anterior ribs and protruding sternum) occurs.

Duration of the attack varies greatly from hours to several days, but is often uniform for a particular child. Persistence of an attack (especially with pyrexia) is usually due to concomitant infection or less commonly to persisting acute anxiety.

Investigation and Assessment

The diagnosis of asthma is clinical. The purpose of investigation therefore is to determine the causation of the attacks, and to assess the prognosis. At leisure, in an interval between attacks, the following items should be considered.

1. History

1.1 Events associated with the onset of an attack. For example whether preceded by respiratory infections or strong emotional stress.

1.2 Variations in the disease pattern since the first attack, including any relationship to new factors such as changes in district or residence, respiratory infections, school, home, pets.

1.3 Association with antigens: house dust, animals, fibres, plants.

1.4 Prognosis. Whether the condition is improving, deteriorating or remaining stationary.

1.5 Clinical Types. Health between episodes. Whether asthma is produced by exertion, laughter or nonspecific factors.

2. Examination. Particular attention should be paid to:

2.1 Presence of overdistension, deformity, lack of expansion—all these indicate poor control.

2.2 Adventitia. Continuous asthma is suggested if rhonchi are present during intervals; persisting localized râles suggest focus of infection.

3. Pulmonary ventilation tests (PEF, FEV_1, FVC (*see* p. 194). Adequate assessment of asthma cannot be made without ventilation studies.

4. Sweat electrolytes (*see* p. 268). Should always be performed on children with continuous asthma to exclude cystic fibrosis. Asthma frequently complicates CF.

5. Radiography of chest should be performed infrequently. Children with asthma tend to have too many X-rays.

5.1 Evidence of over-inflation should be looked for. The ribs are widely spaced and placed at right angles to the sternum. Heart is often long and thin due to a low diaphragm. Increased bronchial markings show thickened bronchial walls enclosing a narrow air space.

5.2 Collapse: mucus plug syndrome. Minor segmental collapse due to mucus plugs is quite common. Rarely may be almost the only evidence that the child is an incipient asthmatic.

6. Skin tests. Because false positive and negative results often occur, tests are unreliable in children. Occasionally useful to confirm the history. Desensitization, which is time-consuming, expensive, unpleasant for the child and potentially dangerous, should never be instituted on the results of skin tests alone.

7. Radioallergosorbent test (RAST). Measure specific IgE antibodies against individual antigens. Test is only of value if the IgE is high.

Differential Diagnosis

Asthma must be considered whenever there is wheezing and evidence of airway obstruction.

Prognosis

Children and young adults usually improve spontaneously at puberty.

The prognosis is far better in asthma commencing before the age of 8–10 years. Fifty per cent become symptom free by adult life, but between 5 and 10% have a severe disability. Most asthmatic children in later life can become fully employed, more than half being symptom-free. The prognosis is related to the clinical type: (1) Intermittent asthma has a much better prognosis than continuous asthma. (2) The advent of bronchitis (infection indicated by persistent cough and sputum) gravely worsens the prognosis, e.g.:

1. Of asthmatics who do not develop bronchitis, almost all become symptomless. No deaths.

2. Of asthmatics who develop bronchitis approximately 20% become symptomless, 40% develop moderate asthma, 30% have severe asthma and 10% die.

Asthmatic deaths. Are very rare in childhood. Most cases are probably due to severe unrecognized status and/or drug overdosage, particularly aminophylline.

Treatment

The management of an asthmatic child must be individualized to each case. The object in the overall, long-range treatment should be to give the patient some periods when lung function returns to normal or near-normal and to eliminate sputum from the lungs.

Treatment between major attacks. Some guiding principles:

Since asthma is likely to continue for many years and much patience is needed by doctor, parents and child, the child should be taught to regard asthma as an inconvenience, not a disease. He should be given every encouragement to live a normal life. Restrictions should be minimal.

The key to the prevention of asthma attacks is to teach the parents, and later the child, the skilled use of the various drugs available, e.g.

1. Disodium cromoglycate (given 3–4 times daily by inhalation). This drug is of particular value in exercise-induced asthma. Cromoglycate should be given regularly for prevention. It is of no value in the acute attack. If any wheeze is present, the administration should be preceded by inhalation of a bronchodilator.

> 1.1 Via spinhaler—dose 1 capsule—can be doubled. Important to ensure capsule emptied by 3 or 4 deep breaths. Use of 'whistle' attachment helpful. Difficult to administer to children under 4 years. Acts by reducing bronchial sensitivity to inhaled allergens.

1.2 Via a mechanical inhaler for young children.

2. Long-acting slow release forms of theophylline may be given twice daily with benefit to children whose attacks are not controlled by cromoglycate alone.

3. Aerosol long-acting steroids are given as topical steroids to the respiratory epithelium. They cause minimal systemic effects and therefore are much to be preferred to oral steroids.

4. Maintenance corticosteroids should very rarely be required in paediatric practice. They should be given only for a few days in continuous asthma if all other drug therapy or manipulation of the environment has failed.

Home management of mild attacks. The key is to teach the parents that early vigorous management with bronchodilator e.g. salbutamol or terbutaline given by inhalation, either metered in the older child with occasional wheeze, or by mechanical inhaler in more severe attacks in the older child, and always by this method in younger children, will prevent most attacks becoming severe. The advent of the mechanical insufflator for use with bronchodilatation, and occasionally with cromoglycate, is one of the most important advances in asthma therapy in recent years.

Oral bronchodilators are of less value but may be adequate for mild wheezing in an infant.

Some accessory therapy

1. Treatment of allergy. Birds or animals should not be kept if the child is known to be sensitive. Offending plants should be removed. House dust (the commonest allergen) should be reduced by good housekeeping. Mattresses should be of rubber or plastic. No feathers in either the pillows or duvet.

2. Treatment of infection. Antibiotics should only be given in asthma if there is undoubted evidence of infection, i.e. moderate pyrexia or purulent sputum.

Postural drainage with preceding bronchodilatation, is very valuable in continuous asthma when infection is present.

3. Breathing exercises help to achieve relaxed breathing during attacks, but do not alter the pulmonary base line.

4. Prevention of concomitant allergic rhinitis by topical cromoglycate or steroid may reduce frequency of asthma attacks. Antihistamines are of little value.

5. Psychological psychotherapy rarely of benefit but commonsense advice to parents and child should be given, aimed for instance at:

    5.1 Persuading child that he is not abnormal.

    5.2 Separating a too close emotional attachment of parent and child by interposing sport, mixing with other children, etc. Especially releasing child from overprotection by mother.

    5.3 Encouraging aggressive attitude towards life and to give outlets for mental and social development.

6. Environment and Institutions. Changes of environment do not help children as much as adults. Some chronic asthmatic children improve in hospital, at boarding school, or in special institutions. Probably due to combination of factors—less exposure to household allergens; regular life; feeling of security; absence of emotional tension or overprotection.

Treatment of acute attacks. Acute attacks are either attacks of intermittent asthma which respond readily to therapy or acute exacerbations of continuous asthma which are more resistant.

Management of more severe attacks. In asssessing the need to hospitalize a child with an acute attack of asthma, many factors need to be considered such as:

1. The severity and pattern of previous attacks.

2. Whether the parents possess a mechanical inhaler to administer bronchodilators.

3. The skill of the parents; the cooperation of the child and various environmental factors.

Failed therapy by inhalation is an indication for intravenous treatment to control hydration and acid–base balance, and to administer bronchodilators and hydrocortisone.

Additional therapy:

1. Postural drainage which should always be preceded by inhalation of a bronchodilator.

2. Oxygen therapy is very useful in severe cases. It should be given intermittently and patient encouraged to respiratory effort to prevent a rising P_{CO_2}.

3. Antibiotics are of no value in uncomplicated asthma.

Bibliography

Kuzemko J. A. (1980) A natural history of childhood asthma. *J. Pediatr.* **97**, 886.
Milner A. D. (1981) Bronchodilator drugs in childhood asthma. *Arch. Dis. Child.* **56**, 84.

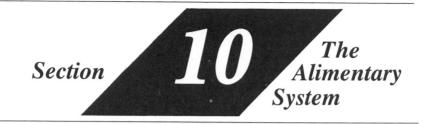
Chapter 65   *DEVELOPMENT OF THE DIGESTIVE SYSTEM*

The Gut

At birth shows relatively greater development of secreting mechanism than of supporting musculature. Stomach very distensile. Most food leaves stomach in 2 h, but may remain more than 8 h. Progress in lower intestine more rapid: some food reaches caecum in 6 h, reaching faeces by 15 h. Transit is often more rapid in pre-term infants, although extreme immaturity is sometimes associated with colonic pseudo-obstruction, perhaps because of incomplete ganglion cell migration.

Gastric Hydrochloric Acid

Secretion high immediately after birth. Falls in first 10 days, remains low up to 6 months, then gradually increases during first year to levels comparable to adults.

Pancreatic Function

Secretion of enzymes relatively low at birth, particularly in pre-term infants. Increases rapidly in few days.

Liver Function

Conjugation of bilirubin is poorly developed at birth, particularly in pre-term infants, but rapidly matures. Bile salt pool is small in pre-term babies. Taurine conjugates predominate.

Intestinal Disaccharidases

Lactase develops in last trimester to maximal levels at term, which decline after infancy, particularly in African and Asiatic races. Sucrase-isomaltase activity well developed at birth, even in pre-term infants.

Composition of Normal Stool

1. Water. 80%
2. Protein. About 8%
3. Carbohydrate. (*a*) As sugar. All absorbed in older child; up to ½% sugar in faeces of normal infants. (*b*) As starch. Usually some present. Starch granules can be demonstrated by blue coloration on addition of iodine to stools.
4. Fat. Appears as neutral fat, soaps and fatty acids. Quantity varies: up to 50% dried weight in breast-fed; up to 30% in artificially fed. Two-thirds of fat is split.

| Chapter 66 | FUNCTIONAL PROBLEMS OF INFANTS AND TODDLERS |

'Colic'

Screaming or crying episodes in young infants are very common and often alleged to be caused by colic, with scant evidence.

The following should be considered:

1. Discomfort from hunger, thirst, wet clothing, tiredness.
2. Poor mother–infant relationship; anxious, irritable mother.
3. Pain from otitis media, oesophagitis, etc.
4. Intestinal obstruction or acute abdomen if:
   4.1 Signs of shock: pallor, or look of apprehension during or just after attack of screaming.
   4.2 Pushing away warmed hand examining abdomen, if persistent.
   4.3 Guarding or rigidity of abdomen.

Management

If no organic cause apparent, reassurance and explanation of the infant's need for contact with relaxed parents is the only measure which frequently helps. Antispasmotics and gripe water of no proven value, very occasionally a particularly difficult baby justifies mild sedation with a drug such as trimeprazine (Vallergan) or Dicyclomine hydrochloride (Merbentyl).

Vomiting

Should be regarded as significant if infant vomits bile or fails to gain weight. Mild vomiting very common, significance often difficult to evaluate.

Causes

1. Air swallowing. A baby when sucking always swallows some air, which is eructed later ('burping'). If large amount, food may come up with air bubble. Common reasons for swallowing air: (*a*) If breast-fed—retracted nipples; poor milk supply; ravenous baby; leaving infant too long at breast; nasal obstruction. (*b*) If artificially fed—small hole in teat; sucking empty bottle; nasal obstruction; underfeeding. (*c*) Crying.

2. Organic causes. (*See Table* 68.1, p. 211) (*a*) Obstruction, e.g. pyloric stenosis; duodenal atresia, etc. (*b*) Oesophageal reflux, with or without hiatus hernia.

3. Symptomatic. Almost any acute or chronic illness will give rise to vomiting in a small child.

4. Reflex. Following violent cough, as in whooping cough.

5. Rumination. A rare disorder in which infant regurgitates food into mouth and retastes it for pleasure. A compulsive habit. Sometimes significant amounts are vomited, to the extent that occasional child fails to thrive.

Constipation

Aetiology

The following causes should be considered:

1. Physiological. Breast-fed babies may only have bowels open every 2–7 days.
2. Dietetic. (*a*) Underfeeding. (*b*) Too little fluid, especially in hot weather. (*c*) Early introduction of solids.
3. Organic lesions. (*a*) Obstructive, e.g. intestinal atresia, meconium plug, intestinal aganglionosis, pyloric stenosis. (*b*) Metabolic, e.g. hypothyroidism, hypercalcaemia, renal tubular acidosis, diabetes insipidus.
4. Occurs with mental handicap, negativism, faulty training.

Symptoms
The following may occur: pain on passing motion, sometimes with blood streaking of stool from laceration of anus; abdominal distension; colic. If very severe, intestinal obstruction occurs with vomiting and visible peristalsis.

Diagnosis
See under appropriate sections.

Treatment
1. That of the cause.
2. *Drug therapy.* Only if essential. (*a*) Fruit juice. (*b*) Milk of Magnesia. Dose will have to be adjusted to individual case. (*c*) Cautiously increasing sucrose content of feeds widely used, often effective.

Toddler Diarrhoea

A common condition in children aged 6 months to 3 years or more, perhaps equivalent to one form of adult 'irritable bowel syndrome'.

Clinical Features
Stools watery or mushy, not particularly offensive; colour yellow or brown, often with mucus but no blood. Usually worse in morning. Stool number varies from 1 to 12 or more daily. *Child continues to thrive*, typically active and otherwise healthy. Onset may follow suspected or documented gastroenteritis. Spontaneous bouts of remission and relapse common.

Investigations
1. Stools negative for pathogens, parasites and reducing substances and do not contain excess fat globules.
2. Jejunal biopsy normal or shows minor abnormalities only on light microscopy.

Aetiology
Uncertain, but some evidence exists for:
   1. Primary disorder of motility: inability to suppress migrating motor complexes (and resultant peristaltic waves) during meals, so that small intestinal transit time is shortened and the colon may be unable to compensate.
   2. Chronic, low-grade infection of small intestine.
   3. Increased secretion of prostaglandins by small intestine.

Differential Diagnosis
   1. Food allergy, particularly to cow's milk, should be suspected if eczema or other atopic features are present.

2. Malabsorption syndromes: usually with associated failure to thrive.
3. Chronic enteric infection, particularly in immunodeficiency states.
4. Ganglioneuroma.
5. Lactase or sucrase-isomaltase deficiency.
6. Giardiasis.

Treatment
1. Reassurance that the condition is nearly always self-limiting by age 4 years.
2. A trial of cow's milk exclusion is worth trying.

Chapter 67   ## FUNCTIONAL PROBLEMS IN OLDER CHILDREN

Vomiting

Very common symptoms of many diseases in childhood. Persistent vomiting should always be regarded as due to raised intracranial pressure until proved otherwise.

The Periodic Syndrome (*Cyclical Vomiting*)
Syndrome characterized by periodic bouts of severe vomiting with ketosis, occurring at fairly regular intervals. Uncommon.

Aetiology
Unknown, but emotional disturbances are frequently associated. Some affected children have migraine.

Treatment
May be symptomatic. Intravenous fluids usually required until vomiting ceases. Sometimes helped by clonidine (Dixarit) or propranolol as prophylactics.

Recurrent Abdominal Pain

Very common symptom in children of school age, affecting up to 10% of children in some series. About 90–95% are psychosomatic.

Clinical Features
Child often serious, conscientious, introspective. Pain usually central or diffuse, not lateralized, varies in intensity, frequency and duration. Probably arises from intestinal pressure changes ('spasm'). Bowels normal or constipated. Vomiting uncommon. May be associated psychosomatic problems, e.g. headache, limb pains or enuresis. Family history of migraine common, also social disturbances, e.g. school problems, divorce, bereavement. Clinical examination usually negative, but must be thorough.

Investigations
Urine should always be examined. Other investigations usually unnecesary, but

barium meal or upper alimentary endoscopy may be required in some cases as peptic ulcer symptoms are often atypical in childhood.

Differential Diagnosis (*Table 67.1*)

Table 67.1.   Causes of recurrent abdominal pain (90–95 % are psychosomatic)

Gastrointestinal tract	Urogenital tract
Recurrent pharyngitis	Hydronephrosis
Peptic ulcer	Pyelonephritis
Bezoar	Renal calculi
Duplication	Renal and suprarenal neoplasm
Intermittent volvulus	Ovarian cyst
Meckel's diverticulum	Dysmenorrhoea
Appendicitis	Mittelschmerz in adolescents
Mesenteric adenitis	Endometriosis
Abdominal tuberculosis	Testicular torsion
Regional enteritis	Testicular neoplasm
(Crohn's disease)	
Ulcerative colitis	*Liver, spleen and pancreas*
Milk protein intolerance	Cholecystitis
Other food intolerances	Cholelithiasis
Lactose intolerance	Familial and other pancreatitis
Dietary indiscretion	Cystic fibrosis
Constipation	Massive splenomegaly
Drugs	*Metabolic*
Anticonvulsants	Hypoglycaemia
Antibiotics	Porphyria
Bronchodilators	Lead poisoning
etc.	Hereditary angioneurotic oedema
	Familial hyperlipidaemia types I, IV, V

Always difficult to completely exclude organic causes but diagnosis can be made with some confidence if history gives positive evidence of psychosocial disturbance, e.g. recent parental divorce, and clinical examination reveals no abnormality.

Management
If no evidence of organic disease and history suggests psychosomatic aetiology, careful explanation should be given to parents and temptation to investigate further resisted. Drug treatment not indicated. Reassurance often very helpful in itself, reducing frequency and severity of bouts.

Chronic Constipation (*Idiopathic Megacolon*)

Common condition. Incidence higher in boys, but difference not so striking as in Hirschsprung's disease.

Main Types
1. *Infantile*. Baby has always had difficulty with motions especially when bottle fed. Motions often hard and craggy; sometimes blood streaked and painful to pass. Length of time between motions gradually increases.
2. *Childhood*. Age 18 months to 4 years. Bowels previously normal. Sudden onset associated with episode such as: new baby, visit to stay with grandmother, admission to hospital, illness (e.g. measles). Sometimes history of pot-forcing,

bribery, smacking, or excessive interest in potting on part of mother, leading to negativism in toddler. Constipation mild at first but may become chronic if: (*a*) Insufficient treatment of mild constipation. (*b*) Fissure-in-ano develops with vicious circle of pain→voluntary suppression of defaecation→constipation with hard, massive faeces→pain on eventual defaecation.

3. In mentally backward children. Severe constipation common. May start at any age from 1 to 5 years. Child never clean, gradually becomes more and more constipated.

4. Associated with physical handicap, e.g. meningomyelocele, amyotonia congenita, postoperative anal stricture.

Clinical features

1. Persistent constipation (obstipation)

2. Faecal soiling. (*a*) Faeces in rectum protrude through anus. (*b*) Diarrhoea. Due to liquefaction of faeces in colon by bacterial action. Liquid seeps past static faeces in rectum. Gives rise to faecal incontinence.

Abdominal Examination. Craggy mass can be palpated in descending colon. If large amount of faeces present, mass tends to be midline from dilatation of sigmoid. Following points should be noted: (*a*) Mass painless. (*b*) Faeces palpable in midline. Rare in right inguinal fossa. (*c*) Faeces can be indented. (*d*) Normal defaeciation rarely sufficient to shift large mass. (*e*) Characteristic picture on straight radiograph of abdomen, or with barium enema.

Examination of Anus. May be forced open by faeces. Circumanal soiling almost invariable unless bowels recently opened.

Digital Examination of Rectum. Rectum loaded with faeces right down to anus.

The 'Potting Couple'

Relationship between mother and constipated child complicated but important.

1. Mother may have originated condition by over-anxiety about bowel action and/or by pot-forcing.

2. When condition established, mother's anxiety understandable and inevitable, especially if faecal soiling present.

3. Child may perpetuate condition as attention-seeking device.

Course

Normally urge to defaecate occurs when rectum is loaded. Children with chronic constipation become accustomed to perpetually loaded rectum. Rectum and lower colon passively dilate to huge size. Constipation alternates with overflow diarrhoea and massive liquid motions with hard lumps in it.

Barium Enema

Not necessary. Reveals grossly dilated colon and rectum; may extend proximally to transverse colon, distally to anal sphincter.

Differential Diagnosis.

From intestinal aganglionosis, *see* p. 217.

Treatment

1. *Initial removal of semi-impacted faeces.* Daily laxative should be given in adequate dosage. Mixture of several aperients often best. Suppositories rarely

required. Olive oil instilled into colon to soften faeces, followed by daily enema until the colon is clear.

2. *Prevention of recurrence* (*a*) Careful training and inculcation of good habits essential. Often best accomplished by stay in hospital with sympathetic nursing staff. Position must be explained to parents and to child if old enough, and cooperation obtained. (*b*) Psychological position must be reviewed and cause of attention-seeking must be remedied. (*c*) Regular laxatives e.g. Senna granules. A softening agent, such as dioctyl sodium sulphosuccinate is an important adjunct, particularly when anal fissure has occurred. Dosage—by trial and error. Should be given two or three times daily for month or so and dosages gradually decreased when good habits formed.

Prognosis
1. In infantile type regular aperients usually required throughout childhood; often for life.

2. In mentally normal children with acquired condition, disease progresses by remission and relapses, remissions gradually becoming longer. Duration from start of active treatment to cure usually 3 months to 3 years depending on psychological background.

3. In mentally backward children little hope of cure until mental age about 7 years.

4. In children with physical handicaps cure may never be possible. Palliative measures such as bi-weekly enemata may be required.

Encopresis

Far less common than enuresis. Characterized by repeated passing of faeces at inappropriate places and times. To be differentiated from *overflow incontinence*, where child's abdomen is loaded with faecal masses (*see* p. 206), which child voluntarily retains. In overflow incontinence stools are fluid and examination of abdomen and rectum discloses masses of faeces. Illness may follow a fissure-in-ano or fear of toilet or be a reaction against parental attitudes, especially inappropriate toilet training. Child strongly resists enemas, suppositories and rectal examinations. Enuresis present in a third.

Children with true encopresis pass regular and formed motions—often achieved control of faeces at appropriate time but relapse. Mothers may be overdemanding and meticulous; often neurotic, requiring psychotherapy.

Management
1. True encopresis. Refer to child psychiatrist.

2. Overflow incontinence. Combination of stool-softening agent, mild laxative and 'informal psychotherapy'. Ultimate prognosis good but symptom may persist for several yeras. Social worker may be helpful if domestic or school problems.

Chapter 68	# *CONGENITAL ANATOMICAL DEFECTS*

Micrognathos

Condition in which mandible is abnormally small. Minor degrees common; gross condition rare. May be associated with cleft palate (Pierre Robin syndrome).

Clinical Features
Tongue falls backwards, causing difficulty in breathing and sucking, especially when supine. Severe cyanotic attacks and choking may occur.

Treatment in Severe Cases
1. Tube feeding.
2. Nurse child prone; this develops mandible by ensuring that lower jaw is protruded to hold teat, also prevents tongue falling back.
3. Dental plate to occlude cleft palate.

Prognosis
If child survives first few months ultimate prognosis is good.

Cleft Lip (Hare Lip)

Varies from small notch to complete cleft. May be unilateral (more commonly left side) or bilateral.

Cleft Palate

Varies from bifid uvula to complete cleft. If associated with bilateral cleft lip, premaxilla (morphologically the prognathos or snout) projects, leading to hideous deformity.

Signs and Symptoms
Diagnosis obvious. Sucking may be difficult or impossible, with regurgitation of milk through nose. Tendency to upper respiratory infection. Otitis media common.

Treatment
1. *Obturator*. Dental plate to occlude cleft made as soon as possible after birth. Larger plates required as child grows. Often gap narrows sufficiently with this treatment.
2. *Orthodontics* of great value from birth to give correct alignment of alveolar segments and reposition of protuberant premaxilla prior to closure of lip at 3 months of age.
3. *Feeding*. Spoon feeding. If suction inadequate even with dental plate.
4. *Preoperative*. Correct respiratory infection. Child must be in good state of nutrition, adequately hydrated. Compatible blood should be available.
5. *Operation*. Performed between 12 and 18 months, before speech commences. Repair may be in two stages.
6. *Postoperative*. Skilled nursing essential. Prophylactic antibiotics. Blood transfusion frequently required. Semi-fluid diet from spoon.
7. *Speech education*. Vitally important, but speech often poor even with surgically perfect repair; probably due to weak musculature.

Tracheo-oesophageal Fistula (Oesophageal Atresia)

Embryology
Trachea develops from primitive gut. At 4th week of fetal life, median

laryngotracheal groove appears on anterior wall of pharynx and oesophagus, deepens, and lips fuse to form tube. Upper end opens into pharynx, lower end develops into lungs. Fusion of lips may be abnormal, leading to various types of atresia and fistula.

Incidence
About 1 : 2000 births.

Pathological Types (*Fig. 68.1*)

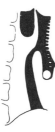 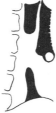 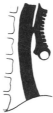 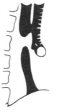 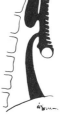

| Esophageal atresia with distal TEF | Esophageal atresia without TEF | TEF without esophageal atresia | Esophageal atresia with proximal TEF | Esophageal atresia with proximal and distal TEF |

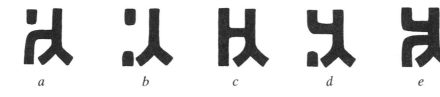

a   *b*   *c*   *d*   *e*

Fig. 68.1. Tracheo-oesophageal anomalies. (*a*) Oesophageal atresia with distal tracheo-oesophageal fistula. (*b*) Oesophageal atresia without tracheo-oesophageal fistula. (*c*) Tracheo-oesophageal fistula without oesophageal atresia. (*d*) Ocsophageal atresia with proximal tracheo-oesophageal fistula. (*e*) Oesophageal atresia with proximal and distal tracheo-oesophageal fistula. (By kind permission of *Pediatric Clinical Gastroenterology* by C. C. Roy, A. Silverman and F. J. Cozzetto.)

1. Upper oesophagus ends as blind sac at level of superior thoracic inlet. Lower oesophagus communicates with trachea, thus allowing air to enter and distend stomach. Commonest (75%).

2. Both parts of oesophagus are blind. Stomach is then empty of air. Less common.

3. 'H' type fistula, third most common.

In cases coming to post-mortem evidence of inhalation of saliva or feed almost always found, especially affecting right upper lobe.

Clinical Features
1. Mother may have hydramnios, as amniotic fluid is not swallowed.
2. The infant brings up frothy saliva from birth.
3. The abdomen is distended with gas (except in Type 2 when no air can reach gut and abdomen is flat).

4. Gastric juice refluxes up distal fistulas into lung causing chemical pneumonitis.

5. *Food should not be given.* If it is, fluid fills blind pouch and excess floods over into trachea, with risk of bronchopneumonia. In cases in which feed has been attempted, cyanosis during feed may be first symptom noticed.

Immediate Management

Adult-sized radio-opaque catheter should be passed into oesophagus. It will only pass about 10 cm (4 in) before reaching obstruction. If a small catheter is used it may coil up in pouch. Radiographs of chest and abdomen taken to demonstrate (1) level of obstruction, (2) whether gut contains gas (excludes Type 2), (3) presence of associated anorectal anomalies intestinal atresia, hemivertebrae or pneumonia.

Surgical Treatment

Operation must be performed as soon after birth as possible, owing to danger of lung collapse due to inhalation of mucus or feed. On no account must any feed be given until diagnosis is established.

Baby is transported to surgical centre with head held up and with repeated suction of blind upper pouch. This is to prevent gastric reflux which is more irritating than saliva.

Prognosis

If infant >2·5 kg, no associated anomalies, no pneumonia on presentation, 95% survive with operation. If infant <2·5 kg with severe associated anomalies or pneumonia, 30% success.

Gastro-oesophageal Reflux *(Hiatus Hernia; Partial Thoracic Stomach; Congenital Short Oesophagus; Oesophageal Reflux; Cardiochalasia)*

Part of stomach located in thorax. Manifested clinically by vomiting from birth. If severe, regurgitated acid causes ulceration of oesophagus with haematemesis and ultimate scarring and stenosis of oesophagus. Identical reflux may occur without demonstrable intrathoracic stomach (hiatus hernia).

Aetiology

Sex. Male: female, 3 : 1.
Age. Symptoms usually date from birth.

Clinical Features

1. *Vomit with feeds from birth.* Copious and sometimes projectile, or minor spills, e.g. two or three vomits may occur during course of feed. Vomiting tends to improve when: (*a*) Child starts to take solid food. (*b*) Greater curvature of stomach elongates to form fundus, thus developing pinch-cock action at lower end of oesophagus. (*c*) Child sits up, and especially when child walks.

Note: Above clinical features *alone* comprise common benign condition of cardiochalasia (uncomplicated oesophageal reflux). Vomiting due to laxity of cardia which allows regurgitation of stomach contents especially when child is lying down.

2. *Failure to gain weight.* Common if vomiting severe. Constipation less common.
3. Screaming may be severe and be presenting feature.
4. Cough from aspiration and apnoeic spells.
5. *Haematemesis.* Usually only small amount with vomit. Occasionally melaena. Indicates oesophagitis and worsening of prognosis.
6. *Anaemia.* Uncommon. Usually due to malnutrition, less commonly to blood loss.
7. *Dysphagia.* Late sign. May be due to spasm from active oesophagitis, or to actual stricture formation.

Investigations
1. *Gastrografin swallow.* Cineradiographic technique of value. May show: (*a*) Free oesophageal reflux but no herniation (so-called 'cardiochalasia). Common in neonates. (*b*) Hiatus hernia. (i) Sliding type, i.e. oesophagogastric junction displaced through oesophageal hiatus. Hernia is retroperitoneal. (ii) Para-oesophageal type, i.e. oesophagogastric junction remains in normal subphrenic location while fundus of stomach herniates past it into peritoneum-lined recess, (iii) Combined type. (*c*) Large loculus of stomach in chest. Usually girls. Usually right side. (*d*) Oesophagitis. Indicated by associated spasm and sometimes filling defect due to an ulcer. (*e*) Stricture formation; sometimes with considerable oesophageal dilatation above it.
2. *Oesophagoscopy.* Gives evidence of oesophagitis with or without stricture.
3. pH monitoring of oesophagus may reveal acid regurgitation.

Complications
1. Oesophagitis.
2. Stricture formation.
3. Pyloric stenosis may coincide with hiatus hernia.

Differential Diagnosis (*Table 68.1*)

Table 68.1.   Differential diagnosis of vomiting in infancy

1. Idiopathic vomiting of infancy. Common, usually responds to thickened feeds. Generally mild, no demonstrable pathology
2. Hiatus hernia/gastro-oesophageal reflux
3. Feeding problems
4. Pyloric stenosis. *Projectile*
5. Surgical causes: atresias, malrotation with congenital duodenal bands, enteric duplication, Hirschsprung's disease, etc.
6. Peptic ulcer
7. Cow's milk protein intolerance
8. Infections: septicaemia, urinary tract, otitis media
9. Raised intracranial pressure
10. Metabolic disorders: Congenital adrenal hyperplasia, phenylketonuria, galactosaemia, hypercalcaemia, uraemia

Treatment
1. Child should be kept upright day and night. Nurse in baby chair.
2. Antacid therapy of value in oesophagitis e.g. an alginate (Gaviscon), which forms surface foam on gastric contents or cimetidine.

3. Thickening feeds with cereal may be useful adjunct. May cause mild diarrhoea.

4. Surgery; fundal plication for severe reflux unresponsive to medical treatment.

Congenital Atresia and Stenosis of Small Intestine

1. Atresia
Most commonly in ileum, less often in duodenum or jejunum. May be multiple. May be associated with cystic fibrosis.

2. Stenosis
Fifty per cent occur in duodenum, varies from complete or almost complete obliteration of lumen to slight narrowing. Often duodenal stenosis/atresia in Down's syndrome.

Clinical Features
1. Persistent vomiting: Commences within few hours of birth. Often projectile; in 90% vomit contains bile.

2. Constipation: Meconium stool small and drier than normal; green colour, but not so dark as usual.

3. Abdominal distension: May be gross. Mainly in upper or lower abdomen, depending on site of obstruction. Visible peristalsis usually observed.

Lesser degrees of stenosis cause milder symptoms, and occasionally may not become manifest until late childhood or adult life.

Investigations

Radiography of abdomen
1. Plain anteroposterior film usually gives most information owing to presence of gas in dilated proximal gut and absence in collapsed distal portion. Fluid levels often present. Film may have to be taken with child lying on one side or upside down if anorectal malformation sought. Usually possible to discover site of obstruction.

2. Gastrografin meal seldom adds further information and can be dangerous as gastrografin is hyperosmolar and causes hypovolaemia. Gastrografin enema shows distal bowel patency, relieves obstruction with meconium plug, and often with meconium ileus; may show 'cone' of Hirschsprung's disease; may show a malrotated caecum.

Differential Diagnosis (See Table 68.2)

Treatment
Surgical, after restoration of fluid and electrolytes, if necessary.

Persistent Meckel's Diverticulum

Remnant of vitello-intestinal duct. Connects free border of ileum about 50–100 cm above ileocaecal valve, to umbilicus. Found in 2% of all autopsies, 3 males : 1 female. Diverticulum usually lined by gastric or pancreatic mucosa. *Can give rise to following complications*:

Table 68.2.   Differential diagnosis of intestinal obstruction in neonatal period

	Congenital intestinal atresia	Infantile intestinal aganglionsis	Meconium plugs	Meconium ileus	Anorectal malformation	Paralytic ileus from peritonitis	Malrotation of gut and volvulus	Pyloric stenosis
Age of onset	First 2 days	2–30 days	Birth	First 2 days	Birth	Birth	Within first month	2–6 weeks
Sex incidence	Equal	Males more common	Equal	Equal	?	Equal	Equal	Males more common
Vomit	Projectile; bile-stained	Bile-stained	Bile-stained	Bile-stained	Occurs late	Bile-stained	Bile-stained	Projectile; no bile
Constipation	Present	Delay in passing meconium	Absolute	Present	Absolute	Absolute	Not complete	Mild
Stool	May be light green stool at first only	Small, may be hard	Nil	Often nil		Nil	Normal	Normal at first, then 'hunger' stool
Abdominal distension	Upper abdomen	Generalized	Lower abdomen	Generalized	Lower abdomen	Generalized	At first upper abdomen, later	Stomach-shape
Visible peristalsis	'Step-ladder'	Large intestine	Large intestine	Slight	Absent at first	Absent, no bowel sounds	Present	In stomach
Special features	Duodenal stenosis especially in mongols	Constriction felt per rectum	White, firm plug at anus	Sweat test positive	May be dimple at site of anus	Due to intra-peritoneal haemorrhage infection, etc.	Barium enema diagnostic	Pyloric tumour palpable

1. Haemorrhage. Occurs in 45 % of cases recognized during childhood. Bleeding often severe, dark at first, but later bright red. Rarely accompanied by abdominal discomfort. Chronic blood loss uncommon.

Note: Massive painless bleeding per rectum in first two years of life usually indicates Meckel's diverticulum.

(Differential diagnosis, *see Table 71.1*, p. 218.)

2. Abdominal pain. (*a*) May give rise to symptoms similar to acute appendicitis—pain, vomiting, fever, leucocytosis. Pain remains para-umbilical, does not shift to right iliac fossa. (*b*) Vague abdominal pain may occur—cause unknown. This pain sometimes precedes haemorrhage.

3. Intussusception. Meckel's diverticulum occasionally acts as starting point of intussusceptum.

4. Obstruction. Usually around a band from tip of Meckel's to root of mesentery, rarely attached to umbilicus.

5. Fistula formation. If patent throughout, fistula with bile-stained fluid may present at umbilicus.

Investigations
Diverticulum not usually visualized radiologically unless screening of small bowel performed by experienced radiologist. Ectopic gastric mucosa demonstrated by localization of i.v. injected radioactive technetium 99. Detectable by gamma-camera if more than 1·5 cm gastric mucosa present.

Enterogenous Cysts (*Reduplication of Intestine; Enteric Cysts*)

Rare condition of reduplication of any portion of alimentary canal can occur from tongue to anus. Can be large or small. Lumen patent, but seldom communicates with gut.

Essential Pathology
1. Often strongly connected to intestine, with no line of cleavage between duplication and intestine. Muscular coat may be common to both.
2. Lined by gut mucosa, but not necessarily same type as contiguous intestine. Often ectopic gastric mucosa, which may bleed or ulcerate.
3. Only occasionally communicates with intestine.

Symptoms
May present with pain or intestinal obstruction. Sometimes lump in abdomen discovered accidentally.

Treatment
Excision. Usually portion of bowel has to be resected.

Anorectal Malformations

Many varieties occur. Most have a fistulous track and are not imperforate. If lesion above puborectalis, even with correction, control will not be normal.

Clinical Features
Neonatal intestinal obstruction with abdominal distension and delayed passage of

meconium, bile-stained vomitus. Meconium or flatus in urine of male with recto-urethral fistula. Meconium at fistulous opening or bluish colour under membrane of low type. Constipation from stenotic ectopic orifice. Associated anomalies: intestinal, cardiac, renal, vertebral—common.

Radiology
Lateral view of pelvis whilst baby held upside down. Level of puborectalis muscle (muscle of continence) indicated by line drawn between symphysis pubis and sacrococcygeal junction. If air at, or above this line it is a high lesion. Marker at anal dimple also gives guide to distance of bowel above skin level. Gas may take 24–48h to reach end of dilated gut and displace meconium. Micturating cystourethrogram may show fistula in male.

Treatment
Seek orifice or incise fistulous track back to anal orifice and dilate. If in doubt, and for all high lesions, transverse colostomy, and at 9–10 months of age definitive procedure by sacroperineal approach to place rectum anterior to the puborectal sling for maximum chance of continence.

Results
Excellent for low lesions. Good to poor control for high lesions: good are continent with a formed stool but incontinent with diarrhoea. Most improve around puberty with muscular and intellectual maturation.

'Microscopic' Anus

Minute hold present through which meconium escapes. May require lens to find it. Anal dimple may bulge when child cries.

Treatment
Dilatation of hole.

Ectopic Anus

Anal orifice displaced anteriorly and may be on perineal surface, within vagina, at base of scrotum or as part of hypospadias in common with urethra.
Note:
1. Ectopic anus usually has sphincter control.
2. Stricture common and dilatation may be required otherwise megacolon develops.

Chapter 69   # INFANTILE HYPERTROPHIC PYLORIC STENOSIS

Common (2–3 per 1000) cause of vomiting in young babies. Not a true congenital malformation, but may be initiated in utero.

Aetiology
Is thought to be multifactorial, with interaction of genetic and environmental factors. Male : female, 4 : 1. Male relatives of female patients particularly susceptible. Occurs in pre-term and term infants alike, more common in firstborn. Autonomic control of gastric emptying may be abnormal. Can be produced in newborn puppies by administration of pentagastrin to mother during pregnancy.

Age of Onset
Second to fifth week of life, but frequently 6–8 weeks old when first seen. Rarely found in first week.

Pathology
Pylorus elongated and thickened to form hard tumour about 1·5 cm long. Greater hypertrophy of circular muscle fibres than longitudinal. Terminates abruptly at duodenum. Normal vascularity reduced by compression. Mucous membrane normal. Secondary effects—stomach dilated; gastritis, oesophagitis.

Pathogenesis
Two elements required before symptoms occur: Pyloric tumour and superadded spasm or mucosal oedema. Asymptomatic 'tumours' have been reported.

Symptoms and Signs
Child usually thrives for first 2–4 weeks of life. Later:
1. *Vomiting*. Projectile; usually after each feed. May become larger in quantity and only occur after 2 or 3 feeds. Vomit not bile-stained, but some blood streaks often present. Vomiting increases in force and volume. No nausea as shown by the fact that the infant will accept another feed immediately.
2. *Constipation*. Often complete. If not, stool may be green 'hunger' stool.
3. *Baby becomes dehydrated and loses weight. Metabolic alkalosis occurs. Rarely, infants become jaundiced, probably because of adverse effects of starvation on bilirubin conjugation.*
4. *Visible gastric peristalsis* (late sign). Resembles golf-ball rolling under skin, from left costal margin to border of right rectus.
5. *Pyloric 'tumour'*. The essential diagnostic sign. Best felt with infant feeding on left breast or resting in mother's left arm if bottle fed. Examiner sits at left side of baby palpating with finger-tips of left hand. Tumour felt as small knob, size and shape of olive which periodically contracts and relaxes, situated just behind right rectus muscle, half-way between costal margin and umbilicus. Middle finger has to be crooked into angle formed by liver and right border of rectus. Best time to feel tumour is after vomiting.

Differential Diagnosis (Table 68.1, p. 211)

Investigations
1. *Electrolytes*. Must always be checked prior to surgery; serum chloride may be low, bicarbonate elevated.
2. *Radiology*. Opaque meal necessary if palpation of mass uncertain. Shows characteristic 'string sign' of contrast medium passing through narrow pyloric canal, and 'double track' due to mucosal oedema. Delayed emptying of stomach.
3. *Ultrasound*. Alternative to radiology, will demonstrate pyloric mass.

Treatment
Ramstedt's operation, after restoration of fluid, electrolyte and acid–base balance as necessary. If surgery impossible, treat with atropine methyl nitrate 1–3 drops of 0·6% alcoholic solution 20 min before feeds, but note that prolonged treatment is necessary and surgery may still be needed eventually. Surgical mortality should be nil.

Chapter 70   **HIRSCHSPRUNG'S DISEASE**
(*Congenital Intestinal Aganglionosis*)

Uncommon condition usually manifested in early infancy. Characterized in untreated cases by intractable constipation, abdominal distension and stunted growth; on macroscopic examination by dilatation and hypertrophy of normally innervated colon; normal appearance of distal colon and rectum devoid of ganglion cells; microscopically by absence of ganglion cells in distal segment. Incidence about 1 in 1000 live births. Males : females, 5 : 1.

Clinical Features
1. *Neonatal obstruction*. Persisting until relieved by colostomy.
   Main Features

   1.1 Vomiting: May commence within 24h of first feed. Persistent. Vomitus contains bile.
   1.2 Constipation: Delay in passing meconium; faeces small in amount.
   1.3 Abdominal distension: Rapidly becomes gross.
   1.4 Visible peristalsis: Usually large-gut type.
   1.5 Rectal examination: Anus may feel tight; usually gush of flatus and faeces follows as finger withdrawn and condition temporarily relieved.
2. *Recurring obstructive episodes*. During infancy until relieved by operation (colostomy or primary definitive operation). Probably largest group.
3. *Attacks of diarrhoea and distension in early infancy (enterocolitis)*. Rare. Easily mistaken for gastro-enteritis and underlying obstruction missed. Cause of attacks unknown. Possibly obstruction with ileocaecal incompetence leads to bacterial overgrowth in small bowel and bile salt deconjugation. No bacterial pathogen found.
   Clinical Picture. Grossly distended abdomen with diarrhoea and vomiting. Untreated—death from fluid and electrolyte loss within hours. At autopsy necrosis of mucosa may be found suggesting vascular lesion.
4. *Presentation in childhood*. Mild symptoms dating from infancy. Rare.
   Clinical Picture

   4.1 Chronic intestinal obstruction with huge tympanitic abdomen, visible and audible peristalsis; gross constipation. Stools: if hard—small pellets; if soft—ribbon-like. Faecal incontinence uncommon, but may occur. Rectal examination: rectum empty, narrowed segment can often be felt higher up.

4.2 *Dwarfism, wasting and anaemia.*
4.3 *Recurrent episodes of enterocolitis* with increased distension, diarrhoea and often vomiting.

Investigations
1. Plain radiograph of pelvis with air as contrast medium—lateral projection may
show the cone of transition from collapsed distal gut to normally innervated
dilated proximal gut in the usual type of Hirschsprung's disease.
2. Barium enema. Special technique: Bowel not prepared. (*a*) Barium watched
running up from undilated rectum into dilated megacolon through typical cone of
transition. Examination then completed, otherwise danger of: (i) Inspissation of
large amount of barium into megacolon with worsening of symptoms. (ii) Rapid
water absorption with fatal water intoxication. (*b*) Emptying of colon never
complete. Barium may remain for 2–14 days.
    Note: In normal neonates evacuation usually complete; may even take place as
barium being administered. In one-third of cases a little barium remains after
evacuation.
3. Rectal biopsy. (*a*) Suction rectal biopsy for submucosal ganglion cells. (*b*) Full
thickness rectal biopsy for intermyenteric ganglion cells. Cholinesterase present
in excess.
    Rectal pressure studies. Failure of normal relaxation of internal sphincter when
rectal balloon inflated.

Differential Diagnosis *(See Table* 68.2, p. 213 and *Table* 70.1)

Table 70.1.   Differential diagnosis of constipation

	Hirschsprung's disease	Idiopathic megacolon	Infantile type of chronic constipation
Age of onset	Birth. Passage of meconium delayed	Usually over 1 year. No delay in passing meconium	From cessation of breast feeding
Sex incidence	90% male	70% male	?
Abdominal distension	Very marked; mainly gas. Peristalsis prominent	Marked, mainly craggy faeces. Peristalsis uncommon	Nil
Pain	Rare	On defaecation	On defaecation
Diarrhoea	Enterocolitis uncommon	Overflow diarrhoea common. Often presenting feature	Nil
Perianal region	Clean	Soiled	Clean
Rectum	Empty; may be spasm	Full	Full
Faeces	Small; hard pellets or soft and ribbon-like	Large; hard *and* fluid. Often blood-streaked	Large; hard, dry
Barium enema	Distension of colon ends some distance from anus	Distension extends to anus	Normal

Treatment
1. Medical. Only until surgical treatment possible. (*a*) Newborn with acute
obstruction: Rectal examination or passing rectal tube often gives temporary

relief. Daily rectal washouts with normal saline. (*b*) Treatment of enterocolitis. *Note*: May occur in untreated case or in apparently successfully treated case. (i) Empty bowel by rectal tube, washout, or even perform colostomy. (ii) Fluid and electrolyte replacement therapy. (iii) i.v. antibiotics
2. *Surgical*. Temporary colostomy at site of transition at time of diagnosis—confirmed by histology—reduces risk of enterocolitis developing. Definitive anastomosis of ganglionated bowel to anal canal at 9–12 months of age or 6 months after defunctioning colostomy in older child.

Congenital Intestinal Hypoganglionosis (Pseudo–Hirschsprung's Disease)

Ganglion cells present but greatly reduced in number. Clinical picture and operative findings similar to Hirschsprung's.

Meconium Plugs

Meconium is a mass of bile-stained mucus composed of mucoproteins and mucopolysaccharides. Contains keratinized epithelial squames derived from infant's skin and ingested with amniotic fluid. Terminal mass of meconium has unpigmented cap which infant may not be able to pass. Can cause intestinal obstruction. Plugs in colon can cause stercoral ulceration, peritonitis and death.

Treatment
Gentle removal of plug.
   Note: (*a*) Ninety per cent of newborn pass meconium within first 24h; 8% in next 12h. (*b*) Failure to pass meconium in first 24h should give rise to suspicion of meconium plug, aganglionosis, or other cause of intestinal obstruction, e.g. meconium ileus.

Chapter 71   *CONDITIONS AFFECTING UMBILICUS*

Anatomy

Contents of Umbilical Cord
   1. One umbilical vein; pierces abdominal wall and runs in free border of falciform ligament.
   2. Two (occasionally only one) umbilical arteries; become hypogastric arteries, which run down anterior abdominal wall separated only by peritoneum from abdominal cavity.
   3. Urachus.
   4. Wharton's jelly.
   After birth vessels normally close within few days, but remain patent to probe for some weeks.

Umbilical Cyst

Uncommon. Composed of Wharton's jelly. May very rarely be large enough to obstruct birth.

Patent Urachus

Usually associated with bladder outlet obstruction. Gives rise to intermittent discharge of urine.

Persistent Vitello-intestinal Duct

Rare abnormal component of cord continuous with Meckel's diverticulum. Produces faecal fistula.

Omphalitis (Infection of Umbilicus)

Serious infection e.g. tetanus neonatorum, rare except in countries where asepsis not practised in care of umbilical cord (*see* Chapter 33). Ascending infection may lead to local lesion, hepatitis, peritonitis, septicaemia.

Treatment
1. *Prevention.* Very important. Umbilical stump should be covered with sterile dressing, or sealed with aerosol plastic dressing.
2. *Antibiotics.* Usually control infection.

Exomphalos (Umbilical Eventration; Omphalocele)

Embryology
Owing to rapid growth of liver and other organs occupying available space in coelomic cavity, a U-shaped loop of gut normally extruded into umbilical cord between sixth and tenth week. This physiological umbilical hernia, normal in fetus, may persist after birth. Prenatally causes raised α-fetoprotein level in amniotic fluid.

Clinical Features
Abdominal contents, usually liver and gut, contained in translucent sac protruding from anterior abdominal wall. Size varies. May rupture during delivery or in early days. Rupture in utero called *gastroschisis*.
   Beckwith Syndrome. Exomphalos associated with macroglossia and visceral enlargement and danger of neonatal hypoglycaemia.

Treatment
   1. Operation within first few hours of life. May be difficulty in repairing gap in abdominal wall, especially if liver in sac. Small lesion closed in layers.
   2. Large lesions. Sac painted with 2% aqueous thiomersal or mercurochrome if primary closure impossible. Eventually spontaneous reduction and epithelization of sac may allow delayed surgical repair. Silver sulphadiazine cream is an alternative to mercurochrome. Some large lesions treated by covering with silastic bag sutured to defect and gradually reduced. Delayed function and recovery of motility requires prolonged parenteral nutrition.

Gastroschisis

Rare developmental disorder. Abdominal contents, without peritoneal sac, extruded from defect in anterior abdominal wall in utero. Umbilical cord has *normal* insertion (cf. exomphalos). Associated with malrotation of small bowel, and sometimes atresia. Treatment: Immediate surgery.

Umbilical Hernia

Very common in normal children (incidence 1 : 10), more often in girls than boys. Cretins almost always have umbilical hernia. Size varies; often 2–6 cm in diameter. On palpation while child quiet, hernia can be reduced easily with gurgling sound. Often contains both bowel and omentum. Palpation of empty sac reveals small opening into abdominal cavity, surrounded by firm ring. When child cries the hernia protrudes again.

Prognosis

Rupture of hernial sac or intestinal obstruction is almost unknown. Spontaneous cure usually occurs by about 4 years of age, hence no treatment indicated.

Umbilical Granuloma

Very common; appears as a warty mass of granulomatous tissue at base of the umbilicus. Usually has an offensive discharge from secondary infection. A ligature should be placed around the base or the granuloma cauterized with silver nitrate.

Chapter 72   # DISEASES OF THE MOUTH

Ulcers

Types
1. Traumatic. From biting mucous membrane; injury from hard objects in mouth, etc. In infants commonly from ill-advised efforts at cleansing mouth by mother. Painful, but heal rapidly.
2. Herpetic (*see* p. 87).
3. Aphthous ulcers. Tend to recur in some children. Common in coeliac and Crohn's disease. Local application of corticosteroids in adhesive base relieves pain and accelerates healing. Carbenoxolone sodium locally also useful.

Thrush (*Candidiasis; Moniliasis*)

Infection with fungus—*Candida albicans.* Common saprophyte of mouth in health. Usually localized infection in mouth, though may spread to the skin and elsewhere.

Lesions
Mouth. Very common in newborn babies. Seen as patches resembling milk-curd,

but firmly fixed to mucous membrane. Usually only a few patches, but may cover the whole mouth. Sloughing can occur with secondary bacterial infection. Treatment: Nystatin 100 000u or amphotericin 100 mg q.d.s. as oral drops or gel. *Skin*. Mainly napkin (diaper) area. Distinguished from ordinary napkin rash by involvement of anal margin and, in girls, labial margin. Does not respond to simple treatment for napkin rash. *C. albicans* can be recovered from stools. Treatment: Nystatin 2% amphotericin 3%, or miconazole ointment as well as oral therapy.

Dental Eruption ('Teething')

A normal physiological process which gives rise to no symptoms except, very rarely, pain with blue swollen gums from an eruption cyst.

Dental Caries

Pathogenesis (*Fig. 72.1*)

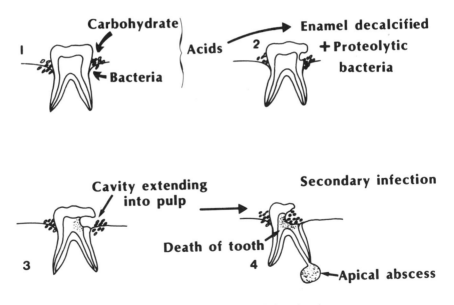

Fig. 72.1. Pathogenesis of dental caries.

Predisposing Causes

1. Diet. Ingestion of fermentable carbohydrates which cling to teeth (e.g. bread, honey, sweets), especially last thing at night.

2. Deficient calcification.

3. Abnormal development of teeth and jaw—resulting in stasis of food particles.

4. Debilitating illness. Because (*a*) Decreased flow of saliva occurs. (*b*) Lack of movement of tongue and teeth. (*c*) Child given soft foods.

5. Cyanotic congenital heart disease.

6. Age. Mainly 4–8 years, and 12–18 years. The latter more serious.

Prevention
1. *Ensure adequate calcification.* (*a*) Calcification of deciduous teeth commences during last 3 months of pregnancy and continues until short time after birth. Calcification of permanent teeth occurs from 6 months to 12 years. Important to ensure that mother and baby have adequate supply of calcium and vitamin D. (*b*) Fluoride promotes calcification and protects teeth. If inadequate natural fluoride in water, deficit can be made up by adding to water supply (if less than 0·3 part per million) or by providing fluoride as tablets to be given daily until the age of 4 years. Optimal fluoride content water 0·3–0·7 ppm. Fluorosis if >2 ppm.
2. *Diet.* Prolonged bottle-feeding promotes caries particularly if the bottle is propped so that the infant goes to sleep sucking it. A pool of milk then remains in contact with the teeth. Ingestion of sticky carbohydrates, cakes and sweets, especially last thing at night, should be restricted.
3. *Oral hygiene.* Teeth should be brushed regularly.

Diseases of the Salivary Glands

Development of Salivation
Three stages occur:

1. Newborn infant salivates little.

2. At about 3 months of age salivation increases. As child has not learnt to swallow it, saliva dribbles from mouth (*drooling*). Often erroneously attributed to teething.

3. From about 1 year drooling should cease. Possible causes of persistent drooling: mental retardation with or without cerebral palsy (commonest); local lesions in mouth; encephalitis lethargica.

Mumps (epidemic parotitis) (*see* p. 85).

Chapter 73   **DISEASES OF STOMACH AND DUODENUM**

Acute Perforation of Stomach

Rare catastrophe in neonate, apparently due to congenital muscular deficiency in wall of stomach. Emergency surgery may be lifesaving.

Peptic Ulcer

Acute Ulcers
1. *Primary.* Rare. Mainly under age of 6 months. Usually no family history of ulcer.

Clinical Features. May present with: (*a*) Haematemesis or melaena which may be very severe. (*b*) Projectile vomiting due to pylorospasm simulating congenital pyloric stenosis. (*c*) Rarely perforation.

Gastrografin meal: Findings similar to those in adults.

Treatment. Symptomatic if possible, but surgery may be necessary.

2. *Secondary*. May occur in stomach, duodenum or lower end of oesophagus, due to: (*a*) Sepsis. (*b*) Long debilitating diseases, (*c*) Severe burns (Curling's ulcer). (*d*) Corticosteroid therapy in older children. Not seen in young children. (*f*) Salicylates.

Chronic Ulcers

Not uncommon. Occur in older children especially if strong family history of peptic ulcer.

Clinical features. Symptoms may be atypical, with bouts of pain unrelated to meals and often of short duration. Night pain uncommon but suggestive. Bleeding may occur.

Investigations. Radiology and endoscopy as for adults.

Treatment. As for adults.

Differential Diagnosis.

Recurrent abdominal pain, *see* p. 204.

Chapter 74   # MALABSORPTION AND FOOD ALLERGY

Steatorrhoea indicates passage of excessive quantities of fat in stools. Failure to utilize fat taken in diet may be due to many causes (*see below*). Fat may appear in stool in large amount and be prominent feature of disease (as in coeliac disease) or only becomes apparent after careful fat-balance studies. Although fat absorption usually predominates, protein malabsorption also present in most patients. Specific malabsorption of fat or carbohydrate occurs when particular enzymes are deficient.

Classification

1. *Impaired digestion of fat*. (*a*) Deficiency of pancreatic lipase: cystic fibrosis, Shwachman's syndrome. (*b*) Deficiency of bile salts: atresia of bile ducts; infective hepatitis.

2. *Impaired absorption of fat (and usually protein)*. (*a*) Inadequate length of bowel: surgical resection; intestinal fistulae. (*b*) Reduced absorptive surface (villous atrophy): coeliac disease, cow's milk protein intolerance, kwashiorkor. (*c*) Decreased transit time: increased gut motility as in some types of diarrhoea. (*d*) Inflammatory disease of intestinal mucosa: intestinal infections; regional enteritis; ulcerative colitis; intestinal infestations—*Giardia lamblia*. (*e*) Obstruction of lymphatics: lymphangiectasia; lymphosarcoma; tuberculosis, Whipple's disease. (*f*) Involvement of intestinal mucosa in systemic disease: nephrosis; Gaucher's disease; Niemann–Pick disease. (*g*) Absence of specific carrier protein: a-beta-lipoproteinaemia.

Table 73.1.   Causes of haematemesis and bleeding per rectum

	Disease	May give rise to following
Newborn	1. Swallowed maternal blood	Haematemesis or melaena. Test for adult haemoglobin
	2. Vomiting of blood-stained mucus soon after birth	Amount of bleeding slight
	3. Haemorrhagic disease of newborn	Haematemesis or melaena. May be severe
	4. Necrotizing enterocolitis	Fulminating rectal bleeding
During first year of life	1. Ingested blood from breast (cracked nipples; abscess)	Haematemesis. Amount may be large
	2. Oesophagitis from reflux	Haematemesis. Usually blood-streaked vomit
	3. Thrush oesophagitis	Haematemesis. Slight amount
	4. Acute peptic ulceration	Haematemesis. Often large
	5. Rectal polyp	Bright red blood per rectum. Amount small
	6. Intussusception	Bright red blood per rectum. Amount large or small
	7. Fissure-in-ano	Bright red blood streak on constipated stool
	8. Meckel's diverticulum with peptic ulcer	Large amount of blood per rectum
Childhood	1. Swallowed blood:	
	a. From epistaxis	Haematemesis or melaena
	b. From teeth	Haematemesis or melaena
	2. Peptic ulcers—usually chronic	
	a. Oesophagus	Haematemesis. May be profuse. Also melaena
	b. Gastric or duodenal	Haematemesis or melaena
	c. Meckel's diverticulum	May be profuse rectal bleeding.
	3. Acute gastritis—poisons, etc.	Haematemesis
	4. Foreign body: Stomach or lower in gut	Melaena; rarely haematemesis
	Inserted into anus	Bright red blood per rectum
	5. Oesophageal varices—cirrhosis of liver	Haematemesis. May be profuse
	6. Blood diseases, e.g.:	
	Henoch-Schönlein purpura	Melaena may be prominent
	Acute leukaemia	Melaena usually slight
	7. Infarction of gut due to mesenteric artery thrombosis, etc.	Melaena often profuse
	8. Haemorrhoids (rare)	Red blood per rectum

3. Cause unknown. Incomplete obstruction, e.g. malrotation, blind loop syndrome: ? aganglionosis; acrodermatitis enteropathica.

COELIAC DISEASE
(Gluten-induced Enteropathy)

Definition
Disorder of absorption caused by damaging effects of dietary gluten upon small bowel mucosa in certain susceptible individuals. Clinical features include wasting, abdominal distension, growth failure, steatorrhoea and anaemia. Spontaneous

clinical relapses and remissions occur but gluten intolerance is permanent. Jejunal villi atrophic but crypts elongated.

Incidence
Rarely presents before age 6 months. Maximal incidence 9 months–3 years. Found in many parts of world, often with racial or tribal variations in neighbouring areas. In UK incidence is in approximate range of 1 : 2000. Very common in West of Ireland (1 : 300).

Aetiology
Genetics. Hereditary susceptibility is involved; 10% of first-degree relatives of proven case are likely to have jejunal mucosal abnormality, often without symptoms. Known genetic associations include possession of HLA-B8 and DR3 tissue antigens, but exact mode of inheritance is uncertain.
Gluten. Glutens of wheat and rye contain specific fractions derived from gliadin components, which are toxic to patients' jejunal mucosa *in vitro*. Exclusion of gluten from diet leads to clinical and histological remission, but reintroduction of gluten eventually produces histological, though not necessarily clinical relapse.
Immunology. Antibodies to gluten and other dietary proteins are often present in serum but probably secondary to mucosal damage. IgA-containing plasma cells found in gut mucosa after gluten challenge. Paradoxically, coeliac disease commoner in children with IgA deficiency.
Pathology. Subtotal atrophy of upper small intestinal villi ('flat mucosa') with lymphocyte infiltration of lamina propria can be demonstrated under dissecting microscope. Electron microscopy shows that enterocyte become more squamous, with disruption of microvilli and changes in cell organelles. Poor correlation between severity of mucosal changes and clinical symptoms. Biochemically, there is reduction of disaccharidases and peptidases in mucosa.
   Note: Villous atrophy, usually less severe, occurs in cow's milk protein intolerance, kwashiorkor, giardiasis and partially treated coeliac disease.

Clinical Features
1. Onset. Insidious. Commences with anorexia, often vomiting, failure to thrive and increasing irritability. Stools noticed to be frequent and loose. Sometimes acute onset resembling gastro-enteritis.
2. Characteristics of well-marked case (now rarely seen). (*a*) Stunted child with generalized wasting, especially of buttocks, which contrast with protuberant abdomen. Rarely oedema due to hypoproteinaemia. (*b*) *On Palpation.* Abdomen tight and inelastic. Ladder patterning of gut may be visible through thin anterior abdominal wall. Liver usually not palpable. (*c*) *Mental Attitude.* Child miserable and fastidious with food.
3. Stools. (*a*) At onset of disease and during relapse (coeliac crisis) stools may be watery and dehydration results. (*b*) More commonly stools large, pale, greasy and offensive. Said to resemble gruel. May or may not be frothy, depending on amount of fermentation present. (*c*) Rarely, child has chronic constipation.
4. Older children may present with growth failure and apparently normal stools.
5. Refractory iron deficiency anaemia is sometimes presenting feature.
6. Rickets occasionally occurs in older children despite slow growth rate.
7. Clinical lactose intolerance occasionally present.

Investigations
1. *Peroral jejunal biopsy* demonstrates subtotal villous atrophy. This is the only investigation of real value. Ideally, diagnosis should be confirmed by two further biopsies: (*a*) After 1 year on gluten-free diet to demonstrate histological recovery, then (*b*) After up to 2 years (or on earlier clinical relapse) on normal diet to demonstrate histological relapse caused by gluten.
2. *Fat absorption.* Steatorrhoea may be shown in two-thirds of cases by daily faecal output of more than 4g/day in child on adequate fat intake (i.e. over 20g/day for child weighing under 15kg; over 40g/day for child weighing over 15kg). Occasionally appetite so poor that adequate intake not reached and child may be constipated. Fat balance rarely indicated: if coeliac disease is suspected a biopsy should be performed.
3. *Whole blood folate.* Normally in excess of 60ng/ml, usually reduced below 50ng/ml in coeliac disease.

Differential Diagnosis
Must be distinguished from cystic fibrosis, cow's milk protein intolerance, giardia infestation.

Course and Prognosis
1. Acute phase of disease usually lasts several weeks. Condition then passes into latent phase. Child stunted. Protruberant abdomen. Frequent large, loose stools. Child may die in acute phase.
2. With treatment by gluten-free diet initial change is usually improvement in mood and activity. Character of stools improves within a few weeks. General condition, weight and height gain all return to normal. If even small quantity of gluten added to diet child may relapse, but some tolerate gluten without symptoms despite histological relapse. In this case, child may not grow to potential height.
3. Increased risk of malignant lymphoma of small gut in coeliac disease of adults. Increase in adenocarcinoma of oesophagus, stomach and small bowel also reported.

Treatment
1. *Coeliac crisis* (rare). If diarrhoea severe, child rapidly becomes dehydrated and serious biochemical imbalance results. Intravenous alimentation may be required with measures to correct electrolyte equilibrium. Corticosteroids may be life-saving.
2. *Most cases.* Child should have normal full diet except that no foods containing gluten may be given, i.e. nothing containing wheat or rye flour. As a substitute for flour, wheat starch may be used. Expert dietetic advice should be given to ensure balanced and varied diet.
3. *Treatment should be continued* throughout childhood and adolescence to realize growth potential, and probably through adult life to prevent malignancy.

Cow's Milk Protein Intolerance

Aetiology
An immunological reaction to cow's milk protein antigens, of which the most important is β-lactoglobulin.

Clinical Features
Similar to coeliac disease; often preceded by persistent vomiting commencing with introduction of cow's milk feeds, so may be from birth. Concurrent eczema increases suspicion but diagnosis is based on response to trial of cow's milk exclusion diet.

Pathology
Jejunal histology resembles coeliac disease, but usually changes are patchy and milder, with partial villous atrophy and lymphocytic infiltration of lamina propria.

Treatment
Elimination of cow's milk from diet, substitute soya milk or semi-elemental feed. Sometimes coexists with coeliac disease, and secondary lactose intolerance, which will require appropriate dietary restriction.

Food Allergic Disorders (*Food Intolerance*)

Many symptoms are attributed to 'food allergy' but with varying degrees of credibility. Some 'allergies' are due to a chemical (rather than a reaginic) response to a food component such as caffeine. Common offending foods include cow's milk, eggs, nuts, shellfish, oranges, wheat, chocolate, soya. Food colourings such as tartrazine are important additives which frequently produce intolerance. Diagnosis depends on prompt remission upon withdrawal of the offending food and relapse on 'challenge' (reintroduction) on at least two occasions.

Clinical Features
Symptoms range from mild, subjective disturbances to anaphylaxis. Commonly eczema, urticaria, conjunctivitis, rhinitis, asthma, migraine, malabsorption, abdominal pain, vomiting, diarrhoea. Some authors claim that behaviour disturbances such as sleep disorders and hyperactivity may respond dramatically to a hypoallergenic diet.

Investigations
    1. Skin tests. May be positive for particular foods.
    2. Serum IgE and RAST (specific antibodies) tests for individual foods may be elevated.
    In practice, these tests have proved unreliable and are positive only when the mechanism is reaginic (IgE mediated).

Treatment
Empirical. When the history is convincing a dietary restriction should be tried. Oral sodium cromoglycate is sometimes a helpful adjunct. Many food intolerances, particularly to cow's milk, are temporary and the food may be cautiously reintroduced after a year or so.

Disaccharidase Deficiencies

(1) Inherited errors of metabolism may result in absence of specific enzyme in small bowel mucosa. Enzymes most often affected: lactase, sucrose/isomaltase. Much more commonly lactase deficiency develops as temporary state after gastroenter-

itis. Distinction between *disaccharide intolerance* (clinical state) and *disacchar-idase deficiency* (by enzyme assay of mucosa) is important: low levels of enzyme do not always produce symptoms. (2) Although lactose deficiency is commonest, other disaccharide and even monosaccharide intolerances may occur after gastroenteritis or occasionally in coeliac disease, kwashiorkor, cow's milk protein intolerance, cystic fibrosis and after neomycin.

Pathogenesis of Diarrhoea
Disaccharide sugar normally split by the missing enzyme remains undigested. Osmotic diarrhoea results, with fermentation by bacteria in colon producing acid and gas stools.

Symptoms
1. Profuse watery, explosive, acid diarrhoea on introduction of offending sugar into diet. Skin of buttocks excoriated.
2. Secondary steatorrhoea.
3. Failure to thrive and electrolyte imbalance.

Investigations
1. Jejunal biopsy Absence or low concentration of specific disaccharidase is the definitive test.
2. Carbohydrate tolerance curves using the appropriate sugar show a flat response of blood glucose to oral load.
3. Stool pH is low, with increased lactic acid output. Reducing substance may be demonstrated with 'Clinitest' or sugar shown on chromatography.
4. Excessive rise in breath hydrogen occurs after a load of the appropriate sugar, due to bacterial fermentation of unabsorbed sugar in the colon.
5. Clinical improvement following removal of offending sugar from diet may be adequate practical diagnostic test in many cases.

Treatment
Dietary exclusion of offending sugar.

Chapter 75   # THE ACUTE ABDOMEN

Appendicitis

Incidence
Commonest abdominal emergency in childhood. Rare below 2 years old. Becomes progressively more common as childhood advances.

Clinical Features
Children over age of 4 years. Signs and symptoms similar to those in adults, except that: localization of pain more difficult; pain may be paroxysmal in character and child runs around and plays between attacks. Vomiting once or twice almost invariable at onset, but rarely persists. Bowels not opened. Tongue coated. Foetor oris.

Children under age of 4 years. Diagnosis often made with great difficulty. Child usually presents with general malaise, lassitude, anorexia, one or two vomits, constipation for 24–48 h. Temperature often 39·5–40 °C (103–104 °F), tachycardia invariable. Diarrhoea uncommon except in pelvic type of appendicitis.

On examination. (*a*) *General.* In early stages child difficult to examine and irritable. *Looks ill.* Later, when peritonitis develops, grey and shocked, lies unheeding. (*b*) *Abdomen.* (i) *Before perforation*; gentle palpation with warmed hand will usually reveal tenderness and guarding, most marked over McBurney's point in right iliac fossa. Evidence of tenderness is child's reaction—wincing, wriggling abdomen away from examiner and *actively pushing away examining hand by child's hands*, this if repeated and definite is most valuable sign. (ii) *After perforation*: Generalized tenderness and guarding may be observed but usually more marked in right iliac fossa. In infants tenderness very difficult to elicit. Guarding may be considerable but often slight. (*c*) *Rectal Examination.* Of great value. Tenderness more marked on right than left side. (iii) After prolonged course appendix abscess may develop and a mass is palpable in the right iliac fossa. *Special Investigations*: (1) Polymorphonuclear leucocytosis of 15–20 000/mm³ usual. (2) Radiograph abdomen for: (*a*) Faecolith. (*b*) Reflex ileus in right iliac fossa around appendix. (*c*) Appendix mass.

Differential Diagnosis
1. *Before perforation*

> *1.1 Food Poisoning.* Pain colicky, fever and leucocytosis rare. Often vomiting and diarrhoea.
> *1.2 Intussusception.* Commonest under 1 year of age. Pain every 5–30 min initially; child may appear shocked immediately after attack, but soon recovers and plays or sleeps. Blood passed per rectum. Often slight pyrexia in late cases.
> *1.3 Urinary Conditions*
> *1.3.1 Pyelonephritis* Pain may be colicky but more usually dull ache. Tenderness in loin over kidney. Pyrexia and leucocytosis present. Pus in urine.
> *1.3.2 Stone in ureter* Colicky pain. No fever. Child not ill. Radiograph may reveal stone.
> *1.3.3 Oxaluria* Oxalate crystals in urine. May follow eating rhubarb, strawberries, etc. Often associated haematuria.
> *1.4 Non-specific Mesenteric Lymphadenitis.* Abdominal pain common in the first 24 h of some upper respiratory infections. Pain less persistent, vomiting slight. Tonsillitis may be obvious.
> *1.5 Periodic Syndrome.* Vomiting before pain. Previous attacks have usually occurred.
> *1.6 Pneumonia.* Especially of right lung. Abdominal pain may be first symptom, but raised respiratory rate and signs in chest occur later. Rectal examination negative. Radiological examination of chest confirms diagnosis.
> *1.7 Rheumatic Fever.* Rarely presents with abdominal pain.
> *1.8 Henoch-Schönlein Purpura.* Abdominal pain can occur several days before characteristic rash and joint swelling. usually, but not always, passage of blood per rectum.
> *1.9* Recurrent abdominal pain (*see* p. 204).

Discussion. Abdominal pain very common symptom in children. May be manifestation of generalized infection (e.g. upper respiratory infection) or local disease (e.g. appendicitis). Requires great skill to differentiate. If in doubt, probably more dangerous to leave appendicitis than to operate unnecessarily. Laboratory tests of little help.

2. After perforation. Peritonitis (*see below*).

Treatment

Surgery. If peritonitis—give plasma or equivalents, resuscitate, rehydrate, nasogastric tube, antibiotics and when stable and improved, 4–6h later appendicectomy. If appendix mass and history less than 4 days, rehydrate, give antibiotics and operate. If abscess and history more than 4 days, may resolve with drip, suction and antibiotic. If toxic or getting worse—drain abscess and 8–12 weeks later remove appendix.

Peritonitis

Aetiology

1. Perforated appendicitis. By far the commonest cause.

2. Other varieties

> *2.1 Primary.* Rare. Usually pneumococcal.
>
> *2.2 Secondary*
>
> *2.2.1 Pneumococcal*: Primary lesion usually pneumococcal septicaemia, empyema or otitis media. Boys affected as often as girls. A rare complication of nephrotic syndrome and liver failure.
>
> *2.2.2 Streptococcal*: Due to septicaemia, skin lesions, may be from vulvovaginitis.
>
> *2.2.3 Gonococcal*: Very rare. Follows vulvovaginitis in girls.
>
> *2.2.4 'Meconium peritonitis'*: An aseptic peritonitis following rupture of intestine in meconium ileus (*see* p. 269).
>
> *2.2.5 Rarely peritonitis follows intraperitoneal haemorrhage.*
>
> *2.2.6* Water skiing in older girls not wearing protective pants.

Clinical Features

Acute onset with prostration, high pyrexia, abdominal pain, vomiting, often diarrhoea. May be signs of infection elsewhere in secondary type. Herpes febrilis and leucocytosis occur in pneumococcal peritonitis. May be slight vulval discharge.

Course. Increasing toxaemia, no localization to right inguinal fossa.

Prognosis

Depends on type of organism and age of child. Very dangerous in young children especially following appendicitis.

Diagnosis

See diagnosis of appendicitis, p. 230.

Treatment
Laparotomy essential if diagnosis in doubt.
Antibiotics. Antibiotics should be given in full doses. Draining of loculated pus may be required later.

Mesenteric Lymphadenitis

Acute Non-specific Mesenteric Lymphadenitis
At laparotomy performed for abdominal pain in childhood, often found that mesenteric lymph nodes are enlarged and appear pathological.
Aetiology. Part of generalized lymphatic reaction to infection, most commonly tonsillitis. Sometimes caused by enterovirus or *Pasteurella pseudotuberculosis*.
Clinical features. Often history of previous attack. Insidious onset, pain usually not very severe, tenderness and guarding often not marked. Vomiting may occur. After 24 h upper respiratory tract infection may develop.

Chapter 76   # INTESTINAL OBSTRUCTION

Classification
Obstruction may be acute, chronic or acute-on-chronic.
In newborn infants. See Table 68.2, p. 213.
In older infants and children
1. *Intussusception. See below.*
2. *Bands and Adhesions*
    2.1 Following peritonitis, abdominal operations or abdominal tuberculosis.
    2.2 Congenital abnormalities of mesentery, or Meckel's diverticulum.
3. *Hernia*
    3.1 External: Inguinal hernia—second commonest cause of obstruction in children under 1 year.
    3.2 Internal: Relatively more common in child than adult due to developmental anomalies.
4. *Malrotation of Gut and Volvulus. See p. 235.*
5. *Meconium ileus*: and 'meconium ileus equivalent' *See p. 269.*
6. *Objects blocking Lumen from Inside*
    5.1 Constipation: See p. 205.
    5.2 Meconium ileus and 'Meconium ileus equivalent': *See p. 269.*
    5.3 Worms: Ascariasis. Not uncommon in some tropical countries.
    5.4 Ingested foreign bodies: Almost never cause obstruction. If object small enough to pass pylorus usually able to traverse remainder of gut. Ninety-five per cent of objects swallowed pass safely through. Main danger from foreign body is perforation of gut or haemorrhage. If object small enough to reach stomach, will almost always reach stool eventually. Pointed objects (open safety-pins, etc.) can

usually be left, but should be removed if radiological examination demonstrates failure to progress for 4 days or if perforation or haemorrhage occurs.

7. *Crohn's Disease*. Uncommon in children.

8. *Pressure from Tumours, Cysts*. Tumour may be simple or malignant.

Intussusception

Definition
Condition of partial or complete intestinal obstruction due to invagination of proximal portion of gut into more distal portion.

Types
(1) Acute (may be recurrent); (2) Chronic; (3) Agonal—uncommon, unimportant, post-mortem finding due to spasms of gut at death. Often multiple.

Acute Intussusception

Aetiology
Age. From 4 to 24 months: commonest 9 months.
Sex. Boys to girls, 3 : 1.
Particularly affects robust, healthy children, often at weaning period.

Pathology
Commonest variety: invagination of ileocaecal region into caecum Less common: colic or ileo-ileal. Invaginated portion called intussusceptum. Portion into which it is invaginated called intussuscipiens. Intussusceptum may extend few centimetres only or as far as rectum. Rarely protrudes from anus. Blood supply of intussusceptum interrupted partially or completely. Affected gut plum-coloured and may or may not be viable. Extremely rarely sloughs off and is passed per rectum, thus effecting spontaneous cure. Mesenteric lymph nodes usually enlarged: non-specific inflammation.

Pathogenesis
Prerequisites:

1. Onset of intussusception initiated and determined in position by some projection from wall into lumen of gut. This projection is carried forward by peristaltic waves, dragging gut wall after it. Hence intussusception may be initiated by:

    1.1 Enlarged Peyer's patches. Most commonly caused by adenovirus infection which can often be cultivated from stool.

    1.2 Local oedema, possibly from allergic reaction.

    1.3 Haemorrhage into bowel wall (cf. Henoch–Schönlein purpura).

    1.4 Intestinal polyps or cysts.

    1.5 Occasionally Meckel's diverticulum.

    1.6 Not uncommon in cystic fibrosis.

2. Abnormally mobile gut due to long mesentery.

Clinical Features

1. Pain. Perfectly normal, healthy infant suddenly has attacks of screaming or whimpering, looks distressed, draws up legs in pain. Attack lasts few minutes, then passes off. Recurs in half to 1 hour at first, later becoming more frequent. Between attacks child will often play or feed, but appears apprehensive. Pain may be minimal or severe enough to cause considerable shock with pallor and collapse. Diarrhoea from irritative focus in bowel, which is partially obstructed, may precede constipation.

2. Blood per rectum. Not constant. Classically, normal motion at beginning of illness followed by stool resembling 'red-currant jelly' (lumps of blood-stained mucus). This sign if present almost pathognomonic.

3. Constipation. Not constant, either because obstruction not complete or because intussusception reduces itself and spontaneous recovery occurs.

4. Vomiting. Often occurs once or twice but not prominent except in neglected cases.

On examination

1. Abdomen rigid and tender during attacks; soft between attacks but appears tender especially over course of colon. Child examined most easily when asleep.

2. Sausage-shaped tender mass usually felt over course of colon. May be felt to harden with onset of pain.

3. *'Signe de Dance'*: emptiness in right inguinal fossa due to migration of caecum into colon. Of doubtful value.

4. Loud borborygmi heard on auscultation.

5. In advanced cases intussusceptum may be felt per rectum. Very rarely projects from anus.

Diagnosis

To be made primarily on history of pain and collapse. Other signs and symptoms may all be absent. If in doubt, barium enema shows characteristic 'lobster-claw' or 'coiled spring' appearance:

1. Central obstruction in lumen of colon.

2. Barium seeps thinly between layers of intussusception beyond obstruction.

3. After evacuation thin coat of barium remains.

Examination under anaesthesia for sausage-shaped mass should only be undertaken in theatre, with all preparations to continue with operation if required.

Differential Diagnosis

1. Other causes of colic:
       1.1 Intestinal: wind; food; Henoch–Schönlein purpura.
       1.2 Urinary: stone in ureter; oxaluria.
       1.3 Mesenteric lymphadenitis; non-specific.
       1.4 Appendicular.

2. Other causes of intestinal obstruction. *See* p. 232.

3. Other causes of bleeding per rectum:
       3.1 Intestinal polyp: haemorrhoids; fissure-in-ano.
       3.2 Henoch-Schönlein purpura.

4. From prolapsed rectum: impossible to get finger up between prolapse and anus. Absence of acute symptoms.

Prognosis
Spontaneous reduction occurs in some cases but active treatment is usually required as early as possible to prevent gangrene of bowel and avoid resection.

Treatment
Reduction of intussusception should be undertaken as early as possible. Delay results in strangulation of blood vessels and danger of gangrene of gut, which may require resection.
   1. Non-operative. If the intussusception has been present for less than 24 h an attempt may be made to reduce it by barium enema under radiological control.
   2. Operative. If barium reduction fails or in difficult cases.
   3. If apparent spontaneous reduction occurs child must be carefully observed afterwards as it may not be complete. Barium enema of value to decide this.

Volvulus

Definition
Condition in which intestine twists round causing obstruction to lumen. Sometimes blood supply of portion of gut occluded, resulting in infarction.

Types
   1. If band or adhesion attached to convexity of intestine, rotation tends to occur with band at apex. Congenital bands are usually found near duodenojejunal flexure ('Ladd's bands').
   2. Associated with malrotation of gut.

Malrotation of Gut and Volvulus

Embryology
Midgut extends from duodenum to middle of transverse colon. At eighth week of fetal life midgut protrudes from peritoneal cavity into physiological umbilical hernia. At tenth week midgut returns to peritoneal cavity and physiological rotation around superior mesenteric artery occurs: in anti-clockwise direction.
   Thus caecum commences in middle of hypochondrium and moves successively up left side of abdomen, into epigastrium, right upper quadrant, and eventually down into normal position in right iliac fossa. Caecum then becomes attached to posterior abdominal wall by peritoneum and intestinal mesentery develops.
   Developmental arrest about eleventh week leads to:
   1. Malrotation of caecum—most commonly lies in right epigastrium, obstructing duodenum. Caecum may be floating free or attached to posterior abdominal wall.
   2. Incompletely developed mesentery.

Possible Results of Malrotation
   1. Duodenal obstruction.
   2. Volvulus of midgut due to inadequate mesentery. Usually revolves in clockwise direction, making one or more revolutions. May give rise to: (*a*) Intestinal obstruction, partial or complete. (*b*) Infarction of midgut.
   3. Frequently both the above occur together.

Clinical Types
1. *Acute intestinal obstruction*. Usually occurs within first month of life.
Clinical features as for other varieties of intestinal obstruction (*Table 68.2* p. 213).
2. *Recurrent attacks of mild intestinal obstruction*. Occur in older children. May
be diagnosed as periodic syndrome, subacute appendicitis, food poisoning, etc.
Barium enema will reveal abnormal position of caecum even between attacks.

| *Chapter 77* | # DISEASES OF THE SMALL AND LARGE INTESTINE |

Intestinal Polyps

Hamartomatous Polyps

Juvenile
1. *Rectal polyp* commonest cause of painless rectal bleeding in infants and
children. Polyp may be viewed and often removed through sigmoidoscope. Polyp
may prolapse; 80% palpable with finger in rectum.
2. *Multiple* (juvenile polyposis). Genetically inherited condition. Multiple
polyps throughout gastrointestinal tract. Not precancerous.
3. *Peutz–Jeghers syndrome*. Rare condition inherited as Mendelian dominant.
Signs: (i) Multiple polyps throughout intestine, particularly small intestine. Not
precancerous. (ii) Pigmentation of buccal mucosa and face.

Neoplastic
1. Solitary is very rare.
2. Multiple familial polyps in large intestine; precancerous. Not seen before
age of 10. Mendelian dominant.
3. Gardner's syndrome or adenomatous polyposis with connective-tissue
tumours, e.g. dermoid cyst, osteoma.

Inflammatory
e.g. ulcerative colitis.

Ulcerative Colitis

Uncommon disease in children in UK. More common in Sweden and USA.
Clinical and histological picture overlaps with Crohn's colitis.

Aetiology
Unknown. Psychological disturbance uncommon (prominent in adults) believed
to be secondary to disease.

Age
Mostly in older age groups but has been reported from 2 years of age. In young
children, haemorrhagic ulcerative proctitis may be a manifestation of cow's milk
intolerance, and responds to milk exclusion.

Pathology

Rectum almost always involved. Mucosa friable, congested and granular. Deep ulcers may alternate with pseudopolyps. Continuous involvement, mainly mucosal, without intervening normal areas. Polymorph infiltrate.

Clinical Features

As for adults. Usually severe disease in childhood. May result in dwarfism. Pseudopolyps of the colon common. Premalignant condition (carcinoma reported from age of 17 years). Occasional fulminating case with toxic megacolon. Rare extracolonic manifestations include arthritis, erythema nodosum and hepatitis.

Diagnosis

Barium enema, endoscopy of bowel and biopsy. Rectum and sigmoid involved in 95%. Findings as for adults.

Differential Diagnosis

From Crohn's disease (q.v.).

Treatment

1. *Medical.* In all except mildest cases, steroids indicated to induce remission, orally or by enema. Maintenance with sulphasalazine. Low-residue diet during relapses. Milk-free diet sometimes helpful.
2. *Surgical.* Colonic resection. Indications are: fulminating disease, frequent recurrence or prolonged relapse, and to prevent malignancy in long-standing cases. Cancer risk increases rapidly after 10 years' history. Most children eventually require colectomy.

Regional Enteritis (*Crohn's Disease; Granulomatous Colitis*)

Rare disease in childhood but incidence increasing in developed countries.

Aetiology

Unknown. Possibly due to unidentified transmissible agent. Cell-mediated immunity impaired.

Pathology

Inflammation of small or large intestine, segmental, may be multiple with normal areas intervening ('skip lesions'), most often involving terminal ileum. Involves whole thickness of bowel. Non-caseating granulomas. Linear fissures or ulceration in mucosa. Fistulas and adhesions may develop between adjacent loops of bowel and other abdominal or pelvic organs.

Clinical Features

Wide range of symptoms and signs, including diarrhoea, bloody stools, abdominal pain, weight loss, anorexia, lassitude and anaemia. Growth failure prominent in children. Low grade fever, iritis and arthritis may occur. Perianal lesions frequent—fleshy masses, fissures, fistulas, abscesses. Linear oral ulcers and cobblestone appearance of mucosa. Subacute intestinal obstruction may occur.

Radiology reveals segmental disease of small or large bowel. Colonic lesions may be biopsied via endoscope. Biopsy of perianal lesions shows granulomas.

Treatment

Low-residue, high-calorie diet. Vitamin supplements including B_{12}. Antispasmodics may help painful episodes. Mild exacerbations may respond to sulphasalazine, steroids helpful in severe bouts and for systemic symptoms. Azathioprine has been used successfully but carries risk of bone-marrow depression. Surgery avoided as far as possible because of risk of recurrence and adhesions. Cancer risk slight.

Bibliography

Janowitz H.D. (1981) Crohn's disease—50 years later. *N. Engl. J. Med.* **304**, 1600.

Chapter 78   # INTESTINAL PARASITES
(Helminth Infestation)

Oxyuris Vermicularis (Threadworms; Pinworms)

Very common. Up to 80% infestation in some communities.

Appearance

Worms look like wriggling white threads ½–1 cm long.

Life Cycle

Normal habitat caecum and appendix. Female migrates down to anus, crawls outside and lays 5000–10000 eggs. These are transferred to mouth, mainly under nails by scratching perineum, then swallowed; hatch in duodenum and pass down to caecum.

Viable in dry conditions for about 10 days. May be present in dust of room. Several members of family may be affected.

Symptoms

Anal and vulval pruritus common, especially at night.

Diagnosis

Worms seen in stool in large numbers. Eggs can be detected by sticking Sellotape gently around anus, then placing Sellotape on microscope slide and examining under microscope.

Treatment

Stringent hygienic measures to prevent reinfestation, and drug therapy with piperazine 50–70mg/kg/24h × 5 or viprynium embonate (pyrvinium pamoate) as single dose of 10mg/kg.

As oxyuriasis is always a family disease the whole family must be treated at the same time.

Ascaris Lumbricoides (*Roundworm*)

Uncommon in countries with good standard of hygiene. Very common elsewhere.

Appearance
Adult worm resembles earthworm but has sharp posterior end.

Life Cycle (*Fig. 78.1*)

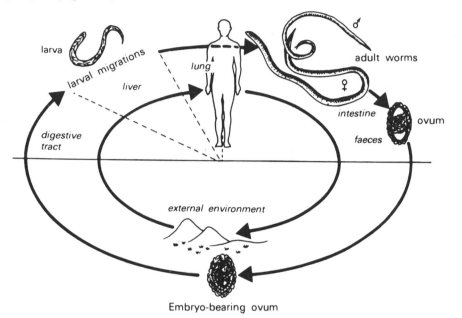

Fig. 78.1. Life cycle of *A. lumbricoides.*

Clinical Features
The condition is first recognized when a worm is passed per rectum. It may occasionally be suspected by the chance finding of an eosinophilia.

Very large numbers of worms are associated with malnutrition, vitamin deficiency, chronic infections due to immunological overload and failure to thrive. Multiple infestations with other worms are common.

Treatment
By improved hygienic measures and appropriate drug therapy: Piperazine as for threadworms, viprynium 10mg/kg daily for 2–3 days, or mebendazole 100mg 12-hourly for 3 days (regardless of age as it is poorly absorbed).

Hookworm Infestation (*Ankylostomiasis*)

Two species of hookworm parasitic to man:
1. *Ankylostoma duodenale.* Mediterranean basin and Asia.
2. *Necator americanus.* Widely distributed in the Americas.

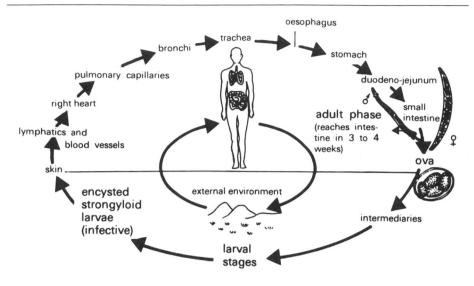

Fig. 78.2.   Life cycle of Ankylostoma.

Life Cycle (*Fig. 78.2*)

Clinical Features
1. Larval invasion. Produces itchy vesicular eruption at site of penetration of skin.
2. Adult worm in intestine. (*a*) Mild infestation. Evidence of chronic blood loss. (*b*) Severe infestation. Severe iron-deficient anaemia, tarry stools, general debility, failure to thrive.

Treatment
Mebendazole 100 mg b.d. for 3 days. Repeated courses may be necessary.

Toxocariasis (*Visceral Larva migrans*)

Caused by infestation by *Toxocara canis*. Very common round worm of dog.

Life Cycle
Puppies infested prenatally through placenta. Larva in lungs at birth. Migrate via trachea into intestinal tract. There mature into adult worms. Eggs evacuated in enormous numbers by puppy at about 3 weeks old. Continues until worms die when puppy about 6 months old. If eggs eaten by bitch, lie dormant until stimulated by new pregnancy. If eggs eaten by man (or more likely by dirt-eating young child), larvae never completely mature and somatic migration occurs.

Clinical Features
Mainly disease of young children. Rare. Low-grade fever, pulmonary infiltration, hepatomegaly, blindness if larvae reach eye via retinal artery.

Diagnosis
By history of possible contact with puppy. Eosinophilia may be very high. Hypergammaglobulinaemia. Serological tests available.

Prevention
No treatment is effective for larval stage in man. Prevention therefore very important—de-worm all puppies at age of 14 days and again at 1 month. Do not let children play where dogs defaecate.
   Note: Danger greatest from young dog to young children.

Trichuris Trichiura (*Whipworm*)

Very common in some parts of the world.

Life Cycle
Ova swallowed from contaminated soil. Adult nematode inhabits caecum but also appendix, colon or terminal ileum. Anterior part of worm embedded in mucosa; rear, whip-like end, free in intestinal cavity. Generally regarded as symptomless but may cause diarrhoea. Often associated with ascaris and other infestation. Characteristic ova can be found in stools and worms can often be seen on sigmoidoscopy.
   Trichuris is very resistant to therapy. Drug of choice is mebendazole 100 mg 12-hourly for 3 days.

Taenia (*Tapeworm*)

Uncommon in children.

Bilharziasis (*Schistosomiasis*)

Rapidly increasing problem because of migration of populations and increased irrigation projects.
   Three species of worm: *Schistosoma mansoni, S. haematobium, S. japonica.*

Life Cycle (*Fig. 78.3*)

Clinical Features
   S. mansoni: Africa, many parts. Mainly rectal involvement, producing blood and mucus in stools, and diarrhoea. Anaemia common. Eventually cirrhosis of liver and portal hypertension from progressive venous occlusion.
   S. haematobium: Africa, especially Egypt. Mainly bladder involvement, producing haematuria and dysuria. Eventually chronic infestation may predispose to cancer. Anaemia common.
   S. japonica: Only in eastern Asia. Similar to *S. mansoni* but more severe.

Diagnosis
Ova found in stools or urine.

Treatment
   1. Praziquantel 40 mg/kg divided doses i.m. once or twice weekly. Rest for 4 hours after drug.

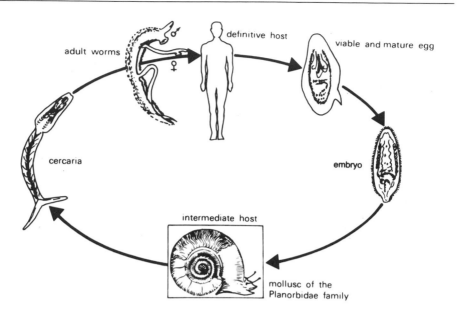

Fig. 78.3. Life cycle of *S. mansoni.*

Prevention
Difficult because of local bathing and toilet customs. Provision of latrines and clean water supply. Attempts to eradicate carrier snails disappointing.

Strongyloidiasis

Infestation with *Strongyloides stercoralis*. This small worm (up to 2 mm) is almost invisible. Larvae from soil penetrate the skin and enter the bloodstream, travel to the lung and via respiratory mucus reach the pharynx, are swallowed and enter the digestive tract. Fertilized female worms then penetrate the intestinal mucosa and lay their eggs in the submucosa. Emergent larvae are excreted in the faeces and live in the soil until the cycle begins again.

Clinical Features
Transcutaneous passage of larvae causes itchy urticaria, transpulmonary passage may produce Loeffler's syndrome, and massive intestinal infestation gives rise to malabsorption and abdominal pain.

Investigations
Marked eosinophilia is characteristic, but obviously not diagnostic. Stools contain larvae.

Treatment
Thiabendazole 25 mg/kg/day for 5 days.

Hydatid disease

Condition caused by larval stage of *Echinococcus granulosus*. Primary host—dog.

Secondary host—sheep, cattle, man. Common in children in endemic areas. Rare in infancy. Cysts commonly develop in lungs, liver or central nervous system. Child may present with chest infection or hepatomegaly or with signs of central nervous system tumour. Life cycle *see Fig. 78.4.*

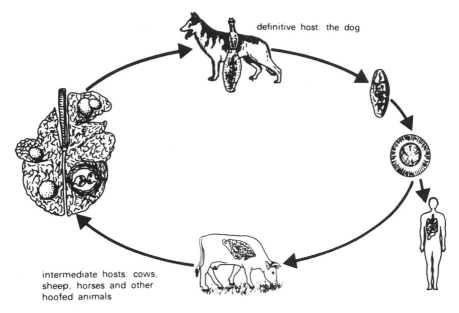

Fig. 78.4. Life cycle of *Echinococcus granulosus* (also known as *T. echinococcus.*)

Hydatid Lung Cysts

Not uncommon in some countries, e.g. Wales. Radiology helpful—may show rounded discrete mass(es); if cyst has ruptured it may show 'water lily' sign—air fluid level with collapsed membranes floating in middle; or cyst may separate from surrounding lung adventitia and a crescent of air be present—the perivesicular pneumocyst. Often multiple. Small pleural effusion may also be present. Casoni test, if positive, is of value; if negative, does not disprove diagnosis. Also complement fixation, bentonite flocculation tests. Treatment: careful surgery to avoid rupturing and thus disseminating cysts.

Giardiasis (*Giardia lamblia infestation*)

Giardia lamblia is a flagellate which inhabits the duodenum of humans in endemic areas. The organisms coat the wall of the intestine, with resultant malabsorption of fat. Common cause of syndrome resembling coeliac disease in many parts of the world. An important cause of chronic diarrhoea in children with immunological deficiencies. Flagellates may be found in stools, but biopsy of duodenum is often required. Often asymptomatic. Giardia may be found in water supplies in some countries

Treatment

Metronidazole 50–200 mg/day × 7 according to age.

Chapter 79

DIARRHOEA AND VOMITING
(*Gastro-enteritis*)

Specific Infective Diarrhoea

Typhoid Fever (*Enteric Fever*); **Paratyphoid A and B**
Typhoid rare in developed countries. Symptoms, signs and course similar to those in adults. Special points to remember are:
1. Usually presents as 'pyrexia of unknown origin (PUO)'. Diarrhoea often slight. May be constipation.
2. Stool often contains blood and mucus. Vomiting not prominent at first.
3. Temperature persists for days without treatment.
4. Spleen usually palpable.
5. Rose spots usually present. Rather inconspicuous. Occur mainly on upper trunk.
6. Salmonella osteomyelitis sometimes occurs, commonly in children with sickle-cell anaemia or other haemoglobinopathy (p. 412).

Diagnosis
1. In early stages organism can be grown from blood or stool, less commonly from urine.
2. Later, rising antibody titre diagnostic.

Treatment
Correct dehydration and electrolyte disturbance. Antibiotics useful especially for septicaemia but can prolong excretion of organism. Growing increase in ampicillin-resistant organisms, but this drug preferable to chloramphenicol in first instance because of less toxic effects.

Bacillary Dysentery
Occasional cause of diarrhoea. Does not commonly affect infants under 6 months. Sometimes occurs in small epidemics, particularly in schools.

Organisms
Shigella sonnei commonest in UK; *S. flexneri* rare; *S. dysenterii* (shigae) very rare; *S. Boydii* very rare.

Epidemiology
Organism conveyed by food, fingers, flies, from faeces of carrier or open case.

Pathology
Chiefly affects large intestine, especially sigmoid colon, rectum and caecum. Terminal ileum occasionally involved. Causes multiple superficial ulcers separated by inflamed mucous membrane. Mesenteric lymph nodes enlarged.

Symptoms and Signs
Fever; abdominal pain; diarrhoea; later vomiting. Tenesmus marked if rectum involved. With Sonnei infection toxaemia rarely great, mild blood-stained

diarrhoea often only indication of infection. Fits can occur. If diarrhoea very severe, dehydration occurs. Stool characteristically contains blood, mucus and pus.

Course and Prognosis
Usually only lasts 3–4 days. Death rare. Chronic dysentery does not occur in children, but symptomless carriers not uncommon.

Complications
Prolapse of rectum as in any severe wasting disease. Typical adult complications—iritis, arthritis, etc.—do not occur.

Diagnosis
Character of stool often enables presumptive diagnosis to be made. Bacteriology of stool gives final diagnosis.

Differential Diagnosis
1. Rectal bleeding.
2. Amoebic dysentery.
3. Appendicitis.
4. Acute ulcerative colitis
5. Intussusception.

Amoebic Dysentery
Disease caused by *Entamoeba histolytica* occurring mainly in developing countries and affecting adults more commonly than children.

Life Cycle
Cysts of Entamoeba contaminating water or vegetables are ingested, lose their outer shell in the terminal ileum to release 'metacystic' amoebae. These form trophozoites which multiply and invade colon wall to produce ulcers and microabscesses, causing dysentery. The amoebae are invasive and can migrate to liver, lungs or even brain, but extracolonic spread is rare in children.

Clinical Features
Malaise, fatigue, anorexia, colicky abdominal pain, diarrhoea or constipation. Acute attacks of dysentery characterized by profuse diarrhoea with blood and mucus. Stools contain amoebae or cysts.

Treatment
Metronidazole, 20 mg/kg/24 h for 10 days.

Staphylococcal Enterocolitis
Rare complication of antibiotic therapy.

Clinical Features
Child who has usually been suffering from some illness requiring prolonged antibiotic therapy develops fever, watery diarrhoea, vomiting, dehydration and shock. May become extremely ill very rapidly. Staphylococci found in stool in large numbers. Death may occur from dehydration.

Treatment
1. Stop original antibiotic.
2. Combat dehydration and shock.
3. Give antistaphylococcal drugs, e.g. flucloxacillin or fucidin.

Gastro-enteritis

Definition
Disease of infants now uncommon in developed countries (but very common elsewhere) carrying high mortality in the past. Characterized clinically by vomiting, diarrhoea, and in severe cases dehydration.

History
In 1893 diarrhoea caused death rate in England and Wales of 0·7 per 1000 population. In 1937, 0·08 per 1000. In 1964, total of 529 deaths of children from gastroenteritis—rate of 0·01 per 1000 population.

Causes of improvement: higher standard of living; better education in cleanliness; use of processed instead of fresh milk.

Aetiology
May be caused by many organisms but two predominate, Rotavirus and *E. coli*.

Rotavirus
A RNA virus about 70–80 nm diameter with a characteristic wheel-like structure which is responsible for up to half of all infective gastro-enteritis in children in various parts of the world. Illness is not usually very severe except in very young infants. May cause epidemics in which vomiting predominates. Diagnosis made from stool by a specific enzyme-linked assay (ELISA) or direct visualization of the virus with an electron microscope. Neonatal infection does not confer lasting immunity.

Escherichia Coli
Various strains of *E. coli* produce diarrhoea by a variety of mechanisms: endotoxins; exotoxins (heat-stable and heat-labile); factors which promote adherence to enterocytes; mucosal damage (structural or functional, with activation of adenyl cyclase in small intestinal cells thus inhibiting absorption and stimulating secretion of fluid and electrolytes); and occasionally mucosal invasion producing a shigella-like illness.

Clinical Features
All gradations of case from mild to fulminating occur.
Mild cases. Diarrhoea may be preceded by vomiting. Stools become more fluid, yellow or green, usually offensive. Baby becomes irritable, refuses feeds. Examination reveals no localized abnormality but there may be slight pyrexia.

Rapid recovery is usual but occasionally diarrhoea becomes persistent: the post-enteritis syndrome (*see below*).
Severe cases. Sudden onset of diarrhoea with or without vomiting. Stools green, liquid almost from the onset, and may be very frequent. On examination the child

is fretful, ill, and draws up its legs as if in pain. Borborygmi may be evident, and dehydration is likely (*see below*). Evidence of extra-abdominal infection should be looked for, e.g. otitis media.

Fulminating cases ('Cholera Infantum'). Sudden onset with copious vomiting followed by profuse diarrhoea. May be high fever. Stools frequent, green, liquid and projectile. Severe toxaemia and dehydration are evident: the child is ill, apathetic, listless, and has a mewing cry. Occasionally convulsions occur. Cheeks sunken; eyes lack lustre and seem deepset; abdomen may be scaphoid, superficial veins collapsed. Tongue and mouth dry. Skin dry and inelastic—when pinched it stays up, instead of immediately springing flat again. Fontanelle depressed and non-pulsating. Pulse often rapid, weak and thready; extremities cold and cyanosed. Urinary output lowered.

Complications

(1) Dehydration and biochemical derangement; (2) Anaemia; (3) Abdominal distension; (4) Impairment of liver function; (5) Venous thrombosis; (6) Infection; (7) Post-enteritis syndrome (*see below*).

Dehydration

Causes. Fluid in large quantity can be rapidly lost by infant with diarrhoea. Vomiting more dangerous, as it not only causes fluid loss but also prevents loss being made good by fluids given by mouth.

Assessment of Severity. Difficulty is that obvious signs of dehydration do not appear until infant has lost more than 5 % of its body weight.

When infant with gastro-enteritis first seen, most valuable indications of severity are:

1. Accurate estimate of weight loss. Inquiry should always be made as to highest known weight.

2. Length of history, frequency of stools and quantity of water passed in them.

Acidosis—Metabolic

Often occurs with dehydration in severe cases, especially if diarrhoea main symptom. Acidosis and dehydration mutually aggravate each other, because, to correct acidosis, large quantities of urine must be passed in order to remove excess acid metabolites, whereas to correct dehydration kidney should excrete small quantity of concentrated urine, thus retaining fluids.

Alkalosis

Far less common than acidosis.

Causes (1) *Vomiting*, with severe loss of hydrochloric acid from stomach. (2) *Therapeutic*, due to over-administration of alkalis.

Clinical manifestations. May cause convulsions or tetany if severe.

Protein Deficiency

Causes. (1) *Prolonged Starvation*; (2) *Liver Dysfunction*.

Clinical manifestations. Usually nil. May led to oedema and possibly lowered resistance to infection.

Potassium Deficiency
Cause. Potassium lost from bowel in prolonged, severe diarrhoea. May also be lost in urine.
Clinical features. When severe case of gastroenteritis first investigated serum potassium often normal or high, but as dehydration and acidosis corrected, figure falls. (1) *Effect of Low Potassium* (i.e. below about 3 mEq/l). Leads to abdominal distension from intestinal ileus. Paralysis not seen. (2) *Effect of High Potassium* (i.e. above about 8 mEq/l). Bradycardia, heart-block, cardiac arrest.
Investigations: (1) *Serum potassium* (2) *Electrocardiogram*: *See* p. 282.
Treatment
Indications. Serum potassium less than 3 mEq/l.
   Potassium can be given as potassium chloride: (1) By mouth—safe. 1–2 g/day. Give in divided doses in feeds. Total required rarely exceeds 6 g. (2) Intravenous route—potentially dangerous, should be given not faster than 1 g in 24 h. If signs of overdosage develop, intravenous calcium gluconate and hypertonic glucose solution said to be of value.

Abdominal Distension
Uncommon complication of severe gastro-enteritis.
Cause. Probably due to low serum potassium.
Clinical features. Abdomen usually noted to be distended when initial dehydration has been corrected. All gradations from mild to severe. In mild case child difficult to feed and may vomit. In severe cases, condition resembles paralytic ileus with: bilestained vomit, absent bowel sounds and even complete constipation. May be associated with signs of liver insufficiency.
Differential diagnosis. Condition must be distinguished from: (1) *Intestinal Obstruction*. Abdominal distension associated with vomiting and constipation but bowel sounds loud, and vigorous visible peristalsis may be seen. (2) *Peritonitis*. May exactly resemble paralytic ileus but in addition there is usually pyrexia and leucocytosis.
Treatment
   1. Correction of fluid and electrolyte disturbance.
   2. Repeated gastric lavage or, if necessary, continuous gastric suction. All feeds and drugs by mouth must be stopped.
   3. Continuous intravenous therapy. Fluid and electrolyte intake must be accurately regulated.
   4. Drugs must be given i.v. or i.m.

Impairment of Liver Function
Occurs late in disease.
Pathology. Findings inconstant. Usually gross fatty infiltration with parenchymatous degeneration. Sometimes also dilatation of sinusoids, cellular necrosis or early fibrosis.
Clinical features
   1. *Enlargement of Liver*. May be difficult to feel owing to coincidental abdominal distension.
   2. *Jaundice*. Rare. Very grave prognosis.
   3. *Haemorrhagic Phenomena*. Rare. Purpura haematemesis, melaena, bleeding, e.g. from intravenous wounds. Possibly due to: (*a*) Prothrombin deficiency from: (i) Inadequate supplies of vitamin K. (ii) Alteration of intestinal flora,

especially following use of antibiotics by mouth, thus preventing synthesis of vitamin K in gut. (iii) Liver damage with lack of synthesis of prothrombin from vitamin K. (*b*) Disseminated intravascular coagulation.

Anaemia
Uncommon complication of severe gastro-enteritis.

Venous Thrombosis

Cause
    1. Primary. Usually as terminal event in severely dehydrated infant. Any large vein may be affected, especially cerebral sinuses, giving rise to convulsions and paralysis.
    2. Secondary to Treatment. Following prolonged intravenous infusions or if certain drugs are administered intravenously, notably penicillin or amino acids.

Infection
1. Thrush. Very commonly found, but rarely severe.
2. Otitis media. Mild catarrhal changes often found if drum of infants with gastro-enteritis examined; drum infected but mobile. Difficult to say in particular case whether middle-ear infection primary or secondary. At autopsy mastoiditis sometimes discovered.
3. Bronchopneumonia. Especially prone to occur following excessive hydration. Basal crepitations commonest sign.
4. Pyelonephritis

Prognosis
Mortality in different epidemics and different centres varies greatly. Depends on:
1. Infant feeding. Breast-fed babies infrequently contract gastro-enteritis.
2. Age. Young babies more susceptible and prognosis worse.
3. Severity. Prolonged mild diarrhoea often carries worse prognosis than fulminating case correctly treated.
4. Complications. (*a*) Biochemical disturbance dangerous if not corrected. (*b*) Abdominal distension serious if it goes on to paralytic ileus. (*c*) Impairment of liver function— jaundice and haemorrhage carry poor prognosis.

Diagnosis and Management
Severity of case must be assessed.
1. Mild case, i.e. *child appears well*: no dehydration; little or no vomiting; taking fluids well; not losing large quantity of fluid in stool. Best treated at home or as outpatient under *constant supervision.* Exceptions: Poor social conditions, e.g.; (*a*) Overcrowding; (*b*) Low maternal intelligence; (*c*) Other infants in the house.
    Note: Disease can worsen dramatically in a few hours. Condition should clear up within a week on appropriate treatment, if it does not, child probably requires hospitalization.
2. Severe Cases. May be long mild history, or short severe one. *Child obviously ill.* Marked loss of weight, stools watery, may be vomiting or refusal of feeds. Complications usually present. Child should be admitted to hospital with cubicle and barrier nursing facilities.

Careful history must be taken, and child examined: (*a*) For parenteral infection. (*b*) Swabs taken of throat and stool. (*c*) Urine for infection. (*d*) Daily weight chart. (*e*) Haemoglobin. (*f*) Serum electrolytes and urea.

Treatment

Principles

1. Replacement of fluid and electrolyte loss. *See* p. 136. (*a*) Correct existing dehydration (and electrolyte imbalance when severe). (*b*) Supply normal basic needs. (*c*) Replace ongoing abnormal losses. (*d*) Resume normal feeding carefully but as soon as possible when diarrhoea ceases. (*e*) Use oral route whenever possible (p. 137).

2. Antibiotics are rarely indicated unless a specific organism (e.g. yersinia, entamoeba) is isolated or child gravely ill and presumed septicaemic.

3. Antidiarrhoeal agents may do more harm than good by slowing transit time and delaying clearance of infecting organism.

Yersinia Enterocolitica

Causes diarhoea and vomiting, accompanied by marked abdominal pain: may mimic appendicitis. Systemic symptoms, e.g. fever, rashes, arthritis also occur.

Treatment
Co-trimoxazole.

Campylobacter Jejuni

Usually less severe in children than in adults. May affect domestic animals; can be acquired from infested food e.g. poultry.

Organism produces an exotoxin. Symptoms include abdominal pain, prostration, severe diarrhoea—often bloody.

Treatment
Erythromycin 40 mg/kg/24 h for 7 days.

Epidemic Winter Vomiting

Not uncommon mild disease of short duration (6–48 h) occurring mainly during the winter months. Manifested by sudden onset of vomiting often starting in the night, occasionally with slight fever or diarrhoea.

Aetiology

Viral. Echovirus, rotaviruses and others have been implicated in various epidemics.

Course

Child recovers without treatment. Family outbreaks common.

Section

11

Diseases
of Liver,
Biliary System,
Pancreas and
Small Intestine

Chapter 80	*JAUNDICE*

Normal Bilirubin Metabolism

Bilirubin is produced from
1. Haemoglobin breakdown.
2. Unknown source in bone marrow.

In Original Form it is
1. Unconjugated, attached to protein.
2. Lipophilic and indirect reacting on van den Bergh test.
3. Not excreted by liver or kidney.

Stages in Excretion
Bilirubin is:

Trapped by liver cell from portal vein blood.

Transformed to water-soluble form—either a glucuronide or sulphate—by microsomal enzymes, e.g. glucuronyl transferase. The water-soluble form is direct-reacting, and can be excreted by the liver or kidney.

Transferred to biliary apparatus—from liver cell across the cell membrane.

Transported along biliary passages to duodenum.

Abnormal Bilirubin Metabolism

1. Excess production of bilirubin—the haemolytic anaemias. Result:
   1.1 Liver transport and conjugating mechanisms unable to cope with load.
   1.2 Bilirubin accumulates in blood.
   1.3 Serum bilirubin unconjugated and so cannot be excreted by kidneys. Stools and urine normal.

251

Examples: Haemolytic disease of newborn, hereditary spherocytosis.

2. Defect in trapping. Unconjugated bilirubin is not fully removed from circulating blood. Stools and urine normal. *Example*: Gilbert's disease.

3. Defect in conjugating bilirubin to glucuronide. Bilirubin accumulates in liver and blood. Stools and urine normal.

Examples:

3.1 Reduced glucuronyl transferase—physiological jaundice in newborn infants.

3.2 Absent glucuronyl transferase—Crigler–Najjar syndrome.

3.3 Glucuronyl transferase inhibition—by steroids. *Example*: Neonatal jaundice associated with excretion of excess maternal steroids possibly pregnanediol in breast milk. Infants develop prolonged, moderate 'physiological' jaundice, disappears when breast feeding stopped. May recur in successive infants.

4. Defect in transporting bilirubin to bile canaliculus. Conjugated bilirubin regurgitates back into blood, appears in urine. Stools may be normal colour. *Examples*: Dubin–Johnson and Rotor's syndromes.

5. Defect in transport along biliary apparatus. Conjugated bilirubin returns to blood, is absent in stools, but is excreted by kidney. Obstructive jaundice. *Examples*: extrahepatic biliary atresia, choledochal cyst, intrahepatic biliary atresia, inspissated bile syndrome.

Dubin–Johnson Syndrome

A rare autosomal recessive disorder in which an unidentified greenish-black pigment is deposited in the hepatocytes.
Clinical Features. Variable jaundice which may begin at any time from birth to adult life. No hepatomegaly. Good prognosis.
Laboratory Investigations
  1. Elevated serum bilirubin, 25–75% conjugated.
  2. No rise in liver enzymes.
  3. Liver biopsy reveals normal architecture, dark granules in hepatocytes.

Rotor Syndrome

Very rare. Similar to Dubin–Johnson syndrome; mild familial conjugated hyperbilirubinaemia, but liver biopsy normal. Prognosis excellent.

Causes of Jaundice in Neonatal Period
  1. Physiological.
  2. Haemolytic disease of newborn (with extra and intra-corpuscular defects). *See* p. 402.
  3. Atresia of bile ducts. *See below*.
  4. Neonatal hepatitis syndrome. *See below*.
  5. Sepsis. *See below*.
  6. Congenital syphilis. *See* p. 102.
  7. Galactosaemia. *See* p. 159.

8. Inspissated bile syndrome
9. Breast milk
10. Non-haemolytic congenital hyperbilirubinaemia
11. Hypothyroidism
12. Excessive bruising

Causes of Jaundice in Infancy
All rare.
1. Infective hepatitis. *See* p. 259.
2. Hereditary spherocytosis, *See* p. 408.
3. Choledochal cyst. *See below.*
4. Masses pressing on bile ducts. Malignant, tuberculous, hydatid cysts, etc.
5. Sepsis, e.g. septic cholangitis, portal phlebitis or sepsis elsewhere.
6. High intestinal obstruction, e.g. volvulus, pyloric stenosis. Probably starvation effect on liver conjugating mechanisms.

Causes of Jaundice in Older Children
1. Obstructive jaundice
 1.1 Extrinsic Obstruction to Bile ducts by malignant disease, choledochal cyst, hydatid cyst.
 1.2 Intrinsic Obstruction to Bile Ducts by:
 1.2.1 Gallstones: Very rare in children. Occasionally pigment stones may be found in acholuric jaundice.
 1.2.2 Roundworms. Very occasionally block common duct.
 1.3 Intrahepatic Cholestasis, e.g. drugs.
 1.4 Congenital Non-haemolytic Hyperbilirubinaemia
2. Haemolytic jaundice e.g. acholuric jaundice.
3. Toxic and infective jaundice
 3.1 Infective Hepatitis. See p. 259.
 3.2 Weil's Disease. See below.
 3.3 Hepatocellular Failure. See below.
 3.4 Suppurative Hepatitis. See below.
 3.5 Malaria

Biliary Atresia

Aetiology
Probably true congenital malformation in some cases. About 25% have other malformations. May also develop in child with neonatal hepatitis syndrome and bile in early stools.

Pathology
Atresia totally extrahepatic in 20% but may be partially or wholly intrahepatic. Portal tracts show inspissated bile, marked fibrosis and bile duct proliferation. Generally much less hepatocellular damage in idiopathic extrahepatic atresia than in neonatal hepatitis. Cirrhosis develops in untreated case.

Note: Histological differentiation between intrahepatic atresia and neonatal hepatitis is very difficult.

Clinical Features
Onset. Gradually increasing jaundice commencing during first 3 weeks. At first may be thought to be physiological, but it fails to clear up in a few days. Colour gradually deepens and child becomes olive green. Jaundice may fluctuate in intensity. Urine and saliva become bile stained. Stools pale and fatty, but not completely colourless owing to excretion of bile into intestine with succus entericus.
On examination. General condition may remain good for a few months. Liver is enlarged. Later spleen also becomes palpable and ascites develops.

Investigations
1. *Liver function tests* give little additional information, except for serial serum bilirubin estimations. In atresia values steadily increase. In hepatitis values fluctuate more.
2. *I^{131} Rose Bengal Test*. Faecal excretion of less than 8% of isotope in 72h following intravenous injection is evidence of biliary obstruction. May be repeated after 3 weeks of cholestyramine (1·0g q.i.d.). No change in atresia, but increase exceeding 10% occurs in hepatitis.
3. *Duodenal Bile Acids*. In complete biliary obstruction (as by atresia) duodenal juice contains no bile acids.
4. *Percutaneous Liver Biopsy* may be helpful but sometimes histology indistinguishable from neonatal hepatitis syndrome, particularly in early stages. Serial biopsy justifiable. If any cirrhosis proceed to laparotomy, cholangiogram and operative liver biopsy.
5. *Laparotomy and Operative Cholangiogram*. If no duct demonstrated proceed to exploration of porta hepatis. If ducts of >150μ found anastomose porta with Roux-en-Y loop of intestine (Kasai operation).

Differential Diagnosis
Neonatal hepatitis syndrome and choledochal cyst.

Complications
1. Prothrombin level low, due to lack of absorption of vitamin K. Haemorrhages may therefore occur.
2. Rickets may develop, due to lack of absorption of fat-soluble vitamin D.
3. Large quantity of fat remaining in gut may combine with calcium, with resultant osteoporosis.
4. Skin xanthomas sometimes seen as late manifestation.

Course and Prognosis
Jaundice gradually deepens. Biliary cirrhosis develops; liver and spleen enlarge. Ascites may appear. Long survival possible with intrahepatic atresia.

Treatment
Depends on anatomical type:
1. If only common duct involved cholecyst-duodenostomy can be performed

with good effect in less than 10%. At operation gallbladder found to be distended with bile.

2. If other parts of biliary system involved curative operation difficult or impossible. Hepatic porto-enterostomy (Kasai) may be tried but must be performed early if it is to succeed. Ascending cholangitis is a common complication. Prognosis is poor but up to 30% survive without jaundice and with few immediate problems, although development of cirrhosis may continue.

Intrahepatic Biliary Hypoplasia
(Alagille syndrome)

Rare familial disorder, dominant with incomplete penetrance and clinical variability, in which hypoplasia or atresia of intrahepatic bile passages occur causing persistent obstructive jaundice. Other features of the syndrome include cardiac malformations (particularly pulmonary artery stenosis) and characteristic facies. No definitive treatment is possible but symptomatic treatment with phenobarbitone, cholestyramine and fat-soluble vitamins is helpful and death from biliary cirrhosis may be postponed for 2 decades or more.

Neonatal Hepatitis Syndrome

Definition
Disorder starting in first 4 months, characterized by conjugated hyperbilirubinaemia and features of hepatocellular damage. Liver biopsy shows cholestasis and liver cell necrosis with inflammatory reaction and often multinucleated giant cells.

Aetiology
Uncertain in 70%. Similar clinical and histological features may result from a variety of conditions.

1. Intra-uterine infection

    1.1 Virus—herpes simplex, Coxsackie, adenovirus, cytomegalovirus, rubella.

    1.2 Syphilis (p. 102).

    1.3 *Listeria monocytogenes.*

    1.4 *Toxoplasma gondii* (p. 111).

    1.5 Hepatitis B antigen—some infants of mothers with HB positive hepatitis in last trimester have liver disease, usually mild.

2. Metabolic disorders

    2.1 Galactosaemia—positive Clinitest, negative Clinistix, galactose in urine (p. 159).

    2.2 Fructosaemia—positive Clinitest, negative Clinistix, fructose in urine (p. 161).

    2.3 Tyrosinosis—positive Phenistix or ferric chloride test. Serum amino acids show tyrosinaemia (p. 149).

    2.4 α_1-Antitrypsin deficiency (*see below*).

2.5 Cystic fibrosis (p. 267).

2.6 Niemann–Pick disease.

3. Sepsis. Septicaemia and urinary tract infection in neonate may be complicated by jaundice and deranged liver function.

4. Umbilical Infection. Ascending infection from septic umbilicus. Portal
pyelophelebitis.

5. Erythroblastosis fetalis. Severe rhesus incompatibility may be accompanied
by signs of hepatocellular damage.

6. Biliary atresia (see above). Clinical picture may be indistinguishable.

Management

That of the underlying condition, where possible. Differential diagnosis from
biliary atresia difficult (*see above*).

α_1-Antitrypsin Deficiency

Normal serum contains inhibitor of trypsin, located in α_1-globulin fraction.
Several genetic variants exist, most important are M, S and Z. Homozygous ZZ
state indicates complete absence of α_1-antitrypsin, detectable on electrophoretic
strip. Biological importance of α_1-antitrypsin uncertain, but absence associated
with some cases of neonatal hepatitis syndrome and hepatic cirrhosis. May also
be asymptomatic. Deficient adults may develop pulmonary emphysema. Liver
biopsy reveals pigmented material in hepatocytes.

Obstruction by Inspissated bile

Following haemolytic disease of newborn bile ducts may become blocked by
inspissated bile or mucus. Conditions should be suspected when jaundice of
haemolytic disease persists unduly and becomes obstructive in type. Jaundice
intermittent.

Treatment

Steroids may help.

Choledochal Cyst
(*Congenital Cyst of Common Bile Duct*)

Very rare condition occurring almost exclusively in girls. Present from birth, but
often not recognized before 5–12 years of age. Symptoms may begin in infancy
and mimic biliary atresia.

Clinical Features

History of recurrent attacks of jaundice and sometimes of 'dragging' pains in
abdomen. Large cystic mass felt in right side of abdomen separate from liver.
Biliary system may become secondarily infected and in older cases liver
sometimes cirrhotic.

Treatment

Surgical: anastomosis of gallbladder or part of cyst with intestinal tract.

Leptospirosis (*Weil's Disease*)

Definition

Very rare disease caused by rat-borne spirochaete, *Leptospira icterohaemorrhagica*. Manifested clinically by fever, muscle pains, headache, haemorrhages and jaundice.

Aetiology

L. icterohaemorrhagica carried by about 40% of rats. Mode of infection: Organism excreted into water in rat's urine. People immersed in this water run risk of being infected. Incubation period: about 10 days.

Clinical Features

Many subclinical cases occur, jaundice being present only in those severely affected.

1. Pre-icteric phase. Sudden onset, often with rigor. Pyrexia, headache, conjunctival suffusion, marked pain and tenderness in muscles and over liver.

2. Icteric phase. Jaundice characteristically orange-yellow colour. Haemorrhages common. Herpes febrilis often occurs and is usually haemorrhagic. Meningeal irritation or lymphocytic meningitis may develop. Anuria is a severe manifestation and renal failure may cause death.

Investigations

1. Blood urea. Raised constantly and early in disease.

2. Urine. Albuminuria common.

3. White blood count. Polymorphonuclear leucocytosis usual, but leucopenia can occur.

4. Isolation of organisms. Can be found in blood during first 6 days. Most successful method is by immediate guinea-pig inoculation.

5. Agglutination tests. Valuable confirmatory evidence but not positive for 7–10 days. Rising titre should be obtained with successive samples of serum.

6. CSF. May show lymphocytic reaction.

Treatment

Ideally commenced in pre-icteric phase. Penicillin or other antibiotics given in large dose. Vitamin K may be of value. Anuria should be treated as indicated on p. 386.

Hepatocellular Failure

Causes

Fulminating hepatitis A; chronic active hepatitis; Wilson's disease; terminal obstructive jaundice; poisons, e.g. chloroform, halothane or carbon tetra-chloride; unknown.

Pathology
Massive necrosis of liver.

Clinical Features
Note: Speed of development of these features varies greatly. May be fulminating or quite slow.
1. Pre-coma. Anorexia, persistent vomiting, headache, fever. On examination:

> 1.1 Circulatory changes and cyanosis marked: hyperkinetic circulation, bounding pulse, tachycardia, low blood pressure and flushed extremities.
> 1.2 May or may not be jaundice. If so, usually profound with haemorrhages.
> 1.3 Liver enlarged at first, later shrunken and not palpable. Ascites and oedema may or may not be present.
> 1.4 Fetor hepaticus: characteristic foetid odour to breath, likened to smell of freshly opened corpse.
> 1.5 Spider naevi. Present in large numbers over upper part of body and arms.
> 1.6 Liver palms: erythema around periphery of palms of hands and soles of feet.

2. Hepatic coma

> 1.1 Mental state: Disturbed consciousness with personality change, irritability, intellectual deterioration, slow, slurred speech, low screaming cry, lapsing into coma.
> 1.2 Neurological abnormality. 'Flapping' tremor very characteristic: arms held out straight, flapping takes place at wrist and at metacarpophalangeal joints; absent at rest. Increased muscle tone leading to rigidity. Deep reflexes exaggerated; plantar response flexor at first, later becomes extensor. Muscle twitching, grasp and sucking reflex present. Hyperventilation and hyperpyrexia terminal.

Investigations
1. Serum ammonia high; serum glucose and potassium may be low.
2. Gross amino aciduria revealed by paper chromatography.
3. Prothrombin time prolonged, fibrinogen concentration and platelets often reduced, fibrinogen degradation products increased.

Prognosis
Usually fatal.

Treatment of Coma and Pre-coma
1. Diet. All food containing protein should be stopped. Glucose given orally, or if necessary intravenously into a deep vein. Vitamins K and B parenterally.

2. Enema and purgation with magnesium sulphate to empty bowel. Oral neomycin to decrease gastrointestinal ammonia formation.
3. Fresh frozen plasma and possibly heparin for control of bleeding tendency.
4. Check electrolytes.
5. Avoidance of sedation, especially with morphine or paraldehyde.
6. Steroids may be of value.
7. Antibiotics required for infection. Particular risk of Gram-negative septicaemia.
8. Exchange transfusion occasionally lifesaving.

Encephalopathy with Fatty Degeneration of Viscera (*Reye's Syndrome*) (*See* p. 339.)

Suppurative Hepatitis

Causes
1. Following portal pyaemia. Primary lesion usually in intestinal tract or umbilicus.
2. Amoebic hepatitis. Very rare in countries with good hygiene. History of preceding amoebic hepatitis may be obtained. Liver tender. Amoebic abscess uncommon in children.

Bibliography

Altman R.P.(1981) Biliary atresia. *Pediatrics* **68**, 896.

Chapter 81   **ACUTE VIRAL HEPATITIS**

Definition
Acute disease caused by a virus manifested clinically by fever, anorexia, vomiting, malaise and jaundice; pathologically by focal degeneration of liver cells.

Aetiology
Sex. Equal incidence.
Virology
1. Virus of epidemic infective hepatitis—virus A, a RNA virus. Incubation period about 2–8 weeks. Virus recoverable from faeces and blood.
2. Virus of serum hepatitis—virus B, a DNA virus. Incubation period 8–26 weeks. Virus recoverable from blood.
No demonstrable cross-immunity between two types.
3. A further syndrome (non-A non-B hepatitis) is clinically indistinguishable from hepatitis B but no virus has yet been identified to account for it. It may also follow blood transfusion.

Epidemiology
Geographically widespread:

1. *Hepatitis A*. Oral transmission: flourishes when sanitary conditions poor; carried by food, water, etc.

2. *Hepatitis B*. Parenteral and oral transmission occur. Introduction of virus by injection of serum, plasma, whole blood, blood products (e.g. factor VIII), or contaminated syringe from infected person who may be in pre-icteric phase or chronic carrier. Can occur at any age, uncommon in childhood outside institutions. Special danger to patients on chronic renal dialysis, and to teenage drug addicts.

HB antigen (HB Ag, 'Australia' antigen) may be outer coat of virus, often present in blood of carriers for many years. These are ineligible to be blood donors. Danger to medical and nursing personnel of accidental inoculation.

Pathology
Histological appearance of liver (mainly determined from biopsy specimens): diffuse hepatitis with acute focal degeneration of parenchymal liver cells; lesion is centrilobular or periportal. Healing by regeneration of parenchymal cells may be complete, but commonly some fibrosis occurs.

Clinical Features
1. *Preceding history*:

1.1 Hepatitis A. Other cases of jaundice, or subclinical cases with malaise, anorexia and vomiting only, may be known in district with or without direct contact.

1.2 Hepatitis B. History of injection or transfusion up to 6 months previously.

2. *Pre-icteric phase*. Lasts 3–7 days.

Onset often fairly acute with anorexia, general malaise, vomiting, headache and pyrexia up to 39 or 39·5 °C (102 or 103 °F). Occasionally abdominal pain, maximal over liver, may be prominent symptom. Liver tender.

Many cases do not pass beyond this phase. In others it is mild or almost non-existent.

3. *Icteric phase*. Lasts about 2–4 weeks. Tends to be longer in hepatitis B than hepatitis A.

Jaundice may be first shown by yellow colour of conjunctivae or sometimes by darkening of urine and pallor of stools. Jaundice can be mild or severe. As colour appears, pre-icteric symptoms often improve.

On examination: tender liver usually palpable 1–3 finger-breadths below costal margin. Spleen may also be enlarged in young children.

Investigations
1. *Urine*. (*a*) Contains bilirubin. (*b*) Urobilinogen increased at onset of jaundice as liver unable to excrete it. Later level falls, as with increasing jaundice no bile enters gut. As recovery takes place, level rises again. After jaundice has disappeared it falls back to normal.

2. *Faeces*. Important to record colour. Become pale because of lack of stercobilin; moderate steatorrhoea. Colour improves as child recovers.

3. *Serum bilirubin*. Raised, up to 350 mmol/l (20 mg%).

4. *Liver function tests*. (*a*) Serum alkaline phosphatase is moderately raised but not as high as in obstructive jaundice. (*b*) Serum transaminase. Aspartate

aminotransferase (AST) may rise over 1000 u/l. (*c*) In fulminant cases: blood ammonia level rises; blood glucose level falls; prothrombin time prolonged.
5. *HB Antigens*. Present in blood from several days before to 3 months after onset of jaundice. The most widely used is HBsAg test, which detects surface antigen of HB virus. Chronic carrier state may occur, particularly after anicteric infection.
6. *Hepatitis A*. Rise in specific Ig M antibody just before onset of jaundice. Diagnose by radioimmunoassay.

Differential Diagnosis
1. In pre-icteric phase diagnosis may be very difficult, especially in endemic cases. Abdominal emergencies or onset of infectious fever may be mimicked.
2. When jaundice present diagnosis not difficult. Inquiry must always be made for history of previous serum administration.
Other causes of hepatitis should be considered, especially:
1. Infectious mononucleosis.
2. Leptospirosis—characteristic features: muscle pain, haemorrhages, herpes febrilis, albuminuria, raised blood urea and leucocytosis.
3. Hepatitis due to drugs and poisons. Jaundice usually severe.
4. Cytomegalovirus infection.
5. Brucellosis.
6. Amoebiasis.
7. Malaria.
8. Yellow fever.

Course
Disease may:
1. Be mild. Complete recovery within few weeks.
2. Be fulminating. Death occurring within a few weeks—syndrome of hepatocellular failure (*see* p. 257).
3. Progress relentlessly to hepatic cirrhosis (*see below*).
4. Progress by several recurrences of jaundice, eventually resulting in hepatic cirrhosis.

Treatment
No specific therapy known. The ill child will usually wish for bed rest but there is no evidence that this influences the cause of the illness.
Diet. Child should be allowed to eat or drink whatever he fancies in initial stages, as long as adequate fluid intake maintained. In practice most children prefer low-fat, high-carbohydrate diet when appetite recovers. Adequate vitamin intake must be ensured.

Prophylaxis
1. General. (*a*) Scrupulous hand washing after contact with infected patients. (*b*) Hygienic preparation of food, washing of uncooked vegetables etc. in endemic areas.
2. Risk of hepatitis B reduced by: (*a*) Screening all donors for carriage of HBsAg by most sensitive method available. (*b*) Use of single donors rather than pooled serum. At present not possible to sterilize blood from virus IH or SH. (*c*)

Sterilization of all needles, etc. between one patient and the next. Disposable equipment safer.

3. Gammaglobulin, 0·06ml/kg body weight (0·03ml/lb) provides passive immunity for at least 8 weeks, probably longer. Must be given before infection or early in pre-icteric phase. Valuable in preventing family epidemics.

4. Specific Hepatitis B vaccine now available.

Chronic Hepatitis (*Chronic Active Hepatitis*)

Rare group of liver diseases, aetiology usually unknown. Similar clinical features occasionally follow known viral hepatitis. Onset abrupt with fever, anorexia, nausea and jaundice, or may be insidious. Amenorrhoea, arthritis, ascites, erythema nodosum may occur. Gammaglobulin raised and positive ANF test. Wilson's disease must be excluded.

Investigations
Elevated IgG, antinuclear factor and LE cells, and prolonged prothrombin time may be found in addition to usual biochemical changes of hepatitis (raised transaminases, bilirubin). Diagnosis depends upon liver biopsy demonstrating *chronic active hepatitis* (inflammatory cell infiltrate, piecemeal hepatocellular necrosis) or *chronic persistent hepatitis* (inflammatory infiltrate but normal liver architecture mostly preserved).

Treatment
Corticosteroids for chronic active hepatitis. In females, *azathioprine* may also be useful.

Prognosis
Usually very good in *chronic persistent hepatitis*, but very variable in *chronic active hepatitis*, which often progresses to cirrhosis.

Chapter 82   # HEPATIC CIRRHOSIS
(*Cirrhosis of Liver; Subacute and Chronic Hepatitis*)

Causes
Frequently unknown.

Genetic
Galactosaemia
Fructosaemia
Glycogenosis   } Carbohydrate metabolism
Hurler's syndrome

Tyrosinosis
Cystinosis
α_1-antitrypsin deficiency $\Big\}$ Protein metabolism
Wilson's disease
Gaucher's disease
Niemann–Pick disease $\Big\}$ Fat metabolism
Cholesterol ester storage disease
Byler's disease
Cystic fibrosis
Hepatic porphyria
Sickle-cell anaemia
Thalassaemia
Haemolytic disease of newborn
Trisomy D
Trisomy E

Non-genetic
Following hepatitis A or B, or neonatal hepatitis
Chronic active hepatitis
Extrahepatic biliary atresia
Choledochal cyst
Ascending cholangitis
Drugs, toxins and radiation injury
Cardiac cirrhosis—chronic congestive failure, constrictive pericarditis
Budd–Chiari syndrome (hepatic vein occlusion)
Veno-occlusive disease (Jamaica, ? secondary to drinking 'bush tea')
Indian childhood cirrhosis—associated with malnutrition
Congenital syphilis

Pathology
Nomenclature not finally decided. Main pathological varieties:
1. Portal cirrhosis (Post-necrotic scarring; multilobular cirrhosis; Laënnec's cirrhosis). Strands of fibrous tissue separate variously sized areas of liver tissue.
2. Biliary cirrhosis (Diffuse hepatic fibrosis; monolobular cirrhosis). Bile ducts dilated; connective tissue increased and encircles lobes; infiltration with inflammatory cells often occurs.
3. Hypertrophic biliary cirrhosis (Hanot's cirrhosis). Gross jaundice; liver green, chronic intrahepatic cholangitis present. Very rare in childhood.
Note: Mixed types usually occur in children.

Clinical Features
Different groups of symptoms and signs predominate, depending on cause. Clinical picture otherwise similar to adults.
1. Syndrome of excretory failure, e.g. in obstruction of extrahepatic bile ducts or pressure from lymph nodes.
   Main Features: jaundice and liver enlargement. Splenomegaly common. Clubbing of fingers.

2. *Syndrome of hepatocellular faiure. See* p. 257.
3. *Syndrome of portal hypertension. See below.*

Investigations
1. *Liver function tests.* Of little value in babies.
2. *Radiography.* May be possible to demonstrate oesophageal varices.

Prognosis
1. Syndrome of excretory failure. Prognosis poor.
2. Hepatocellular failure. Prognosis poor.
3. Portal hypertension (*see below*).

Treatment
Removal of cause if possible. Good mixed diet should be given. If portal hypertension present portacaval anastomosis or similar operation often attempted. Results disappointing.

Indian Childhood Cirrhosis

Virtually confined to the Indian subcontinent, where it is locally common. Aetiology unknown but may be related to excessive ingestion of copper.

Clinical Features
Initially fever, anorexia and irritability, with an enlarged firm liver and often splenomegaly. There is rapid progress to cirrhosis, usually within 6 months, accompanied by evidence of portal hypertension. Death is usually from decompensated liver failure.

Pathology
Liver biopsy in the early stages shows swollen hepatocytes containing hyaline bodies. In the later stages dark granules which stain positively for copper are seen, and the normal liver architecture is distorted by wide bands of fibrous tissue.

Portal Hypertension
(Syndrome of Portal Obstruction)

Aetiology
1. *Extrahepatic portal venous obstruction*
   1.1 *Neonatal Cavernous Malformation.* Portal vein replaced by leash of small veins. Most cases are secondary to umbilical sepsis. Rarely follows exchange transfusion.

1.2 Acquired

1.2.1 Sequel to hepatic cirrhosis. Due to slow portal blood flow.

1.2.2 Post splenectomy. Especially if platelet count was raised.

1.2.3 Schistosomiasis

1.2.4 Veno-occlusive disease

2. *Intraheptic portal venous obstruction.* Rare in children. Usually due to hepatic cirrhosis (causes, *see* p. 262).

Clinical Features

Presentation:

1. Sudden unexpected haemorrhage from gastrointestinal tract. Bleeding mainly from oesophageal varices. If a slow bleed there is melaena only; if a rapid bleed haematemesis and melaena.

Note on collateral circulation: Veins which connect portal and systemic venous systems enlarge. These can be divided into: (*a*) Those which give rise to no symptoms: e.g. on bare area of liver. (*b*) Those which give rise to symptoms: (i) Oesophageal veins—the most important. Oesophageal varices develop and may rupture to give rise to profuse haematemesis. This is often presenting feature of disease. (ii) Veins around umbilicus—giving rise to caput medusae. (iii) Haemorrhoidal veins—causing piles, very rare in children.

2. Chance finding of enlarged liver and spleen. Sometimes associated with pancytopenia due to hypersplenism.

Note on hypersplenism: If spleen enlarged, from whatever cause, hypersplenism may develop, i.e. abnormal splenic activity resulting in reduction in number of red blood cells, white blood cells, platelets, or all three.

3. Associated with liver failure. Spleen big, ascites and oedema may be prominent, due either to portal obstruction or to associated hypoproteinaemia. Failure may be precipitated by a haemorrhage.

Note on essential clinical difference between intra- and extrahepatic obstruction: (*a*) Intrahepatic obstruction—signs and symptoms of portal obstruction: liver hard, and at first large but later may be small. Hepatocellular changes prominent. (*b*) Extrahepatic obstruction—signs of portal obstruction only. Liver normal. No hepatocellular changes.

Investigations

1. Radiography. Barium swallow may demonstrate oesophageal varices.

2. Upper alimentary endoscopy. Identified oesophageal varices and source of bleeding.

Note: Bleeding in portal hypertension often from acute haemorrhagic gastritis even when varices present.

3. Intrasplenic pressure. Bears close resemblance to portal venous pressure.

4. Percutaneous splenic portal venography. Splenic puncture gives splenic pulp pressure. Dye studies demonstrate portal venous system and collateral circulation. General anaesthetic required in children. Method simple but not without risk.

5. Wedge hepatic pressure. If catheter passed from peripheral vein and

'wedged' in liver, this approximates to portal pressure. Normal if block extrahepatic.

Differential Diagnosis of Palpable Spleen

1. Physiological

 1.1 In neonatal period spleen frequently palpable.

 1.2 In young children spleen often palpable for no apparent reasons and without apparent ill-effect.

2. Bacterial infection

 2.1 Septicaemia

 2.2 Bacterial endocarditis

 2.3 Syphilis

 2.4 Typhoid

3. Protozoal infection

 3.1 Malaria

 3.2 Kala-azar

4. Blood disorders

 4.1 Hereditary spherocytosis

 4.2 Acute leukaemia

 4.3 Chronic leukaemia

 4.4 Thrombocytopenic purpura

5. Disorders of reticulo-endothelial system. Hodgkin's disease.

6. Mechanical due to back-pressure. Portal hypertension.

7. Disorders of metabolism

 7.1 Gaucher's disease

 7.2 Niemann–Pick disease

 7.3 Hand–Schüller–Christian syndrome (Histiocytosis X)

 7.4 Amyloid disease

Prognosis

1. If due to extrahepatic causes main danger is haematemesis from rupture of oesophageal varices.

2. If due to intrahepatic causes additional danger of parenchymal failure.

Treatment

1. Emergency treatment for bleeding oesophageal varices:

 1.1 Sedation

 1.2 Blood transfusion. Slow drip of packed cells advised.

 1.3 Intravenous vasopressin (Pitressin) infusions lower portal venous pressure and control bleeding in 50% of cases.

 1.4 Balloon tamponade using Sengstaken tube can be used but carries risk of aspiration of stomach contents during insertion.

2. Catastrophic haemorrhage: Perform oesphageal transection.

3. Surgery for portal hypertension.

 3.1 Direct injection of varices. Very useful procedure in children.

 3.2 Portacaval or splenorenal anastomosis. Difficult in small children and should be postponed until at least 6 years old when anastomosis of 1 cm can be achieved.

For selection of cases for surgery *see* textbooks of surgery and liver disorders.

Chapter 83   ## DISEASES OF PANCREAS AND SMALL INTESTINE

Cystic Fibrosis (*Fibrocystic Disease of Pancreas; Mucoviscidosis*)

Definition
Genetic disease manifested by chronic pulmonary infection, pancreatic insufficiency and elevated sweat electrolytes.

Incidence
In most Caucasian populations, varies between 1 : 1500 and 1 : 2500. Carrier rate about 1 : 20. Much less common in other races.

Aetiology
Autosomal recessive inheritance. Basic metabolic error unknown. Serum factor, present in patients and heterozygotes, inhibits ciliary movement in isolated rabbit trachea, and factor present in saliva and sweat inhibits sodium reabsorption in rat parotid duct. Elevated sweat electrolytes and increased calcium of submaxillary saliva and other glycoprotein-rich secretions suggest abnormality of ion transport across cell membranes.

Pathology
Different organs may be maximally affected in different cases.
1. *Pancreas.* Acini and ducts dilated and partly filled with inspissated material: producing so-called cysts. Later, atrophy and fibrosis occur. Islets of Langerhans not affected.
2. *Lung.* Tenacious mucus blocks smaller bronchi, resulting in small areas of collapse, surrounded by compensatory emphysema. Lung susceptible to secondary infection, especially with staphylococcus; bronchopneumonia, bronchiolitis, bronchiectasis or lung abscess may occur.
3. *Liver.* Focal biliary cirrhosis may occur in older children, probably owing to blockage of intrahepatic biliary system by inspissated material.
4. *Intestine.* Meconium ileus (*see* p. 269).
5. *Salivary glands.* May show dilatation of acini.
6. *Vas deferens.* Obliterated in fetal life, hence virtually all affected males are sterile.

Clinical Features
1. *General appearance.* In early stages baby small and fails to gain weight despite voracious appetite. Abdomen is slightly distended. In later stages—probably due partly to chronic chest infection—infant becomes severely wasted, with thin thighs and buttocks over which skin hangs in folds. Abdomen distended. Ribs often splayed out and Harrison's sulcus prominent. Appetite fails.
2. *Intestinal manifestations.* Stools appear normal at first, especially in breast-fed baby. From a few weeks of age stools characteristic owing to fatty appearance and foul smell. To doctor or nurse acquainted with the disease the smell is almost diagnostic. At first stools are small, frequent and loose, but later become larger and putty-like, with high fat content.
3. *Pulmonary manifestations.* Child has frequent attacks of 'bronchitis'. Cough

often spasmodic in character and resembles pertussis although whoop does not occur. Emphysema develops but is slight. Repeated respiratory infections occur throughout life. Ultimately bronchiectasis and fibrosis develop. Asthma frequently coexists.

Note: Either intestinal or pulmonary symptoms may predominate.

4. *Other manifestations*. (*a*) Occasionally child presents with heat exhaustion from salt loss due to sweating. (*b*) Salivary gland involvement occurs but usually of no clinical importance. (*c*) Prolapse of rectum not uncomon. (*d*) Nasal polyposis and sinus involvement very common. (*e*) Fine hepatic fibrosis or fatty liver common but not important. Frank cirrhosis with or without portal hypertension develops in about 5 %. (*f*) Fingers clubbed in most cases.

Late case. Occasionally mild case escapes detection for years. Severe case ends with respiratory failure and cor pulmonale. May have exudative retinopathy. Increased incidence of diabetes mellitus in older patients probably due to impairment of blood supply to pancreas.

Investigations

1. *Screening*. Over 90 % have elevated serum immunoreactive trypsin at birth, which can be detected in dried blood spots. Trypsin in blood probably reflects pancreatic damage. Confirmatory sweat test is required in positive cases. About 65 % can also be detected by increased albumin content of meconium but both false positive and false negative evidence is high with this test.

2. *Sweat electrolytes*. Patients with cystic fibrosis excrete sweat with higher sodium and chloride content than normal controls, i.e. sodium over 70 mEq/l or chloride over 60 mEq/l. Sweat sample of over 100 mg obtained by pilocarpine iontophoresis required for accurate analysis. If clinical features indicate cystic fibrosis but sweat electrolytes are normal, test must be repeated.

3. *Fat excretion*. Degree of steatorrhoea greater than in coeliac disease.

4. *Pancreatic enzymes*. Reduced or absent tryptic activity in duodenal juice. *Note*: Up to 20 % may have adequate pancreatic function in early infancy.

5. *Chest radiography*. Patchy collapse, prominent thickened bronchi, cystic changes all occur.

6. *Sputum culture*. In early cases, *Staphylococcus aureus* or sometimes *H. influenzae* most important pathogen, but later *Pseudomonas aeruginosa* usually predominates. Sputum rarely obtainable from young infant, throat swab much less useful. Treatment should nevertheless be given in absence of culture.

Prognosis

The prognosis is usually one of progressive lung damage and respiratory impairment but the rate of deterioration is variable between individuals and quite unpredictable. Mean life span gradually increasing with improved treatment, and now approaches 20 years; increased numbers are living into their fourth decade. Some die in infancy or childhood despite early diagnosis. Probably natural variation in severity is more important determinant than therapeutic measures.

Treatment

1. *General management*. As with all children afflicted with a disease which carries a poor prognosis the parents require constant support and every effort should

be made to bring the child up in as normal a manner as possible, both physically and psychologically.

2. Diet. Low fat, high calorie, extra vitamins, sometimes supplements of medium-chain triglyceride (MCT) oil. Elemental diet occasionally useful for limited period, e.g. following surgery for meconium ileus, or to aid growth after severe chest infection.

3. Intestinal manifestations. Pancreatin replacement therapy. Dosage should be regulated to obtain optimum result. Excessive dosage causes oral and perianal excoriation.

4. Pulmonary manifestations. Regime to be adopted varies with age of child, severity of pulmonary involvement and type of organism present in sputum.

> *4.1 Physical Therapy.* Postural drainage, percussion and exercise encouragement to cough. *This is the single most important measure.*
>
> *4.2 Treatment of Exacerbation.* Intermittent courses of antibiotics to counteract predominant organism in the sputum. Eradication of *Ps. aeruginosa* impossible but a course of i.v. antibiotics such as a combination of a β-lactam antibiotic (carbenicillin, piperacillin, azlocillin, ticarcillin, ceftazidime or cefsulodin) and an aminoglycoside (gentamicin, tobramycin, netilmicin or amikacin) in full dosage for 10–14 days is usually beneficial.
>
> *4.3 Continuous Prophylactic Therapy.* Oral flucloxacillin, erythromycin or fucidin during the first two years or more are sometimes used but opinion varies as to the real value of antibiotic prophylaxis.
>
> *4.4 Aerosol Therapy.* Equipment required: compressed air pump, ultrasonic nebulizer. Gentamicin 0·5–1·0 g and carbenicillin 80–100 mg (separately) q.i.d. in 3 ml diluent can be administered in this way. Aerosol pumps can also be used to deliver bronchodilators or mucolytics (acetylcysteine, propylene glycol) to lungs. Effectiveness questionable.
>
> *4.5* Coexisting bronchospasm requires routine bronchodilator therapy. Sometimes allergic aspergillosis produces bronchospasm and requires nystatin, amphotericin or ketoconazole.

5. Electrolyte balance. Extra salt required in hot weather.

6. Hepatic manifestations. Treated on individual merits (*see* p. 263).

Meconium Ileus

This is a manifestation of cystic fibrosis occurring in 10–15 % of newborn infants with cystic fibrosis. Meconium is inspissated in the terminal ileum. Symptoms and signs of acute intestinal obstruction result.

Pathology
Meconium in gut inspissated and thick owing to lack of pancreatic enzymes.

Clinical Features

Onset: Within few hours of birth symptoms of complete intestinal obstruction occur, infant vomits; abdominal distension develops; no stools may be passed or only a little thick meconium. Intestinal perforation may occur in utero or after birth. Ileal atresia sometimes occurs, mechanism uncertain.

Differential Diagnosis. See p. 213.

Investigations

Radiological examination of abdomen may show: (1) Little gas in lower abdomen; (2) Gas under diaphragm if perforation has occurred; (3) Calcification of peritoneum following intra-uterine perforation; (4) Gas bubbles in meconium gives appearance of faeces; (5) Gastrografin enema shows 'microcolon'.

Treatment

  1. *Gastrografin enema.* Hygroscopic enema draws water into bowel and may loosen meconium to allow wash-out. Intravenous fluids necessary to avoid dehydration. Procedure may be repeated if first attempt unsuccessful.

  2. *Surgery.* If enema fails, ileum opened and inspissated meconium removed. Bishop–Koop operation provides temporary ileostomy.

Shwachman–Diamond Syndrome

Rare autosomal recessive manifested by fatty replacement of pancreas leading to pancreatic insufficiency, with chronic or cyclical neutropenia, tendency to chest infections and sometimes metaphysial dysostosis. Resembles cystic fibrosis but sweat test negative. Tends to improve with age.

Congenital Chloridorrhoea (*Congenital Alkalosis with Diarrhoea; Familial Chloride Diarrhoea*)

Definition

Very rare metabolic error, characterized by chronic diarrhoea with marked faecal loss of chloride and metabolic alkalosis. Absorption of chloride in lower gut severely impaired. Autosomal recessive inheritance.

Clinical Features

Infants often premature with abdominal distension and neonatal jaundice. Polyhydramnios frequent. Recurrent bouts of severe watery diarrhoea with severe dehydration in early infancy, faecal losses of chloride increase later and child becomes alkalotic and hypochloridaemic.

Investigations

  1. *Faecal chloride* levels elevated (50–200 mmol/l, normal 6–17 mmol/l).

2. *Urinary chloride* very low, potassium high, pH low.
3. *Serum chloride* may be low.
4. *Metabolic alkalosis* after first few months.

Treatment
Oral potassium supplements (potassium chloride 2–14 mmol/kg/day) will maintain electrolyte balance but do not affect the diarrhoea.

Intestinal Lymphangiectasia

Congenital malformation of lymphatics of small intestine resulting in protein-losing enteropathy. The large dilated lymphatics rupture frequently into the bowel lumen with loss of protein-rich lymph.

Clinical Features
Failure to thrive, abdominal distension, diarrhoea and oedema. Laboratory findings are hypoproteinaemia, decreased immunoglobulins, lymphopenia and steatorrhoea.

A-Beta-Lipoproteinaemia (*Bassen–Kornzweig Disease; Acanthocytosis*)

Definition
Autosomal recessive disease characterized by steatorrhoea, acanthocytosis, retinitis pigmentosa and progressive ataxia.

Pathology
Beta-lipoproteins transport cholesterol in plasma as chylomicrons. Absence leads to low plasma lipids; fats absorbed into gut mucosal cells unable to leave and remain as vacuoles in jejunal biopsy. Abnormal red cells (acanthocytes) due to abnormalities of cell membrane lipids. Progressive degeneration of posterolateral columns and spinocerebellar tracts.

Clinical Features
Failure to thrive, with steatorrhoea and abdominal distension commencing in first year. Later child develops weakness, progressive ataxia and nystagmus. Deep tendon reflexes are lost. Retinitis pigmentosa appears in adult life.

Investigations
1. *Plasma cholesterol* less than 1·5 mmol/l (60 mg/dl)
2. *Absence or severe deficiency of beta-lipoprotein*
3. *Faecal fat elevated*
4. *Jejunal biopsy* shows epithelial cells engorged with fat droplets.
5. *Acanthocytosis* of red blood cells (bizarre shapes, thorny projections and shortened life).

Treatment
No known cure. Dietary fat should be given as medium-chain triglycerides (MCT) which do not require lipoprotein for transport.

Neonatal Necrotizing Enterocolitis

Definition
Uncommon fulminating disease of pre-term and newborn infants characterized by widespread necrosis of large and small bowel.

Aetiology
Unknown, possibly due to ischaemia. May follow exchange transfusion or complicate Hirschsprung's disease. Gram-negative or Clostridial invasion of damaged gut usually present: may be cause.

Clinical Features
Most often seen in pre-term infants. Abdominal pain, tenderness and distension, bloody diarrhoea, vomiting and fever are initial symptoms. Bowel may perforate, peritonitis, bacteraemia, circulatory failure rapidly follows. Prognosis grave.

Investigations
Radiography of abdomen shows gut distension and intramural gas bubbles (pneumatosis intestinalis). Free air in portal system and peritoneal cavity if perforation has occurred. Blood culture usually shows gram-negative bacteraemia.

Treatment
Stop oral feeds, give gastric suction. Intravenous nutrition, fresh frozen plasma to keep serum albumin and clotting factors in adequate concentration. Antibiotics including metronidazole for gram-negative organisms. Surgery for perforations.

Acrodermatitis Enteropathica

Definition
Rare condition of infants characterized by chronic diarrhoea, alopecia and dermatitis of extremities, mouth and anus.

Aetiology
Uncertain. Zinc sulphate is curative, but not due to simple zinc deficiency. Probably due to congenital absence of zinc-binding ligand which facilitates zinc absorption.

Clinical Features
Onset usually follows weaning from the breast. Intractable diarrhoea with vomiting and weight loss followed by severe dermatitis with vesicles, pustules

and crusting, most marked around mouth and anus, and on extremities. Conjunctivitis and corneal opacities may occur. Prognosis very poor unless treated.

Treatment
Zinc sulphate (200–500 mg/day) by mouth highly effective in curing all clinical manifestations. Diodoquin (di-iodohydroxyquinoline) 1–4 g daily used formerly, also effective in most cases, probably because of zinc contained in product.

Chapter 84   **THE INFANT AND CHILD'S HEART IN HEALTH**

Normal Development

Cardiac development commences at 3 weeks' gestation and is complete between 7 and 8 weeks. Most structural anomalies occur as a result of 'insults' or 'arrested development' within this period.

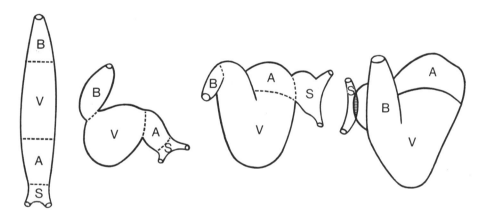

Fig. 84.1. The early stages of development of the heart. A, Atrium; B, Bulbus; S, Sinus venosum; V, Ventricle. (Modified from Pichon.)

The heart commences as a tube (*Fig. 84.1*) which develops constrictions dividing it into bulbus cordis, common ventricle, atrium and sinus venosus. Bulbus is outflow ('arterial' end) and sinus venosus inflow ('venous' end). Tube elongates and bends to form S-shaped loop with two curvatures not in same plane: bulbus in front, atrium and sinus venosus above and posteriorly.

Development of dividing septa converts the tube structure into the basic heart form:

1. Bulbus cordis into: (*a*) Distally: truncus arteriosus and hence the proximal aorta (AO) and pulmonary artery (PA). (*b*) Mid-portion: into left and right ventricular outflow tracts (conus cordis). (*c*) Proximally: right ventricle (RV), separated from the left ventricle (LV) by the development of the muscular interventricular septum.

2. Common atrium by downgrowth of septum primum leaving defect at its lower edge (ostium primum) (*Fig. 84.2*). Later a higher defect develops (ostium secundum) prior to the development of a second atrial septum parallel and to right of the first (septum secundum). A defect in this septum (foramen ovale) permits functional communication between right (RA) and left atria (LA) in fetal life (*Fig. 84.2*).

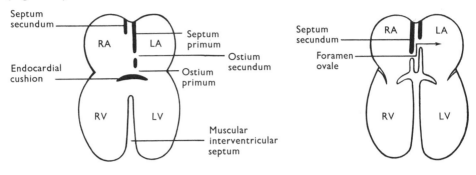

Fig. 84.2.   Further stages in development of the heart showing (*a*) atrial septa, and (*b*) foramen ovale.

3. Opening between atrium and ventricle (atrioventricular canal) is completed from either side by areas of mesenchymal tissue (superior and inferior endocardial cushions). Fusion of this tissue forms the mitral and tricuspid orifices and essential parts of both valves. Fusion above with septum primum completes atrial septation and below ventricular septation.

4. Great arteries: A considerable proportion of the early paired arterial system, consisting of 2 dorsal aortic and 6 pairs of connecting aortic arch vessels, degenerates. Only 3 arch pairs persist, i.e:

Third arch forming common carotid arteries.

Fourth arch forming central aortic arch and initial right subclavian artery.

Sixth arch forming right and left pulmonary arteries and ductus arteriosus.

Of the paired dorsal aortae:

The right becomes part of right subclavian artery.

The left becomes the thoracic descending aorta.

5. Great veins. (*a*) Systemic veins, orginally bilateral. Some degenerate (but may persist as various anomalies). Of right and left veins only right persists, as the superior vena cava (SVC). If left persists, retains connection to sinus venosus and drains to coronary sinus. Inferior vena cava (IVC) is formed from amalgamation of a complex of venous systems.

(*b*) Pulmonary veins from each lung (principally two from each lung) unite to form common pulmonary vein and hence to left atrium (LA). This common vein and proximal part of its 4 branches is eventually incorporated into wall of LA.

Fetal and Neonatal Anatomy

Anatomical differences between normal fetal and postnatal cardiovascular systems:

1. Ductus venosus—connects umbilical vein and IVC, thus short-circuiting liver.

2. Foramen ovale—opening between right and left atria.

3. Ductus arteriosus—connects pulmonary artery and aorta.

Fetal Circulation

Oxygenated blood from placenta enters single umbilical vein. Part flows through liver, most passes direct to heart through ductus venosus. Both enter heart via IVC. Blood entering right atrium from IVC divides (*Fig. 84.3*):

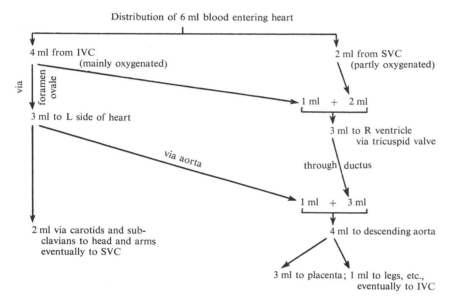

Distribution of 6 ml blood entering heart

4 ml from IVC (mainly oxygenated)

via foramen ovale

3 ml to L side of heart

2 ml from SVC (partly oxygenated)

1 ml + 2 ml

3 ml to R ventricle via tricuspid valve

via aorta

through ductus

1 ml + 3 ml

2 ml via carotids and sub-clavians to head and arms eventually to SVC

4 ml to descending aorta

3 ml to placenta; 1 ml to legs, etc., eventually to IVC

Fig. 84.3.   Distribution of blood entering right atrium.

1. First stream flows directly across chamber, out through patent foramen ovale, into left atrium, through mitral and aortic valves to aorta. Most of this more oxygenated blood goes via carotid and subclavian arteries to head and arms, some goes down descending aorta.

2. Second stream mixes with that from superior vena cava, flows through tricuspid and pulmonary valves into pulmonary trunk. Approximately 7% only flows to the lungs (due to the high pulmonary vascular resistance), the majority passing through the ductus arteriosus to the aorta.

3. Finally, mixture of oxygen and deoxygenated blood flows down aorta, to both internal iliac, hypogastric and umbilical arteries; also supplies blood to lower part of body.

Circulatory Changes after Birth

1. Ductus venosus—obliterates to a fibrous thread within weeks.

2. Foramen ovale—following increased pulmonary blood flow after birth and decreased RV pressures, left atrial pressure becomes slightly higher than RA pressure, results in 'valve-like' closure of the foramen ovale due to apposition of septa primum and secundum. Remains potentially open should RA pressures exceed LA pressures until functional closure becomes permanent due to fibrosis at approximately 2–4 years. Anatomical depression persisting on right atrial wall called fossa ovalis.

3. *Ductus arteriosus.* Once lungs are aerated, they require blood flow, therefore purpose of ductus to shunt blood away from lungs to aorta is obsolete. (*a*) Functional closure commences from pulmonary end within minutes of birth due to direct muscular action. Mechanism complex, initiated and maintained by several agents including Po_2 and circulating prostaglandins. (*b*) Anatomical closure by fibrosis occurs within weeks.

4. *Regression of pulmonary vascular resistance.* Following inspiration and aeration of lungs, the pulmonary arteriolar vascular bed changes to accommodate increased pulmonary blood flow. Fall in vascular resistance starts within hours of birth and continues until the pulmonary resistance is approximately one-tenth of the systemic vascular resistance. This regression usually complete within 3–6 weeks.

Chapter 85	# EXAMINATION OF THE CARDIOVASCULAR SYSTEM

Before a child is disturbed by being undressed he should be observed to see whether he is cyanosed. The respiration and, if possible, the heart rate should be counted. If it is likely that undressing will make him cry the heart should be auscultated. More will be learned by listening through the shirt to a quiet child than with the chest bared in a crying one. After he is undressed closer inspection should be made for:

1. Precordial bulge and rib insuction. The respiratory rate should be checked. Normally it is around 40 in newborns. It should be compared with the heart rate and should be significantly less even in heart disease. If it is higher there is the possibility of a primary pulmonary problem.

2. Cardiac ventricular impulses. Normal (or increased) right ventricular impulse may be detected at the lower end of the sternum and a left ventricular impulse at the apex.

3. Abnormal pulsation may be present over the chest wall, e.g. over the region of the outflow tract.

4. Engorged veins indicating increased jugular venous pressure; these are difficult to detect in a young infant, but it should be possible to see whether they fill when the infant is propped up.

5. Prominent arterial pulsation in the neck is suggestive of aortic run-off lesions, e.g. patent ductus arteriosus (PDA), aortic regurgitation or A–V fistulas.

6. Thrills may be palpated over the chest wall, suprasternal notch or neck. This suggests blood flow forced through a narrow orifice, e.g. ventricular septal defect (VSD) or narrowed aortic/pulmonary valve.

7. Non-cardiovascular congenital anomalies often coexist with congenital heart disease.

8. The radial, femoral and dorsalis pedis pulses should be examined routinely. In particular it should be observed whether there is absent or delayed femoral pulsation compared with the cardiac apex beat; asymmetry of pulsation. The character should also be observed, e.g. whether it is collapsing.

The heart rate fluctuates greatly within normal limits:

Fetal heart rate	140/min
Neonate	120–130/min
6 months	about 120/min
1 year	about 110/min
5–10 years	about 90/min

Auscultation

In infants the first and second sounds are equal in intensity. In later childhood the first sound is louder at the apex, the second sound louder at the base.

The first sound consists of two components, although commonly heard as one. The first component is mainly due to closure of the atrioventricular valves.

Intensity of the first heart sound is increased when the heart beats forcibly, e.g. with exercise, fever, anaemia, or in mitral stenosis and is decreased when there is some degree of fat, muscle or fluid interposed between the heart and the stethoscope; or when there is an atrioventricular conduction time lag, as indicated by a prolonged P–R interval on the electrocardiogram. This is sometimes found in acute rheumatic carditis.

The second sound is due to closure of the semilunar valves: first component mainly aortic; second component mainly pulmonary. Two components can usually be distinguished by auscultation during inspiration. Referred to as splitting of second sound. Split normally less than 0·04 sec. Split lengthens with full inspiration because increased filling of right ventricle prolongs right ventricular systole.

Note:

1. The intensity of sound depends mainly on aortic component which may mask pulmonary component. When pulmonary component loud (in pulmonary hypertension), or when there is a loud murmur at the base of the heart, the split may be heard best at bottom of sternum.

2. The split is widest in complete right bundle-branch block, the commonest cause of which is increased right-sided flow (atrial septal defect or anomalous pulmonary venous return with shunt from left to right). In these cases the split does not increase with inspiration.

The split is absent in Fallot's tetralogy.

A third heart sound is found in 20% of normal children.

An ejection sound ('click') may be heard early in systole. This is always abnormal. If heard maximally in the pulmonary area it is probably due to dilatation of the pulmonary artery as in post-stenotic dilatation or pulmonary hypertension. If maximal at the apex it is probably caused by valvular aortic stenosis.

Murmurs

Systolic murmurs fall into two groups:

1. Midsystolic ejection murmurs: Rise to crescendo in midsystole. Usually harsh. *Cause*: Forward flow of blood through pulmonary or aortic valves.

2. Pansystolic regurgitant murmur: Murmur of same intensity throughout systole. Usually blowing. *Cause*: Shunt from left to right through ventricular septal defect or regurgitation through incompetent tricuspid or mitral valve.

Diastolic murmurs fall into three groups:

1. Ventricular filling murmurs: Commence at time of physiological third heart sound. *Cause*: Mitral or tricuspid valvulitis or stenosis; relative stenosis due to high rate of flow across tricuspid or mitral valve from atrial septal defect, ventricular septal defect, anomalous pulmonary venous return or patent ductus arteriosus.

2. Atrial systolic murmurs: Crescendo presystolic murmur, maximal at time of the first sound. *Cause*: Mitral stenosis.

3. Regurgitant murmurs from incompetent pulmonary or aortic valves. Pandiastolic and diminuendo in character.

Murmurs can be graded according to their intensity. This is particularly of value to follow the progress of a changing murmur.

Grade 1: Just audible on careful auscultation.

Grade 2: Obvious but soft murmur.

Grade 3: Intermediate betwen 2 and 4.

Grade 4: Thrill palpable.

Grade 5: Very loud murmur. Audible with stethoscope chest piece just off chest.

Grade 6: Murmur audible without stethoscope.

They should be expressed as 3/6 etc.

Conduction, e.g. into axilla depends mainly on the loudness of the murmurs.

Blood pressure

May be difficult to measure in infants. The sphygmomanometer cuff must be of appropriate size e.g.

Newborn	2·5 cm (length 8–10 cm to encircle upper arm)
6 months to 1 year	5 cm
1–13 years	9 cm

In infants the blood pressure can be measured (*a*) by using a Doppler transducer. This measures the systolic pressure only. (*b*) by the flush method which gives the mean pressure.

Method: The arm or leg is rendered bloodless by elevating and squeezing. Sphygmomanometer cuff applied proximally and inflated above probable systolic pressure. The cuff is slowly deflated. A flush is observed as the blood returns to the limb. The mercury level at this point gives the mean pressure only. Approximate normal readings are:

Neonate	about 60 mmHg
6 months	about 75 mmHg
1 year	about 80 mmHg
5–10 years	about 90 mmHg

Chapter 86   # ECG ABNORMALITIES

P Waves

1. Tall 'peaked' P (>2 mm) in Lead II indicates right atrial enlargement.

2. Broad 'notched' P in Lead II, with partial or total inversion in VI suggests left atrial enlargement.

3. Inverted P in Lead I suggests incorrect lead connections, dextrocardia or ectopic atrial rhythm.

QRS Complex

1. If >0·10 sec in children, or >0·12 sec in adults indicates delayed interventricular conduction, i.e. bundle-branch block (BBB).

2. Lead VI will normally differentiate left from right bundle-branch block. If the dominant portion of the QRS complex is up*R*ight (above the isoelectric line) then *R*BBB is likely—the converse reflecting *L*BBB.

3. Abnormalities of interventricular conduction may exist without a wide QRS complex. The left bundle branch has anterior and posterior branches. A block in either one of these is referred to as anterior or posterior hemiblock. If either combined with right bundle-branch block then patient is in danger of developing complete heart block.

Right ventricular hypertrophy. Following observations all suggestive:

1. Right axis deviation.

2. V1—Tall R wave, i.e. more than 20 mm. S–T depression indicates right ventricular strain.

3. V6—Deep S wave, i.e. more than 12 mm (birth–1 month).
more than 6 mm (1–6 months).
more than 5 mm (6 months–16 years).

4. V1—R/S ratio of: more than 7·0 (birth–3 months).
more than 4·5 (4–11 months).
more than 2·5 (1–2 years).
more than 2·0 (3–5 years).
more than 1·5 (6–16 years).

5. Presence of q in V1.

6. q/R ratio in aVR more than 1·0.

Left ventricular hypertrophy. Following observations all suggestive:

1. Left axis deviation.

2. V6—Tall R wave, i.e. more than 20 mm. S–T depression indicates left ventricular strain.

3. V1—Deep S wave, i.e. more than 20 mm.

4. V1—R/S ratio of : less than 0·8 (birth–12 months).
less than 0·2 (1–5 year).
less than 0·1 (6–16 years).

5. Inversion or flattening of T waves in V5 and V6. Tall T in V6 may indicate left ventricular dilatation rather than hypertrophy.

Combined ventricular hypertrophy

1. Right and left ventricular hypertrophy patterns both present. R and S large and equal in V3–V4.

2. Signs of right ventricular hypertrophy plus: (*a*) q of 1 mm or more in V5 or V6, (*b*) Inverted T in V 6 (with positive T in right chest lead).

Systolic and diastolic overloading. Definition:

Systolic overloading = increased resistance to expulsion of blood during systole.

Diastolic overloading = increased volume of blood filling ventricle in diastole without increase in pressure.

1. Systolic overloading of right ventricle: V1 – Rs, qR, qRs, rR or R pattern with sharply inverted T, or upright T in infancy. Found in e.g. pulmonary stenosis; Fallot's tetralogy, pulmonary hypertension due to increased vascular resistance.

2. Systolic overloading of left ventricle: V5–6—Initial q followed by tall broad R with ventricular activation time (VAT) more than 0·04 sec, plus flattened or inverted T and in gross cases depression of S–T segment.

Found in e.g. aortic stenosis; coarctation; systemic hypertension.

3. Diastolic overloading of right ventricle; V1—RsR′. RSr′ or rSr′ pattern. Plus right axis deviation (or left axis deviation in septum primum defects). VAT more than 0·03 sec.

Found in e.g. atrial septal defect; common atrioventricular canal; ventricular septal defect; anomalous pulmonary venous return; pulmonary valve insufficiency; right ventricular failure.

4. Diastolic overloading of left ventricle: II, III, aVF, V5, V6—Deep Q, tall delayed R. Tall peaked upright T. V2 and V3—Deep S. Found in e.g. patent ductus arteriosus; ventricular septal defect; single ventricle; tricuspid atresia; mitral or aortic valve insufficiency.

S–T Segment

End of QRS to start of T wave. Vertical deviation 0·2 mV either side of iso-electric line is abnormal.

Elevation suggests myocardial necrosis—pericardial injury (concave elevation).

Depression—myocardial (usually endocardial) ischaemia via coronary artery disease or ventricular overload.

Q–T Interval

Onset of QRS to end of T wave. Normally varies with heart rate. *See* under Electrolyte Changes reflected in the ECG (*below*). Prolongation occurs in carditis. Shortens with digoxin treatment.

T Wave

Inverts over anterior standard and lateral chest leads with subendocardial ischaemia. (This mainly accounts for the T wave changes seen in ventricular hypertrophy.)

Widespread flattening or inversion with pericardial disease or postoperatively where pericardium has been opened.

Electrolyte Changes Reflected in the ECG

1. Potassium

      1.1 *Low*: Wide, low or inverted T, prolonged Q–T interval. Depressed S–T segment. Low-voltage wave.

      1.2 *High*: Elevated T. Long P–R interval. Wide QRS.

2. Calcium. Q–T varies inversely with blood calcium. If blood calcium high, Q–T shortened; if low, Q–T lengthened but note that Q–T also varies with age and heart rate.

ECG Changes with Digitalis

1. In abnormalities of rhythm, e.g. paroxysmal tachycardia, slowing of heart rate with reversion to normal rhythm.

2. Changes in S–T segments and T waves: those previously iso-electric or elevated become depressed. Those previously depressed are elevated. Changes most obvious in leads with tall R waves.

Note: S–T changes tend to be straight and angular, but often difficult to distinguish from myocardial changes.

3. Shortening of Q–T interval. Includes digoxin toxic effects.

Note: Toxic effect exaggerated by low serum potassium.

Endocrine Influence on ECG

1. *Hypothyroidism*. Slow sinus rate. Generalized low voltages. Widespread flattening or inversion of T waves.

2. *Hyperthyroidism*. Sinus tachycardia or atrial fibrillation. Rate does not slow on treatment with digoxin.

Atrioventricular Conduction Disturbances

Introduction

Block caused by prolongation of time taken for impulse to travel from sino-auricular node (pacemaker) down bundle of His to ventricle.

Types

1. *First degree*. P–R interval longer than expected from patient's age and heart rate.

    Causes

        1.1 May occur in normal children.

        1.2 Rheumatic carditis; myocarditis.

        1.3 Congenital heart disease, e.g. Ebstein's disease or corrected transposition.

        1.4 Digitalis therapy.

2. *Second degree*. Occasional P wave not conducted to ventricles. May occur as: (*a*) Wenckebach phenomenon, i.e. P–R interval lengthens progressively until one QRS beat is dropped. (*b*) Mobitz block—a persistent fixed block between P waves and QRS, e.g. 2, 3 or 4 P waves for each QRS. May alternate, e.g. varying 2 : 1, 3 : 1 block.

3. *Third degree*. Complete heart block. A random relationship between P and QRS complexes. May be:

        3.1 High block—QRS complexes are narrow, indicating pacemaker to be in A–V node or nearby.

        3.2 Low block—slower rate with wide QRS complexes, or

        3.3 Unstable—varying ventricular pacemaker site.

    Rate—in complete heart block—tends to be more rapid in congenital type (under 1 year: rate 60–70 common; later: rate under 40).

Prognosis

1. *Congenital complete heart block*. Child usually suffers no disability.

2. *Block due to acute rheumatism*. Rarely persists after acute attack over.

3. *Block due to diphtheria*. Never persists after acute attack over.

4. *Due to surgery*. Never recovers. May need electrical implanted pacemaker.

Rhythm Disturbances

Extrasystoles. Less common in children than in adults. Found with normal hearts but more frequently if heart abnormal.

Diagnosis. Rhythm usually becomes normal when heart rate increases with exercise, excitement or fever.

Prognosis and treatment. Depends on underlying cause.

Sinus arrhythmia. Rate accelerates during inspiration, slows during expiration. Benign condition. So common as to be normal in childhood. May be extreme, heart almost appearing to stop; clinically can mimic atrial fibrillation. More obvious on deep respiration. Usually disappears in adulthood.

Atrial fibrillation and flutter. Very rare. Occasionally occurs in older children with fully developed mitral stenosis. Congenital form reported. Digitalis toxicity may precipitate cardiac failure. Signs, etc. as for adult.

Ventricular tachycardia/fibrillation. Very rare. May be the mode of syncope in some forms of congenital heart disease, e.g. severe aortic stenosis.

Chapter 87   # CONGENITAL HEART DISEASE—GENERAL

The incidence is difficult to assess because an anatomical lesion may be present without giving rise to signs or symptoms. Signs present in infancy and childhood may disappear in later life, or new signs develop. Overall it is estimated that there are approximately 7 cases per 1000 live births.

Age at Presentation of Symptoms

If within hours or days of birth: probably severe defect, e.g. the 'atresias'.

If within the first few weeks: probably intact heart with serious anatomical anomalies, e.g. transposition, severe tetralogy.

At 1–3 months: large left-to-right heart communications when pulmonary resistance has fallen permitting massive left-to-right shunting and cardiac overload (e.g. large VSD).

Milder defects are symptomatic and detection is usually by routine medical examination.

Clinical Features

Physical growth varies greatly from child to child. Height and weight are a good index of the severity of a lesion. Central cyanosis is due to admixture of venous and arterial blood. Clinically it can be distinguished from peripheral cyanosis because in central cyanosis the tongue is always blue as it remains warm. The presence or absence of cyanosis forms the basis of the classification of congenital heart disease. Additional signs found with cyanosis include: conjunctival and retinal vessel congestion, the papillae of the tongue are enlarged, dental caries is common and finger and toe clubbing occurs. In addition, in severe cases, the child may sit in a squatting position. The degree of cyanosis varies greatly from child to child and in the same child from time to time. It may increase in cold weather or if the child is fatigued or when cyanotic attacks occur (*see* p. 294).

Clubbing of fingers and toes develops gradually over the years. The cause is unknown, possibly due to hypertrophy of subcutaneous tissue secondary to increased number, congestion and dilatation of nail bed capillaries.

Stages of clubbing
1. Filling in and heaping up of nail bed.
2. Beaking of nail.
3. Swelling of end of finger. Bony structures not involved in this type. Sometimes possible to get 'dipping sensation' on pressing down nail bed.
The most common paediatric cause of cyanosis apart from congenital heart disease is cystic fibrosis.

Heart Failure

Common Causes
1. In first few days of life—severe congenital defects, e.g. hypoplastic left heart syndrome.
2. First week or two—complex defects, e.g. coarctation + VSD + PDA; truncus arteriosus; anomalous pulmonary venous return.
3. Six weeks to 3 months—left-to-right shunts, e.g. VSD; PDA.
4. Three months to 1 year—(*a*) cardiomyopathy, e.g. endocardial fibro-elastosis, (*b*) tachyarrhythmias (may be related to myocarditis), (*c*) anomalous coronary artery (arising from pulmonary artery), (*d*) manifestations of systemic disease, e.g. glycogen storage, (*e*) severe anaemia.
5. Children over 1 year—myocarditis; cardiomyopathy (e.g. rheumatic heart disease); subacute bacterial endocarditis. Congenital defects are very unlikely to present with or develop heart failure after first year of life.
The diagnosis of heart failure in infants may be difficult as there are no pathognomonic signs. The following observations are of value:
1. Tachycardia.
2. Tachypnoea. *Note*: if the respiratory rate is similar to or greater than heart rate in neonates, this suggests a pulmonary rather than a cardiac problem.
3. Heart size. This can be assessed radiographically but it is misleading in neonates.
4. Neck veins—only of value in older children.
5. Lung crepitations—but also occur in respiratory illnesses.
6. Hepatic enlargement—very valuable sign. The liver enlarges or decreases rapidly with the state of heart failure (but beware of the easily palpable liver pushed down by respiratory illnesses).
7. Peripheral oedema—occurs occasionally. Rarely pitting. Usually reflected by weight changes.

Treatment
As for adults but note:
1. Nasogastric feeding is of value in infants as it relieves the work load.
2. Digoxin is a very valuable drug in paediatrics. However, one must be aware of toxicity. The dosage should be monitored by ECG changes and serum digoxin levels. Be *very* careful to place decimal point in prescription correctly.
3. Diuretics, e.g. Frusemide; thiazides are of value. Beware of overdosage.

Physiological Murmurs

(*Syn*. Functional; innocent; insignificant; non-organic; non-pathological)

These are murmurs which have no known anatomical basis and are not dangerous to the patient. They are usually quiet systolic murmurs, localized to a small area, and of short duration.

Types of Physiological Murmurs

1. Generalized, soft, or very soft, systolic murmurs are heard in about 50 % of normal children. They become more obvious with fever or anaemia.

2. Venous hum is best heard over the aortic area and up into the neck. It is a soft, continuous murmur with diastolic accentuation. Varies with position of head. Diminished by pressure on jugular vein.

May be confused with murmur of patent ductus arteriosus.

Note: Important to recognize physiological murmurs so that child is not subjected to unnecessary investigations with danger of cardiac neurosis to child and parents, but in practice it is impossible to be dogmatic about any murmur. For instance, loud murmurs may be found with minimal pulmonary stenosis; physiological-type murmur may be found with atrial septal defect. Symptoms more important than sounds. Echocardiography very helpful in excluding organic disease. If any doubt exists, advise child to receive antibiotic, e.g. penicillin prior to tooth extraction (*see* p. 302).

Chapter 88   **SOME TYPES OF CONGENITAL HEART DISEASE**

General Classification

I.   Acyanotic: no shunt present.

II. Acyanotic: left-to-right shunt present.

III. Cyanotic: right-to-left shunt present.

Note: Mixed lesions may occur. Only the commoner types are described here.

I. Acyanotic Group (*No shunt*)

Pulmonary Stenosis

There are four types of pulmonary stenosis:

1. Valvular. Common. Mostly due to thickened valves which may be tricuspid, bicuspid or dysplastic. In latter, no recognizable cusps; often occurs with Noonan's syndrome.

2. Infundibular. Hypertrophy of RV outflow tract muscle. Anomalous muscle bands can divide RV, resulting in 'two-chambered' RV. Usually occurs in association with valvular pulmonary stenosis.

3. Pulmonary Atresia. Severest variety, incompatible with life unless associated with patent ductus or bronchial collaterals.

4. Pulmonary Arterial Branch Stenosis. Often multiple. May be a sequel of intra-uterine rubella.

Clinical Features

In mild stenosis there are no symptoms, but a murmur is detected on routine examination. A systolic thrill and murmur are located in the second left interspace if valvular, or in the third or fourth interspace if infundibular. The murmur is loud (Grade 4–5/6), harsh and ejection in type. It overlaps the second heart sound. Is usually conducted through to the back.

The first sound is normal but may appear split owing to an ejection click heard in the pulmonary area. The second sound is diminished, single, although it may be split rarely.

In severe stenosis the child may be tired but the lesion is usually not severe enough to cause dyspnoea. There is a very loud murmur, grade 4–6/6, harsh and ejection systolic in time. It obliterates the second sound. It is maximal at the 2nd or 3rd left interspace and widely conducted. There is a marked thrill. If the second sound is heard, it appears single. Giant 'a' waves in the neck veins are common and indicate right ventricular hypertrophy. If the atrial septum is not fused (i.e. a patent foramen ovale is present) it may become stretched, allowing a right-to-left shunt at atrial level. The child will then exhibit some cyanosis.

Chest radiography is within normal limits in mild pulmonary stenosis. With increasing severity RA becomes prominent with dilatation of main pulmonary artery (poststenotic dilatation). Proximal pulmonary arteries usually normal. Overall lung vascularity is normal (since no cardiac shunt present, pulmonary flow must equal systemic), however, proximal vessels larger than peripheral ones. Cardiac catheterization and angiocardiography are required to determine the severity of the stenosis.

Treatment
If the systolic gradient, as measured between the PA and RV on a 'withdrawal' trace during cardiac catheterization, is greater than 50 mmHg, surgery should be advised. The time of surgery depends upon the age and severity and is usually done between 2 and 8 years.

Aortic Stenosis
May be valvular, subvalvular or supravalvular
Valvular
Congenital in origin in which case there are only two effective cusps (bicuspid valve). Less commonly the condition is rheumatic.
Subvalvular
Subvalve 'diaphragm' membrane beneath aortic valve.

Hypertrophic cardiomyopathy—abnormal movement of anterior leaflet of mitral valve during systole approximates to a bulging hypertrophied interventricular septum to virtually occlude outflow tract, producing simultaneously mitral regurgitation.
Supravalvular stenosis may occur in children with mental retardation, hypercalcaemia and elfin-like facies (*see* p. 145).

Clinical Features
Clinical features of aortic stenosis are minimal unless stenosis is severe, in which case the condition may present as syncope. Occasionally the child may complain of 'angina-type' chest pain. In severe cases there is evidence of left ventricular hypertrophy.

Investigations

Echocardiography
Bicuspid valves easily detected by eccentric valve closure.

Detection of increased size of LA, LV.

Abnormal mitral valve motion meeting ventricular septum indicates hypertrophic cardiomyopathy.

Management
Aortic stenosis is usually well tolerated for the first 8–10 years of life. Thereafter, if severe, sudden death a reality. Prone to bacterial endocarditis. Surgical relief advised if gradient is $\simeq 100$ mmHg, or less if signs of cardiac decompensation exist.

Coarctation of Aorta
The only common congenital anomaly with differential racial incidence: rare in Negroes. Males predominate when coarctation is sole anomaly. Coarctation can be considered under the headings of infantile (preductal) or adult type.

Infantile type: the constriction is proximal to the site of the ductus arteriosus. It is usually severe and associated with patency of the ductus and a VSD.

Adult type. The constriction is just distal to the site of the left subclavian artery and ductus which is normally closed. The condition is commonly associated with a bicuspid aortic valve.

A collateral circulation is poorly developed or even absent in preductal coarctation as little blood passes through the arch of the aorta in fetal life. There is therefore no occasion for it to develop prenatally. In postductal coarctation a collateral circulation develops prenatally as the main route for blood to the lower part of the body lies through the coarcted segment. Anastomoses therefore occur between: (*a*) the internal mammary arteries, and epigastric arteries from the internal iliac; and (*b*) the branches of the subclavian artery in the neck and scapular region, and the intercostal arteries.

Clinical Presentation in Infants
Preductal coarctation presents in neonatal life with heart failure. Since the descending aorta is mainly supplied from the pulmonary artery through a patent ductus, when the ductus starts to close the child rapidly deteriorates with heart failure and increasing metabolic acidosis and oliguria.

Diagnosis by cardiac catheterization must be early and accurate.

Clinical Presentation in Older Children and Adults
Coarctation is usually asymptomatic. Diagnosis is made by routine detection of the murmur or hypertension. Signs become more prominent with increasing age and severity. The LV impulse increases, and there is difficulty in detecting the femoral pulses. These are weaker than, and delayed, compared to the radial pulse if felt simultaneously. Normally leg blood pressure is slightly higher than arm blood pressure. (*Note*: palpation of the femoral pulses is an essential part of the routine examination of any infant or child.)

On auscultation an ejection click is frequently heard indicating a bicuspid aortic valve. Murmurs are very variable. There is usually a systolic ejection murmur from the aortic valve or coarcted segment. Collateral vessels produce systolic murmurs audible all over the chest which, if loud, run into diastole. The collateral vessels may be seen or felt in upper part of trunk. May become more obvious if child touches toes when standing.

Investigations
1. ECG may progress to signs of LA and LV overload.
2. Chest radiography. Signs of LA and LV enlargement develop if the coarctation is severe. Rib notching, by intercostal vessels eroding the bone, sometimes found in older children.
3. Echocardiography reveals LA and LV enlargement and bicuspid aortic valve if present.

Adult type coarctation is asymptomatic until a sudden cardiovascular event occurs, e.g. cerebrovascular accident secondary to hypertension, rupture of aorta, bacterial endocarditis or heart failure. Life expectancy is 20–30 years of age unless treated.

Treatment
Infants. Diagnosis should be made early with precise anatomical demonstration. The child should receive immediate medical management for cardiac failure. It is wise to proceed to surgery at the first sign of deterioration or sooner if facilities permit. A few hours of deterioration with onset of acidosis virtually precludes successful surgery.
Older children. Do not usually suffer heart failure. Balance the degree of hypertension to age and size of child. Avoid operation before age 5 years if possible since surgery then carries only a small risk of re-coarctation.

Anomalies of Great Arteries
Are usually asymptomatic but sometimes one vessel compresses the trachea and/or oesophagus. So-called 'constriction ring'. Tracheal compression produces dyspnoea, wheezing, stridor and recurrent respiratory infections. Oesophageal narrowing results in dysphagia.

Dextrocardia
Dextrocardia may be discovered clinically but the diagnosis is usually made radiologically when the cardiac shadow is found to be predominantly on the right side in a PA chest radiograph. The possible alternatives then are:
1. Dextrocardia. Normal heart, lung and viscera, but all positionally reversed (mirror image of normal) = situs inversus. In the very rare Kartagener's syndrome there is situs inversus plus bronchiectasis and sinusitis.
2. Dextroversion. The heart is rotated but the other viscera are normally positioned. Dextroversion is associated with severe congenital heart lessions, also sometimes anomalies of the spine or gut.
3. Dextroposition. Shift of the heart to right, secondary to lung or chest cage disorders.

II. *Acyanotic Group* (*Left-to-right shunt present*)

Ventricular Septal Defect (VSD)
The commonest congenital heart lesion. The defect is normally in membranous or upper ventricular septum just beneath aortic valve. May also occur lower, in muscular septum. Multiple defects may occur.

Large Ventricular Septal Defects

No murmur may be apparent at birth, but as the pulmonary vascular resistance starts to fall (as is normal) left-to-right shunting occurs. The shunting increases until pulmonary blood flow becomes several times greater than the systemic flow. This has two results: (1) The heart is overloaded, resulting in heart failure which presents as tachypnoea, failure to thrive, etc. (2) Congested lungs are more prone to infection so that bronchitis or even pneumonia is often the initial presenting feature.

Signs

Cardiomegaly; loud pansystolic murmur and thrill in the 4th left interspace with a mid-diastolic flow murmur at the apex; loud second sound if considerable pulmonary hypertension; plus signs of heart failure, if present.

Investigations

ECG. Biventricular voltage increases with left atrial enlargement.

Chest radiography. Generalized cardiac enlargement. Increased pulmonary vascular markings.

Echocardiography. Left atrial, left and right ventricular enlargement. Enlarged pulmonary artery. Scanning from ventricular septum to aorta may reveal defect in ventricular septum.

Management

1. Digoxin controls the heart failure in the majority of cases. Despite theoretical control of failure, recurrent respiratory infections and failure to thrive remain clinical problems. However, after age of 1 year there is usually spontaneous improvement. Medication can be reduced or discontinued, although stature remains small.

2. Pulmonary hypertension: Exists in large VSDs (ventricular pressures must equalize if defect is large), but pulmonary vascular resistance remains low with consequent large left-to-right shunt until age of 1½–2 years. At this time either the VSD will be getting progressively smaller spontaneously enabling the PA pressure to fall, or the defect remains large, with progressive increase in pulmonary vascular resistance. Therefore, children with VSDs, having been in heart failure during first year of life, should be watched for clinical evidence of developing pulmonary hypertension—loud P2; decreasing murmur; changes in chest radiography and ECG indicating greater right-side predominance.

3. Defect remains large: at re-study (1½–2 years) if pulmonary pressures similar to systemic, surgical closure should be recommended at that stage, to prevent development of pulmonary vascular disease.

4. Surgical management: If unable to control heart failure at any time, surgery should be undertaken.

Small Ventricular Septal Defects

These are symptomless; usually detected by finding a systolic murmur on routine examination. X-ray, ECG, and echocardiography are all usually normal. The defect may close spontaneously.

Note:

1. Pulmonary stenosis may occur with VSD. Initially mild, the stenosis can progress until shunt becomes right to left. Clinical features then resemble tetralogy of Fallot (p. 294).

2. VSDs are usually in upper membranous septum immediately beneath aortic valve. Occasionally support for the septal leaflet of aortic valve is inadequate, such that cusp prolapses. This may partially occlude the VSD and produce aortic regurgitation. Clinically a murmur suggesting patent ductus develops in a child previously thought to have a VSD only.

Patent Ductus Arteriosus (PDA)

This is the second commonest congenital heart defect with a sex ratio of females : males of 3 : 1. Normally the ductus closes within the first few weeks of life. Spontaneous closure may be delayed, but rarely occurs beyond 12 weeks. Delayed closure is common in premature babies particularly if respiratory distress syndrome exists. Clinically a murmur develops within the first few days of life as pulmonary resistance falls. This results in shunting from aorta to pulmonary artery. Initially only an ejection systolic murmur is heard. This later becomes continuous, depending on the rate of fall of pulmonary resistance. The calibre of the ductus influences the clinical course.

Clinical Features

Pulses are more easily palpable than normal because of the wide pulse pressure, i.e. collapsing pulse. Blood pressure also reveals wide pulse pressure. The LV impulse is pronounced and the apex beat may be displaced.
Second sound. The pulmonary component of the second sound may be increased and even palpable. This indicates the degree of pulmonary hypertension.
Murmur. The murmur is characteristic. Initially there is a loud ejection systolic murmur often with a thrill at the second left interspace. Later, the murmur runs through the second heart sound occupying most of diastole. This is the classical machinery murmur, systolo-diastolic in type. There may be an additional mid-diastolic flow murmur at the apex.

In large PDA, as the pulmonary resistance falls to normal, the magnitude of the left-to-right shunt increases. Heart becomes overloaded, developing failure at 2–4 months. However, a large PDA may not produce frank failure, but the child may suffer from repeated respiratory infections, slow motor development and tiredness (although this may not be appreciated until after the ductus has been tied).

Small PDAs are asymptomatic and detected at routine examination.

Diagnosis

It may be difficult in the first year of life to distinguish a PDA from other causes of a continuous murmur such as:

Large VSD. Aorto-pulmonary window. Truncus arteriosus.

Venous hum. These may be heard in older children and are usually detected equally well beneath both clavicles (ductus louder beneath left). Check persistence of murmur with child upright and then supine. Venous hum usually disappears on positional change. Obstructing jugular vein usually abolishes hum.

Mixed aortic valve disease, surgically created shunts, ruptured aortic valve sinus or coronary artery malformation can also mimic patency of the ductus.

Management

In the neonatal period nothing more may be required than observation. If heart failure or deterioration of respiratory distress syndrome (RDS) ensues, digitalization and diuretics are indicated. Very occasionally immediate surgical ligation is required for deteriorating failure with RDS. Prostaglandin synthetase inhibitors, e.g. indomethacin may be useful. Helpful to reduce fluid intake for few days.

Six Months. If failure can be controlled medically this should be continued until about six months of age. Beyond this time spontaneous closure unlikely, so surgical closure indicated. Risks of surgery at this age are negligible.

In the older child PDA should be closed surgically as soon as detected even if the shunt is small, to prevent the risk of bacterial endocarditis.

Reversed Shunt. Occasionally a large PDA is associated with established, fixed pulmonary vascular disease. The blood flow through the ductus may then reverse, running from pulmonary artery to aorta. The child becomes cyanosed. At this stage surgical ligation is contraindicated.

Atrial Septal Defect (ASD)

Types
1. *Ostium secundum defect.* This is not uncommon although symptoms are inconspicuous in childhood. There is a central defect of variable size at:

The site of the fossa ovalis. Although this is present from birth, the volume of the shunt increases over the first few years of life.

Sinus venosus defect. Situated high in septum, often associated with partial anomalous pulmonary venous return.

2. *Ostium primum defect* (endocardial cushion defect), occurs at the lower end of the septum. May be isolated, or associated with other components of A–V canal syndrome such as VSD, mitral or tricuspid valve defects.

3. *Persistent foramen ovale.* Valve-like closure of the foramen ovale occurs after birth because LA pressure is marginally higher than RA. Closure becomes permanent by fibrosis between the ages of 1½ and 5 years. The foramen may remain probe-patent into adult life. Should the RA pressure at any time exceed LA pressure, e.g. as in pulmonary stenosis, or transiently in breath-holding attacks, the flap valve opens thus functioning as an ostium secundum septal defect, and permitting right-to-left shunting with cyanosis. Persistent foramen ovale is not an ASD in the true sense of the term.

Ostium Secundum Defect
This is the common type of ASD. In young children it is usually asymptomatic, being detected on routine examination by a parasternal heave of right ventricular overload; sescond heart sounds widely fixed and split, i.e. no variation of splitting with respiration; ejection systolic murmur in the pulmonary area due to increased pulmonary blood flow; mid-diastolic murmur over the lower sternum due to increased flow through tricuspid valve.

The ECG shows a right axis deviation (90–160°) with a partial right bundle-branch block, i.e. biphasic complex in Leads V1 Rsr[1], indicating right ventricular volume overload. This is a progressive development; it is not present at birth but develops along with development of shunting.

Investigations
Chest radiography demonstrates an increased heart size from right ventricular enlargement. This is seen well on the lateral film beneath the sternum. The pulmonary artery and proximal branches are prominent with pulmonary

plethora. However, the LA is of normal size, being decompressed through the atrial defect. The aorta may appear small and the SVC shadow is often inconspicuous.

Echocardiography indicates dilatation of the RV; reversed motion of the interventricular septum, but a normal LA size.

Course

ASD is asymptomatic in childhood, unless associated with other defects. This is because pulmonary resistance remains low until mid-adult life. Bacterial endocarditis is virtually unknown. Surgical closure should be performed between the ages of 6 and 10 years or as soon as detected thereafter.

Ostium Primum Defect

Signs and symptoms are as for a secundum defect. However, the condition tends to present earlier with fatigue and respiratory infections. This depends on the degree of associated mitral regurgitation. The ECG characteristically reveals left axis deviation ($-60°$ to $-180°$) with counterclockwise frontal QRS loops and a right bundle-branch block pattern in Lead VI. The defect is confirmed at cardiac catheterization.

Management

As for secundum atrial defect. The only difference centres around degree of mitral regurgitation. Six to 10 years is optimal age for corrective surgery.

Complete Atrioventricular Canal (Endocardial Cushion Defect)

In this condition there is a central cardiac defect involving a lack of the lower atrial septum, a high VSD and clefts of both the mitral and tricuspid valves which results in regurgitation. The condition is commonly found in Down's syndrome. It usually presents with heart failure during the first year of life, associated with recurrent respiratory infections and failure to thrive.

On examination there are a fixed wide splitting of the second heart sound, a pan-systolic murmur of VSD and mitral regurgitation, diastolic apical flow murmur, and often signs of heart failure.

ECG shows counterclockwise loop with left axis (-60 to $-180°$). P–R interval often prolonged. Rsr[1] in Lead VI.

Chest radiography shows a diffuse cardiac enlargement and pulmonary plethora.

Progress

There is often uncontrollable heart failure in the first year of life. Even if this can be controlled medically, pulmonary hypertension and vascular disease develop much earlier than with simple VSD. Down's syndrome children develop pulmonary hypertension before normal children with the same disorder and may survive early period better.

Anomalous Pulmonary Venous Drainage

May be total, in which case all systemic venous return, plus the pulmonary venous return, drain into the right atrium. Life depends on the presence of an ASD (or stretched foramen ovale) to permit filling of the left heart and systemic circulation. These cases develop heart failure and varying degrees of cyanosis, but often no murmur of note. The prognosis is very variable.

Partial anomalous venous drainage accompanies some cases of ostium secundum ASDs, but may occur as isolated defect. Drainage is anomalous from one lung only (commonly the right), affecting one or more veins of the lung. Usually drain to SVC, RA or beneath the diaphragm to IVC. Usually asymptomatic and chance finding.

Eisenmenger's Complex and Syndrome

These conditions are important and not uncommon. Eisenmenger's complex occurs when, owing to a shunt through VSD pulmonary hypertension develops to systemic level due to high pulmonary vascular resistance. This results in a reversed or bi-directional shunt. Historically, the Eisenmenger's complex was described first. In Eisenmenger's syndrome the shunt occurs at any level: aorto-pulmonary level through a PDA or similar lesions, or even at atrial level. In Eisenmenger's complex pulmonary hypertension may have existed since infancy. In Eisenmenger's syndrome the pulmonary resistance was initially lower, with left-to-right shunting, but due to the high flow the pulmonary vascular bed reacts pathologically, with thickening and obstruction of the small vessels. As a result high resistance develops giving rise to a right-to-left shunt and cyanosis.

Management is symptomatic. It is too late for surgery.

III. Cyanotic Group (*Right-to-left shunt present*)

Fallot's Tetralogy

Commonest cyanotic defect compatible with life at age 2 years without previous surgical intervention. There is a spectrum of severity, each basically comprising:

1. Pulmonary stenosis which may be valvular or infundibular but usually both. This is produced by anterior displacement of the conal septum. Pulmonary stenosis is the main determinant of severity, the most severe having pulmonary atresia.

2. Ventricular septal defect.

3. Aorta 'overriding' VSD. A quarter of cases have a right-sided aortic arch.

4. Right ventricular hypertrophy which results as a consequence of the other lesions.

Haemodynamics

Because of the right ventricular outflow obstruction part of blood flows through VSD into aorta, resulting in varying degrees of cyanosis.

Symptoms

Symptoms are initially absent. Later dyspnoea develops on effort, e.g. with feeding.

Cyanotic episopdes ('blue spells') occur. The child, while normally pink at rest, develops episode of extreme pallor, hyperpnoea and severe cyanosis, limpness and rolling up of eyes, with transient unresponsiveness. Such spells are extremely dangerous and require urgent treatment, e.g. morphine or β-blocker.

Signs

1. Cyanosis (p. 284). (*a*) Severe tetralogies may be cyanosed from birth. (*b*) Others remain pink but develop cyanosis as ductus closes and pulmonary stenosis gradually increases in severity. (*c*) Those with mild pulmonary stenosis may never appear cyanosed (so-called 'acyanotic tetralogy'). Cyanosis does not impede mental development.

2. *Growth* is usually retarded.

3. *Pulses*. Normal (unless large ductus present).

4. *Heart* pulsation is increased at the lower sternum from RV enlargement. The second sound is usually single and louder than normal, i.e. the aortic component only is audible. There may occasionally be an ejection click. The characteristic murmur is ejection systolic which is related to the pulmonary stenosis. The louder and longer the murmur the less severe the tetralogy. If the murmur reduces in intensity or disappears on crying, this indicates spasm of infundibular muscle obstructing the right ventricular outflow. Such children are at risk of cyanotic (hypoxic) episodes.

Complications

Cyanotic episodes constitute the major threat. Cerebrovascular accidents are associated with polycythemia and increased viscosity of blood leading to cerebral thrombosis. Haemoglobin may be up to 20 g/dl. Cerebral abscess also occurs but endocarditis is rare.

Investigations

ECG. Right axis deviation (120°). Tall P in Lead II (RA enlargement). Tall R in Lead VI with rapid transition to R/S complex in Lead V2 (plus other changes of RV enlargement, *see* p. 281).

Chest radiography. In the PA view there is an uptilted apex (so-called 'coeur-en-sabot'). The main and peripheral pulmonary arteries are diminished. Right-sided aorta is present in one-quarter of cases.

Echocardiography shows RV enlargement, small pulmonary outflow tract, VSD and overriding aorta.

Cardiac catheterization with angiocardiography is confirmatory.

Treatment

If the child is severely cyanosed at birth or within first year, the pulmonary flow can be improved by systemic–pulmonary artery shunt. Heart failure is extremely uncommon because the RV can be decompressed through the VSD. Digoxin therapy therefore is of little value.

Over the age of one year primary surgical correction should be performed. This impies: relief of pulmonary stenosis by muscle resection; pulmonary valvotomy; 'patching' of outflow tract if severe; and closure of VSD.

Transposition of Great Arteries

This is the commonest cyanotic disorder in newborns.

Anatomically the aorta receives blood from right ventricle with the pulmonary artery being supplied by left ventricle. This usually implies that aorta lies anteriorly to pulmonary artery.

Functionally, two separate circulations exist: systemic and pulmonary. Without some interconnection, the disorder is incompatible with life. Life exists initially because there is a stretched patent foramen ovale and patent ductus. Without surgical treatment death occurs within first month.

On examination cyanosis is usually present from moment of birth. There is a soft ejection systolic murmur if ductus only exists, but a pansystolic murmur if a

VSD is present. The second sound is usually loud and single and is due to an anteriorly placed aorta. Heart failure may develop within the first few weeks of life.

Diagnosis and Management

The diagnosis is established by echocardiography. However, cardiac catheterization is required so that balloon septostomy may be performed. This consists of enlarging the ASD or patent foramen ovale by withdrawing a Rashkind catheter with inflatable balloon at its tip from left atrium to right atrium, so tearing atrial septum. This permits mixing of circulation, often sufficient to allow reasonable life until about 1 year of age (although moderate cyanosis usually persists).

Corrective surgery by Mustard's intra-atrial baffle procedure is performed at about one year of age.

Tricuspid Atresia

In this condition cyanosis usually occurs within the first month. The murmurs are not diagnostic, the second sound is usually single and congestive heart failure is common.

The ECG is diagnostic with evidence of left axis and LV hypertrophy in presence of cyanosis (because right ventricle is diminutive). Large P waves in standard Lead II (because of right atrial enlargement).

Initial treatment is surgical by balloon atrial septostomy. Functional correction is by the Fontan procedure after 5 years.

Pulmonary Atresia

Presents with cyanosis from birth, the pulmonary blood supply being totally dependent on patency of the ductus. It is usually associated with under-development of the right ventricle. Congestive heart failure occurs early, murmurs are minimal and that of the ductus only.

Hypoplastic Left Heart Syndrome

Common condition but should only be considered as a diagnosis in first month of life. It is always associated with mitral atresia and/or aortic atresia. No satisfactory surgical intervention is available.

Ebstein's Disease

In this condition components of the tricuspid valve are displaced (at varying levels) into right ventricle so that part of right ventricle becomes 'atrialized'. May present in infancy with congestive heart failure and cyanosis. May improve with medical management and time. Other cases present in childhood or adolescence with decreased effort tolerance and cardiomegaly. Clinically, there is a pansystolic murmur of tricuspid regurgitation. Superficial scratch sound in diastole.

Chapter 89

ACQUIRED HEART DISEASE IN CHILDHOOD

Myocarditis

This falls into two broad groups:
1. Secondary to an identifiable cause, e.g. (*a*) bacterial, (*b*) rheumatic, (*c*) viral—Coxsackie, influenza, etc.
2. No identifiable agent—includes presumed intra-uterine infections.

Presentation
The onset of cardiac failure at any age in the absence of congenital heart lesions. Cardiac arrhythmia may or may not be present. Pyrexia is variable. On auscultation a pericardial friction rub may be heard. Frequently there are no murmurs or only a soft pulmonary flow murmur. When the child is in gross failure, functional regurgitation of the mitral and tricuspid valves may produce a pansystolic murmur. Third and fourth heart sounds are frequent (summation gallop). Sudden death may occur before heart failure has been established.

Investigations
ECG—generalized low voltage with widespread 'T' wave inversion and S–T segment depression. Conduction disturbances and ectopic beats of multifocal origin.
Chest radiography reveals cardiomegaly and evidence of heart failure.

Congestive Cardiomyopathies

These may occur at any age with symptoms and signs of congestive heart failure. Medical treatment should be instituted immediately for heart failure and following this attempts should be made to exclude a responsible agent. If no anatomical defect is detectable, e.g. an anomalous coronary artery, but there is a large poorly contracting heart the diagnosis is likely to be cardiomyopathy.
The majority, particularly in infants will be:

A. Endocardial Fibro-elastosis
In this condition the endocardium is thickened, white and associated with poor muscular function. Aetiology is unknown. The condition may occur in identical twins. No surgical treatment is available. Medical management for heart failure should be prolonged for at least two years. A few cases improve, such that eventually heart size returns to normal.

B. Glycogen Storage Disease Type II
One of the few congestive myopathies which can be diagnosed during life (*see* p. 164). This is done by skeletal or liver biopsy. The majority of cases die within the first six months of life.

C. Other Diseases Presenting like Congestive Cardiomyopathy are:
1. Coronary artery disease—either anatomical defect, i.e. anomalous origin from pulmonary artery, or obliterative due to premature atherosclerosis or arteritis.

2. *Constrictive pericarditis.*

Rheumatic Fever

This classic disease is now uncommon, although it is still important in some parts of the world. It is commoner in urban populations with crowded poor circumstances. It may manifest itself as:

1. Carditis. Rheumatic heart disease.
2. Arthritis. Also called acute rheumatism, juvenile rheumatism, acute polyarthritis.
3. Sydenham's chorea. St Vitus's dance.
4. Nodules now very rare. Seen only in longstanding neglected cases. They are small, hard, non-tender lumps occurring over the bony prominences. They are always manifestations of active disease.
5. Erythema marginatum: a non-specific phenomenon. The rash is frequently only present for a few hours. It starts as faint red circles which spread and coalesce to form irregular crenated patterns. It is not diagnostic of rheumatic fever.

The name rheumatic fever includes all of the above.

Clinical Features

There is often a history of preceding sore throat occuring 10–14 days previously. Various types of this disorder may occur:

1. Polyarthritis, which is usually acute and sudden, with high fever, very painful joints, and pancarditis. More commonly there is mild arthralgia (painful joints) with no signs of inflammation. The child may not complain for a time and remains ambulant.

2. Insidious with carditis. Particularly occurs in young children. History of general malaise, anorexia, failure to gain weight. Evening pyrexia. Carditis may only be discovered on routine examination.

3. Chorea may coexist with carditis, but very rarely with polyarthritis.

The child appears ill, and easily fatigued, sweats readily. The weight is stationary or drops. Fever is not usually high—37·2–39°C (99–102°F), and is often not raised in chorea. Tachycardia is prominent.

Polyarthritis

Classic Attack

History. Large joints affected (ankle, knee, elbow, wrist) in any order and combination. Arthritis 'flits' from joint to joint, remaining for a few hours or days in each before another is attacked. Rarely more than three joints affected simultaneously. Small joints less commonly involved.

On examination joints acutely painful on active or passive movement. Uncommonly may be red, slightly swollen, hot to touch. Effusion rare.

Atypical Attack

More common. Only one or two joints transiently affected.

Associated Features

Carditis is the most important feature, *see* p. 300.

Chorea (Sydenham's Chorea; St Vitus's Dance)
This condition commences insidiously between the ages of 5 and 15 years. Girls : boys, 3 : 1.
   Probably two types of chorea:
   1. Rheumatic—associated with all the usual signs and symptoms of rheumatic fever (except arthritis).
   2. Simple—occurs alone without manifestations of rheumatic fever. Notably, no carditis, no fever, ESR normal.
   Child is restless and fidgety, frequently drops things. Schoolteacher may complain of deteriorating handwriting.

Movements
Quasi-purposive. Movement of a high order, but fragmented and do not serve any useful purpose. Writhing and plucking movements of arms common, the whole arm taking part. Movements of legs less complicated. Movements of face usually bilateral—smiling, grimacing, frowning, or protruding tongue. Respiration jerky and irregular. Speech difficult and jerky. May be clucking noises. Associated movements often marked, thus protruding tongue causes writhing movements of arms or legs. Movement worse when excited. Disappear during sleep. Voluntary movements are interrupted by involuntary, giving rise to incoordination.
   Following features may also be noticed:
   1. Muscular weakness. Common, with marked hypotonia and inability to maintain posture. On command to hold out hands, arms shoot out, hands droop, with flexion at wrist and hyperextension of metacarpophalangeal joints owing to hypotonia. Rarely: (*a*) Hemichorea: One side of the body often more affected than other. (*b*) Paralytic chorea: Normal hypotonia of disease may be so exaggerated as to result in paralysis. Rarely complete, usually some twitching movement.
   2. Reflexes. May be brisk or (due to weakness) absent. Often show prolongation of contraction, e.g. sustained or pendulum knee jerks occur.
   3. Mental state. Child often emotionally labile, laughs and cries easily, disobedient and difficult to control, especially in convalescent stages when general condition improving. Markedly different from child with rheumatic arthritis.
   4. Carditis. Most important.

Differential Diagnosis
   1. Abnormal movements seen in various organic conditions such as: athetosis, encephalitis lethargica, hepatolenticular degeneration, cerebral tumour. But confusion with chorea improbable.
   2. Tics or habit spasms (*see* p. 351). Occasionally follow attack of true chorea—choreiform movements having become a habit. Typically consist of constant repetition of one or two sterotyped movements. Child can demonstrate the movement on request.

Course and Prognosis
Lasts between 6 weeks and 3 months. Initial severity no guide. Often difficult to judge end of disease as movements may become habit and persist. If heart unaffected in first attack, unlikely to be affected in subsequent attacks.

Carditis (Acute Rheumatic Heart Disease)
This condition is more frequently associated with arthritis than with chorea. May

occur alone. It is the possibility of heart damage that makes rheumatic fever important disease. Arthritis or chorea by themselves never lethal nor permanently incapacitating.

Clinical Features

At the onset of carditis all other signs tend to become more marked. Child appears more ill, pyrexia higher, heart rate more rapid, pallor increased; may be dyspnoeic or have precordial pain.

Myocarditis. The essential lesion in acute rheumatic fever is the myocarditis. Here the heart sounds are muffled; apex beat feeble; tic-tac or gallop rhythm with tachycardia of 120–150 occurs. Less commonly bradycardia. Area of cardiac dullness increases to right of sternum and apex beat moves down and out. Enlargement is due to dilatation (too rapid for hypertrophy). Easily mistaken for pericarditis with effusion.

When the heart dilates a soft, generalized functional-type systolic murmur commonly occurs. As condition progresses murmur at apex follows definite sequence of events:

1. Systolic murmur at first generalized, becomes maximal at apex, louder and may be conducted into axilla.

2. Lengthening of physiological third heart sound into localized mid-diastolic murmur.

3. Occasionally presystolic murmur develops, especially with rapid heart rate. Systolic murmur usually remains throughout.

4. As condition improves, diastolic murmur passes through above stages in reverse order. Systolic murmur may appear or remain.

5. If complete recovery does not occur, murmurs gradually evolve into those of chronic rheumatic heart disease, most commonly mitral stenosis and aortic regurgitation.

Complications

1. Some degree of heart failure is not uncommon in the acute phase of the disease or as an end result of chronic rheumatic heart disease.

2. Pericarditis is rare except in mild subclinical degrees. May be dry (with a friction rub) or with an effusion.

Investigations

1. *Antistreptococcal titre* is raised. This is useful evidence of preceding streptococcal infection.

2. *Erythrocyte sedimentation rate* (ESR). Non-specific test of great value. Is increased while the condition is active. Should be measured weekly as evidence of activity.

3. There is often radiological and ECG evidence of carditis.

Differential Diagnosis of Rheumatoid Arthritis, *see under* Juvenile Rheumatoid Arthritis (p. 442).

Course and Prognosis

Classically rheumatic fever proceeds by relapses and remissions. The relapse may occur during convalescence or years later. Each attack increases the risk of damage to the heart.

Carditis. Possible outcomes:

1. Most commonly the child recovers from the attack completely.

2. Activity seems to disappear rapidly, arthritis being minimal or absent, but yet chronic cardiac damage results. When the social circumstances are poor and care inadequate, the carditis may smoulder on for months with periodic bouts of greater activity. The danger of permanent cardiac damage is then very great.

Indications of activity are very important as signs of active carditis have to be clearly detected. Difficult to assess in some cases.

> *Clinical*
> 1. Lassitude; failure to gain weight; loss of appetite.
> 2. Pyrexia.
> 3. Tachycardia. High sleeping pulse rate especially valuable. Should be charted. May be bradycardia. Return of sinus arrhythmia may indicate cessation of activity.
> 4. Heart. Increasing enlargement, or failure to return to normal size. Muffled heart sounds.
> 5. Arthritis; erythema marginatum, nodules always indicate activity.
> *ECG.* Prolonged P–R interval does not always return to normal even when activity abated. Indicates lessened activity if it does so.
> Erythrocyte sedimentation rate (ESR) return to normal of great value. Raised rate may be the only indication of persistent activity.
> Summary. Greatest reliance should be placed upon presence of: fever, high sleeping pulse, extending murmurs, raised ESR, stationary or falling weight.

Treatment of Attack

All cases with arthritis or chorea must be assumed to have active carditis. Treatment of β-haemolytic streptococcal infection by adequate penicillin dosage should be commenced even before confirmation of its presence. There is no specific treatment for acute rheumatism, but salicylates and corticosteroids both cure the arthritis, promote well-being and reduce evidence of activity. The effect on the carditis, however, is unproven. 1–3 weeks after cessation of therapy with salicylates or corticosteroids 'rebound phenomena' may occur, i.e. recrudescence of symptoms. These may include arthritis, carditis, pyrexia, or increased pulse rate. More commonly a raised ESR is the only manifestation of rebound.

Salicylates should be given in all cases. Since the optimum therapeutic dose is very near the toxic dose, dosage should be monitored by serum levels. *Note*: Children rarely complain of ringing in ears. Overdosage is indicated by deep sighing respiration which must be looked for.

Corticosteroid therapy should be given in addition to salicylates in all cases with carditis.

Prophylaxis

For the prevention of relapse regular prophylactic penicillin should be given to eliminate further streptococcal infections.

Chronic Rheumatic Heart Disease

This is now very rare in childhood.
Manifestations of carditis are:

	In acute disease	In chronic disease
Myocarditis	Important	Not important
Pericarditis	Important	Moderately important
Endocarditis	Not important	Very important

Subacute Bacterial Endocarditis

This condition is now rare in childhood. The clinical manifestations are as seen in adults. It is essential that all children with congenital or rheumatic heart disease who undergo dental extraction or receive surgery to the nose or throat should be given adequate prophylactic antibiotic cover.

Chapter 90	# DISORDERS OF RATE AND RHYTHM

Paroxysmal Tachycardia

In children over 1 year of age paroxysmal tachycardia presents in a similar way to that in adults. Children under 1 year of age present with a sudden onset of listlessness and irritability. Tachypnoea often with slight pyrexia. Heart failure with lung crepitations may develop if paroxysm established for several hours (usually 24). This condition, therefore, can mimic bronchopneumonia if significance of rapid heart rate is not appreciated. If untreated may be fatal. It is difficult to assess the heart rate clinically if it is over 180/min. ECG monitoring is vital. The rate will be found to be somewhere between 180 and 300. Regular P waves are usually not visible. When the rate has returned to normal the ECG may show an underlying picture of Wolff–Parkinson–White syndrome (*see below*).

Treatment
Carotid sinus, or eyeball stimulation is valuable in older children but cannot be used for babies. In these, Digoxin is usually effective, although it may take some time to work. It has the advantage that any associated heart failure is also treated. β-blockers may be required or cardioversion (direct current countershock). After the initial episode anti-arrhythmic medication must be continued for several months. Digoxin is usually the most valuable.

Wolff–Parkinson–White (WPW) Syndrome

There is a normal conduction pathway between SA nodes, A–V node, His bundle and branches, plus *one or more accessory pathways by-passing the A–V node*.

Physiology
Excitation enters ventricles in abnormal way producing some delay in ventricular

depolarization (reflected by widened QRS complex). Heart rate may remain normal despite abnormal conduction, but intermittently depolarization may travel retrogradely to atria returning to ventricles via the normal or abnormal route. A recirculating excitation situation is then established producing tachycardia.

Clinical Picture
The child is initially asymptomatic but prone to attacks of paroxysmal tachycardia throughout life, but especially during infancy.

Electrocardiographic Findings
1. During episode findings are of supraventricular tachycardia—often with aberrant conduction (i.e. may resemble ventricular tachycardia). ECG not diagnostic of WPW syndrome during tachycardia.
2. When the heart rate is normal the ECG shows a short P–R interval and widened QRS.
Note: Short P–R = <0·12s, wide QRS = >0·12s, the wide QRS usually has a slurred initial component = delta wave.

Bradycardia

This is usually asymptomatic. Sinus bradycardia (slow sinus rhythm approx 60/min) is often found in fit, healthy, young individuals. Note that the rate may remain abnormally slow even when stimulated by illness, e.g. appendicitis. Heart rate may also be abnormally slow in such conditions as cretinism, myocarditis, etc.

Hypertension

Owing to the importance of hypertension in adults, efforts are being made to discover cases early so that it can be prevented. However, it is rare in childhood. Mass screening measures are required to catch a few cases. It is questionable whether these are justifiable. Routine blood pressure estimations are required if there is a family history of hypertension. Some causes of childhood hypertension are: secondary to kidney lesion, coarctation of aorta, poisoning, adrenal causes, e.g. phaeochromocytoma or steroid enzyme defect or dysautonomia (Riley–Day syndrome) or tumours, encephalitis, etc. Idiopathic ('essential') hypertension is very rare in childhood (*see* p. 390).

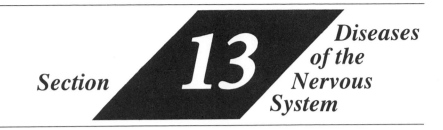

Section **13** **Diseases of the Nervous System**

Chapter 91	*HISTORY TAKING AND EXAMINATION OF THE NERVOUS SYSTEM*

In children, examination of the central nervous system (CNS) is mainly concerned with observation of *function*. It is therefore intimately associated with the examination of mental and physical development and behaviour. To a large extent the examination has to be unstructured and throughout the interview the examiner must be subtly watching the child and his reactions to his parents, strangers and the environment. Nevertheless, while the examiner must be an opportunist and pick up clues wherever he can, he must retain in his mind a logical schema for examination, relevant to the age of the child, to be applied as far as he is able.

History

The history commences with a description of the child's problem as seen by the parents, followed by:

1. The obstetric history, especially details of the pregnancy, labour and delivery. The birth weight and gestational age are often relevant, as is the immediate postnatal state, especially the presence of cyanosis or fits, activity, and tone sucking.

2. In young children a developmental history should be obtained and a quick developmental examination performed. This should be more thorough if any abnormality is found. In older children enquiries should be made about scholastic accomplishment. Formal intelligence testing may be required.

3. Questions should be asked relevant to any injury or fall, history and family history of convulsions, history of meningitis, encephalitis or drugs which might affect the CNS.

4. Family history, consanguinity, current behaviour pattern and motor skills are also relevant. The feeding history may be important.

Examination

The Head

The head circumferance should be measured and charted on a centile chart. It should be examined for the size and tension of the fontanelles, whether the sutures are closed and for any abnormal lumps or depressions. On percussion a 'cracked-pot' sound may be heard in a child in whom the sutures are splayed because of raised intracranial pressure. A systolic murmur may be heard over the cranium. This is not uncommon in young children. In older children it may indicate a vascular abnormality.

Skin

A search should be made for café-au-lait spots, especially in the axillae; adenoma sebaceum, abnormal pigmentation or hypopigmentation, or ichthyosis.

Cranial Nerves

I. This is difficult to test in young children—try orange or chocolate.

II. Is tested by the ability to follow light or a toy with the eyes. Formal visual field testing is only possible in an older cooperative child. However, some inkling of vision loss may be obtainable. Acuity usually requires the help of a skilled ophthalmologist. Fundi examination is important but may be arduous. The pupil often requires dilating. General anaesthesia is rarely necessary. Babies held upright against their mother's shoulder usually open their eyes.

III and IV. Test movements by getting child to follow object. Squint common in children. May be concomitant or paralytic. Third nerve paralysis causes ptosis, lateral deviation, big pupil.

V. *Motor*. Ability to bite can be tested. Unilateral lesions difficult to determine.

VI. *Sensory*. Examination can be crudely assessed by reaction to touch or pinprick. Corneal sensation can be demonstrated by testing corneal reflex.

VII. May require prolonged observation to notice minor facial weakness in baby. Corner of mouth drawn up on unaffected side. In upper motor neurone lesions only the lower face is involved.

VIII. Deafness is very important in children and hearing should always be tested.

IX and X. Rarely involved separately. Nasal speech should be noted and palatal paralysis should be looked for as the tonsils are being examined. As children hate having this done it should always be left until last.

XI. Weakness of trapezius.

XII. Tongue protruded to affected side.

Sensory System

Sensory system is almost impossible to investigate accurately until the child is old enough to cooperate, but reaction to stimuli, e.g. cotton wool or pin can be noted.

Motor System

1. Weakness of muscles. In young babies movement of limbs may be observed. Painful stimuli may have to be applied to encourage movement. Older child should be watched playing and walking, if possible unobserved by child. The gait is rarely natural if the child realizes he is being watched.

In babies a limb may be kept still because of pain or discomfort, i.e. with osteomyelitis or arthritis—so-called 'pseudoparalysis'.

Trunk muscles can be tested by watching child bend down or sit up. Weakness of abdominal muscles shown by movement of umbilicus up or down on rising from lying to sitting posture.

2. Observe gait, speech, behaviour, postures, abnormal movements or paralysis. Note level of consciousness.

3. Tone must be examined by moving the limb passively. No objective tests of tone are available. Assessment therefore is purely subjective and depends on the experience of the examiner to disregard superadded voluntary movement. Young hypertonic babies keep the hands tightly clenched. In older babies, hypertonicity of the upper limbs can be gauged by watching the baby trying to grasp an object. Characteristic 'open hand' approach observed in hypertonic child.

4. Tremor or athetoid movements must be looked for. Athetoid movements rarely diagnosed with certainty before 7 months. Before the movements develop the child is characteristically hypotonic.

5. Co-ordination is tested by the ability to perform fine movements.

Reflexes

Deep Tendon Reflexes. Present from birth. May be brisker than normal during neonatal period. To elicit baby's knee jerk, heel must be on couch. Front of tibia should be tapped all the way down to ankle to elicit 'overflow'. Abdominal and cremasteric reflexes develop about the 3rd–4th month. Extensor response resembling positive Babinski reflex is obtained up until about 18 months of age, or when the child starts to walk. It is possible to confuse a grasp reflex in the toes with a flexor plantar response.

Investigations

1. Lumbar puncture. Usually easy in child. Rarely has to be done under narcosis. Spinal cord in infant extends to L3. Puncture must be below this. Before lumbar puncture, fundi must always be examined for papilloedema. If intracranial pressure is raised, lumbar route may be dangerous owing to risk of 'coning' of medulla.

2. Ventricular puncture can be performed when fontanelle open and lumbar puncture contraindicated.

Normal cerebrospinal fluid, *see Table* 91.1, p.308.

3. Subdural puncture should be performed if haematoma or effusion suspected.

4. Radiography of skull.

> 4.1 In young children, evidence of raised intracranial pressure is shown by widening of the sutures. It is difficult to place an age on this. If a very slow-growing space-occupying lesion is present, the sutures can separate as late as 6 years. Erosion of the clinoid processes, and 'beaten silver' appearance of the vault are only found in older children with longstanding raised pressure. Neither are helpful signs unless gross.
>
> 4.2 Premature fusion of the sutures is seen in craniostenosis.
>
> 4.3 Abnormal calcification may be found in some chronic lesions, e.g. craniopharyngioma, toxoplasmosis, Sturge–Weber syndrome, epiloia and cytomegalovirus infection.

5. CT scan (computerized axial tomography). This investigation has almost completely taken the place of air studies as in paediatric CNS investigations.

6. Brain scan. Can be useful in diagnosing tumours, brain abscess, encephalitis and subdural haematoma.

7. Ultrasound examination of brain extremely useful if fontanelle open.

Table 91.1. Differential diagnosis of cerebrospinal fluid

	Pressure (recumbent)	Appearance	Cells per cmm	Protein	Sugar	Organisms
Normal	Under 175 mm of fluid	Clear; Colourless. No clot	0-4. Lymphocytes	0·1-0·25 g/l (10-25 mg per cent)	2·5-5·0 mmol/l (45-100mg per cent)	Nil
Acute pyogenic meningitis	Increased	From hazy to obvious pus. Clot	1000-10000. Polymorphs	0·45-5·0 g/l (45-500 mg per cent)	1·65-2·2 mmol/l 1·8-2·5 initially. Absent later	Usually present in smears. Requires culture for diagnosis
Aseptic (virus) meningitis	Slight increase	Clear or hazy	50-1500. Polymorphs at first, later lymphocytes	0·5-1·0 g/l (50-100 mg per cent)	Normal	Nil. Virus cultured with difficulty
Poliomyelitis	Normal	Normal. Clot rare	10-250. Polymorphs at first, later lymphocytes	Progressive rise to 3·0 g/l (300mg per cent)	Normal	Nil
Tuberculous meningitis	Increased	Clear or hazy. Colourless. Spider web clot on standing	50-250. Mainly lymphocytes	0·5-2·5 g/l (50-250 mg per cent)	1·1-1·65 mmol/l initially. Down to 0·55-1·1 mmol/l later	Tubercle bacilli found with difficulty in centrifuged deposit
Aseptic reaction: brain abscess etc.	Usually increased	Clear or hazy	Nil to 500. Polymorphs or lymphocytes may predominate	0·3-2·0 g/l (30-200 mg per cent)	Normal	Nil
Cerebral tumour	Increased. Sometimes 400+ mm	Clear; may be yellow	0-50	0·3-10·0 g/l (30-1000+ mg per cent)	Normal. Occasionally absent	Nil
Guillain-Barré syndrome	Normal	Normal	Normal	Raised ++	Normal	Nil

Chapter 92	VASCULAR LESIONS

Chronic Subdural Haematoma

This condition should be urgently considered in any young child who presents with fits, drowsiness, progressive hydrocephalus of recent onset or focal CNS signs. The condition occurs particularly in pre-term infants or in children with a history of recent injury to the head. However, this information is not always forthcoming in non-accidental injury. Fundal examination may reveal preretinal (subhyaloid) haemorrhages.

Pathology
The blood is encysted between thick membranes formed from the adjacent dura and arachnoid. The majority of haematomas occur over the cerebrum. They contain bloodstained fluid of characteristic appearance. The haematoma may be very extensive. Sixty per cent are bilateral. For reasons unknown, the haematoma gradually increases in size, due possibly to continued bleeding from granulation tissue, or osmosis through the wall which acts as a semipermeable membrane.

Investigations
  1. The skull may transilluminate more on the affected side.
  2. Radiograph may reveal fracture of the skull. Unless the possibility of non-accidental injury can be eliminated, radiographic skeletal survey of all bones should be performed to search for other fractures.
  3. Subdural aspiration. This is the essential diagnostic measure. If a haematoma is present bloodstained or xanthochromic fluid will drip out. The protein content of the fluid is high (1–6 g/dl).
  4. CT scan.

Treatment is by repeated aspirations or surgery.

Thrombosis

Lateral Sinus Thrombosis
Not uncommon cause of CNS lesions, especially VIth nerve palsy and hemiplegia in a child who is severely dehydrated for any reason (e.g. gastroenteritis) or is polycythaemic (e.g. cyanotic congenital heart disease). Also follows middle ear/mastoid infection.
    The prognosis is poor. The child may die or have permanent brain damage if he recovers.

Chapter 93	NEUROCUTANEOUS DISORDERS

Sturge–Weber Syndrome (*Encephalotrigeminal Angiomatosis*)

Uncommon congenital condition with cutaneous naevus and leptomeningeal telangiectasis resulting in some or all of the following clinical manifestations:

Vascular naevus on face (Port-wine stain). Predominantly unilateral and occurring over the skin distribution of the ophthalmic division of the trigeminal nerve. Changes, including calcification, occur in the meninges when the upper part of the face is involved.

Convulsions are usually focal motor fits on the opposite side to the port-wine stain. These occur frequently and are hard to control.

Hemiplegia and occasionally homonymous hemianopia occur on the opposite side to the intracranial lesion.

Mild mental retardation is common.

Buphthalmos with infantile glaucoma can occur in either eye; the fundus is dark red, and the retina may detach.

Investigations
1. Radiology of the skull. After the age of about 18 months, 'tram-line' calcification can sometimes be seen over the cerebral cortex underlying the vascular malformation.
2. Electro-encephalogram shows unilateral depression of cortical activity, with or without abnormal discharges.
3. CT scan.

Treatment
Anti-epileptic drugs are required to control the convulsions. Surgery occasionally required.

Neurofibromatosis
(Von Recklinghausen's Disease)

Not uncommon disease inherited as Mendelian dominant.

Clinical Features
Café-au-lait spots are the key to the diagnosis. Appear at birth, but become more numerous with age. Irregular areas vary in size from a millimetre to several centimetres. Appear mainly over trunk including the axilla, the so-called 'sign of the axilla'. Identical patches of pigmentation are frequently seen in normal persons but if so usually fewer than five in number, less than 2 cm in diameter, and never occur in the axilla. Pigmented lesions are often the only manifestation of the disease until adult life. Depigmented areas may also occur.

Neuromas. Neurofibromas, the most characteristic lesion in adults are uncommon in childhood. Multiple, various sizes, soft or firm, may be along course of peripheral nerve, along deep nerves, e.g. vagus, spinal nerve root, etc. leading to neurological symptoms.

Bony lesions are a common manifestation in childhood. They may occur:
1. In long bones, leading to cysts, appearance of fibrous dysplasia, fractures, etc.
2. In the spine, resulting in scoliosis and kyphosis, scalloped spine appearance on radiography.
3. In the skull, resulting in deepening of the middle cranial fossa, elevation of the wing of the sphenoid, and sometimes pulsating exophthalmos.

Rare Manifestations are:
Diffuse and focal gliosis leading to mental retardation, diabetes insipidus, macrocephaly, etc.

Tuberous Sclerosis (*Epiloia*, *Bourneville Disease*)

Autosomal dominant condition with variable penetrance and expression.

Clinical Features

1. Skin lesions

1.1 Hypopigmented macules. Found on trunk or limbs and usually present from birth. Oval or leaf-shaped.
1.2 Adenoma sebaceum. Characteristic of tuberous sclerosis. Red or brown nodules appearing after a few years in a butterfly distribution across the face.
1.3 Shagreen patches. Areas of thickened skin with a texture like orange peel generally found over the lumbar region.
1.4 Periungual fibromas. These develop in late childhood or adolescence and present as fibrous nodules around finger and toenails.

2. Epilepsy. Convulsions occur in the majority of patients and usually commence as infantile spasms during the first year of life. Later psychomotor or grand mal seizures.

3. Mental retardation of some degree occurs in more than half the patients. Behaviour problems are common.

4. Tumours. Small, benign, glial nodules occur throughout the brain and usually become calcified. Benign tumours composed of fibrous tissue, fat and muscle have been found in many internal organs such as the kidneys, liver and lungs. Rhabdomyoma of the heart is a recognised cause of death.

Investigations

Radiology reveals the intracranial calcification, which may be confirmed by computerized tomography. The diagnosis is otherwise made by the clinical combination of the characteristic skin lesions and epilepsy with or without mental retardation.

Treatment

Symptomatic. Genetic counselling is important.

Chapter 94   # NERVE LESIONS

Congenital Lesions of Cranial Nerves

Seventh Nerve Palsy
May be present at birth. It is usually assumed at first that the injury is caused by

the birth, perhaps at forceps delivery. If the palsy persists the cause may be agenesis rather than injury especially if the lesion is upper motor in type.

Nystagmus
Roving nystagmus is associated with, and possibly caused by, a defective retinal fixation point due to blindness, astigmatism or albinism. It may also occur as a genetically determined condition. The child is accustomed to the eye oscillations and they do not cause symptoms. In spasmus nutans the condition is associated with head nodding.

Nuclear Agenesis (*Moebius' Syndrome; Congenital Facial Diplegia*)
Rare congenital condition in which there is paresis of muscles involving the face, eye movements, tongue and soft palate. May be uni- or bilateral. In infancy stridor and micrognathos may be prominent; swallowing may be difficult. Child has appearance of mental backwardness with lack of facial movement, drooling and poor speech, but usually mentally normal.

Strabismus (*Squint*)
Common condition occurring in approximately 2 % of all children.

Classification
The squint may be:
1. Concomitant (commonest). The angle of deviation remains unchanged whatever the direction of gaze. May be convergent (commonest), or divergent.
2. Paralytic. Very important as this may be the earliest evidence of a serious CNS lesion such as a cerebral tumour.

Management
Early referral to an ophthalmologist.

Horner's Syndrome (*Lesion of cervical sympathetic*)
May be congenital or as a result of birth injury.
Classic signs are ptosis, miosis, enophthalmos, hypohidrosis and poor iris pigmentation. Not all of these may be present in every case.

Acute Infective Polyneuritis (Guillain–Barré Syndrome)

Not uncommon disease. The cause is usually unknown, but it may follow a virus infection.

Clinical Features
Usually commences with acute onset of symmetrical muscle paralysis. The legs are often involved maximally at first, with less involvement of the arms. A few days later the arms may be worse and bulbar muscles and muscles of respiration are involved. Assisted respiration may be required for a while.
Muscles become tender with cramping pains, deep reflexes are abolished but cranial nerve weakness is rare and sensory involvement may be slight. Over a matter of weeks or months recovery occurs and is usually complete.

Polyneuropathies

Causes
1. Infections
   a. Virus infection, e.g. rubella, mumps, glandular fever.
   b. Leprosy.
   c. Diphtheria.
   d. May follow tetanus antitoxin and other vaccines.
2. Deficiency disorders. Beri-beri.
3. Refsum disease (Heredopathia Atactica Polyneuritiformis). Autosomal recessive, rare form of hereditary ataxia caused by inability to oxidize phytanic acid, which accumulates in late childhood resulting in progressive ataxia, polyneuritis, retinitis pigmentosa, progressive nerve deafness, ichthyosis. CSF protein raised.
   Treatment. Diet low in phytanic acid (contained in all green vegetables).
4. Poisons
   a. Metals, e.g. lead, arsenic, mercury, thallium.
   b. Organic Substances, e.g. dinitrobenzol.

Lesions of Nerves Arising from Lumbar Plexus
1. Congenital Lesions. Most important are those caused by some variety of spina bifida (*see* p. 314).
2. Injury to Nerves. Sciatic nerve paralysis can follow injection into buttock, especially in newborn.

Chapter 95   # DISEASES OF THE SPINAL CORD

Spina Bifida (*Neural Tube Defect*)

The spinal cord is formed from the neural groove, lateral folds of which join dorsally to complete the neural canal. Congenital failure of fusion of the dorsal folds is associated with defective closure of the vertebral canal. The cause is unknown and is multifactorial. There is probably a genetic factor. The highest incidence is in the Welsh and Irish, often associated with anencephaly. There is a considerably increased incidence of either in subsequent pregnancies.

Prevention
Alpha-fetoprotein is a normal protein produced in fetal life which escapes into the amniotic fluid in open neural tube defects and in exomphalos this may be reflected in raised maternal blood levels. Population screening is possible at 14 weeks in some centres, using maternal alpha-fetoprotein, or ultrasound for fetal spinal examination. Raised serum alpha-fetoprotein should be followed by amniocentesis and examination of liquor, or by ultrasound. Preconceptional vitamin supplementation may reduce the incidence of neural tube malformations when given to mothers who had a previous affected child.

Spina Bifida Occulta

This is a common incidental finding on radiography of the lower lumbar vertebrae. Usually there are no symptoms although occasionally there may be a tuft of hair, area of pigmentation or naevus over the site of the defect. A sinus may track down from the skin to connect with the CNS or meninges. A dermoid cyst may be present at the bottom of the track. Very rarely a projection from the vertebra pierces the spinal cord resulting in neurological lesions of the lower limbs (diastematomyelia). If the nerves are tethered (myelodysplasia) this may produce a neurological deformity, such as dwarfing, coldness or blueness of the leg or foot.

Meningomyelocele and Meningocele

A meningomyelocele is a sac which protrudes from the spine at the lumbosacral region (much less comonly at the thoracic or cervical region). The sac is partly covered by skin which may be defective in parts. It contains the opened spinal cord and nerve fibres are attached to the sac wall. The sac can be transilluminated.

A meningocele, which is considerably less common, contains CSF only. The prognosis is better, but differentiation from meningomyelocele may not be possible except at operation.

In meningomyelocele the nerves passing through the sac are damaged causing:

1. Motor, sensory and autonomic disorders in lower trunk, lower limbs, bladder and anus. Sometimes there is an area below the lesion where the cord functions reflexly leading to signs of upper motor neurone lesions with spasticity. In 5% of cases only half the cord is involved causing one leg to be paralysed and other normal—usually with severe kyphosis.

2. Muscle weakness and imbalance cause deformities of the feet—calcaneovarus, dislocated hips and genu recurvatum, knee and hip flexion.

3. Sensory loss below the lesion causes anaesthesia, poor circulation to the legs, pressure sores and ulcerated feet.

4. Bladder function.

> 4.1 Lesions involving S2–S4 (calf, foot and anus weak) are associated with a weak or paralysed bladder, with dribbling incontinence (about 80% dribble), distended bladder (about 20% retention with overflow), and vesico-ureteric reflux.
>
> 4.2 Lesions where S2–S4 show reflex activity (e.g. spastic calf and toe flexors, exaggerated anal reflex), reflex bladder occurs but co-ordination of detrusor and external sphincter is poor causing incomplete emptying and trabeculated bladder. Progresses to ureteric reflux and hydronephrosis. This in turn is followed by urine infection, pyelonephritis and uraemia.

5. The bowel function is often impaired. Motility, rectal sensation and anal function are poor or absent. The natal cleft disappears and the anus is patulous. It should be tested with a pin for the presence or absence of sensation. Prolapse of the rectum and vagina may occur due to weak pelvic floor muscles. Chronic constipation and soiling common.

Associated Deformities

1. Hydrocephalus (*see also* p. 316)
This is associated with meningomyelocele in 90% cases, although head circumference is usually not above 97th centile at birth. The hydrocephalus is

present from birth although it may not be recognizable clinically during first few weeks of life.

2. Arnold–Chiari Malformation

This consists of a prolongation of the tonsils of the hypoplastic cerebellum and elongation and kinking of the medulla through the foramen magnum. As a result the upper cervical nerve roots run upwards instead of downwards. The malformation probably occurs in all cases of meningomyelocele and some cases of meningocele.

It is the usual cause of the hydrocephalus since CSF can pass down through the 4th ventricle to the spinal cord but cannot pass back through the foramen magnum to be absorbed over the vault.

Other abnormalities may occur, such as skull lacunae, syringomyelia and non-CNS lesions, such as abnormal ribs or kidneys, or congenital heart disease.

Progress and Complications of Meningomyelocele (*Table* 95.1)

Early rupture of the sac may occur, and whether it does or not, meningeal infection is very common especially with *E. coli, B. proteus* or *Ps. pyocyanea.* Cerebral damage then results from ventriculitis or hydrocephalus. This causes cerebral palsy—hemiplegia, diplegia, mental retardation and optic atrophy.

Table 95.1.   Complications of meningomyelocele

Neurophysiological complications		Musculoskeletal complications	
Hydrocephalus	90%	Scoliosis	50%
Internal strabismus	25%	Lordosis	20%
Laryngeal stridor	25%	Dislocated hips	40%
Urinary tract abnormalities	25%	Joint contractures	90%
Cryptorchidism	25%	Hypoplasia of lower limbs	100%
Anal tone diminished	75%	Pathological fractures — legs	25%

Management

Early surgical closure of skin defect reduces the incidence of CNS infection and increases chance of survival but doubts arise as to whether this is a good service to every child and family. Before any operation is performed to close the sac, careful examination is required to evaluate the following:

1. The head circumference should be measured and the tension and size of the fontanelle assessed. Ultrasound examination is performed to assess whether hydrocephalus is already present. Serial head circumference and ultrasound measurements will be required to determine the progress.

2. Sensation in trunk and legs, using pin or paper clip.

3. Posture and spontaneous movements of legs. Extent and power of trunk and leg movements after stimulation. Elicit and outline paralysis, hypotonia and spasticity.

4. Exaggerated reflex activity.

5. Test knee, cremasteric and anal reflexes.

6. Other congenital malformations.

7. Child's general condition.

8. Environmental background.

It is recognized that the prognosis is poor if the following criteria are not met:
1. The lesion should be capable of closure without extensive flaps.
2. Spontaneous knee flexion and extension should be possible, e.g. the neurological lesion is below L3, L4.
3. No significant hydrocephalus present at birth, i.e. head circumference 2 cm above the 90th centile for age merits exclusion from operative treatment.
4. No kyphoscoliosis.
5. No severe associated anomalies of the heart or gut.

Policy for management requires full discussion and agreement between parents and all professionals.

Closure of the lesion is usually followed by the need for ventriculo-atrial, or ventricular peritoneal shunt to control postoperative hydrocephalus.

Postoperative Management

The child will need frequent assessment by the many specialists who constitute the spina bifida team. Skilled counselling for parents and constant support for child imperative.

Parents should be told the risks of recurrence in subsequent pregnancies. Antenatal monitoring (*see* p. 313).

Late Management

The child may require: revision of valve, sometimes frequently; urinary diversion procedures, orthopaedic procedures, etc.

Cases not suitable for primary surgery should be kept under constant review. If hydrocephalus develops in the absence of infection a shunt may be necessary.

Chapter 96   **HYDROCEPHALUS**

Normal Physiology of Cerebrospinal Fluid Circulation

Fluid is formed by choroid plexus mainly in lateral ventricles; it passes through interventricular foramina (foramina of Monro) into 3rd ventricle; through cerebral aqueduct (aqueduct of Sylvius) into 4th ventricle; from there, by way of foramina in roof of 4th ventricle (foramina of Luschka and Magendie), it passes into cerebral and spinal subarachnoid space.

Absorption

CSF reabsorbed into bloodstream by arachnoid villi which project into venous sinuses. (Pacchionian bodies not present in children.)

Pathogenesis of Hydrocephalus

Types:

1. Non-communicating

(Obstructive or internal hydrocephalus). CSF accumulates in ventricles because of obstruction within ventricles or at outlets. Ventricles dilate.

2. Communicating

(External hydrocephalus). CSF free to escape from ventricles. Block is either peripheral or due to impaired absorption.

3. Overproduction of CSF by choroid plexus papilloma (rare).

Causes of Hydrocephalus

1. Non-communicating (Obstructive)

1.1 Aqueduct obstruction may be caused by:

1.1.1 Congenital aqueduct stenosis or replacement by several small channels—'forking'. May occur alone or with spina bifida.

1.1.2 Haemorrhage or inflammation may block the aqueduct or it may be compressed by a posterior fossa lesion, e.g. subdural haematoma.

1.2 Tumour displacing CSF pathways. Colloid cyst of 3rd ventricle may arise near the foramen of Monro and block it intermittently like a 'ball-cock'.

1.3 Block to outlet of 4th ventricle: causes ventricle to dilate into a large cyst.

1.3.1 Congenital—the Dandy–Walker malformation.

1.3.2 Postnatal—caused by infection or haemorrhage.

2. Communicating Hydrocephalus

2.1 Postinfective obliteration of subarachnoid spaces by fibrous reaction. May follow bacterial meningitis, especially *E. coli*, pneumococcus, or tuberculosis. Also toxoplasmosis, cytomegalovirus and posthaemorrhagic.

2.2 Blockage in storage diseases, e.g. mucopolysaccharidosis and histiocytosis X.

2.3 With skull bone lesions, e.g. underdevelopment of posterior fossa in achondroplasia or platybasia.

2.4 Intracranial venous sinus thrombosis.

2.5 Vitamin A intoxication.

2.6 Arnold–Chiari malformation (*see under* Spina bifida, p. 315).

Clinical Features

Hydrocephalus should be anticipated in any child who has meningomyelocele; any vascular accident, especially subdural haematoma; cerebral tumour; toxoplasmosis; meningitis or brain abscess.

Whenever hydrocephalus is expected, head circumference should be measured every 2 weeks and plotted on a chart for comparison with average figures.

On examination the head looks large in comparison with the rest of the body. Brow is often prominent, except in Dandy–Walker lesion, when occiput is big. The fontanelle is fuller and bigger than normal. The sutures are splayed open, scalp veins dilated. The eyes are deviated downwards. Whites of eyes may be visible above cornea—so-called 'setting sun' sign. A cracked-pot note is sometimes elicited on percussion of skull. Optic atrophy may occur if the sutures are fused. The skull may transilluminate.

Associated Features

1. Signs of Raised Intracranial Pressure (see p. 341).
These are surprisingly few in infants as the skull is not a rigid box and widening of the sutures allow the brain to expand.

2. Pressure on Cranial Nerves
   II. Optic atrophy common, with or without papilloedema. Blindness often progressive.
   II, IV, VI. Squint common. May be nystagmus.
   Paralysis of other cranial nerves can occur.

3. Limbs
Spasticity, weakness, incoordination especially in legs. Little loss of sensation.

4. Mental State
Varies with degree of severity. Mentality often surprisingly good even in cases with very little cerebral cortex remaining. Forty per cent have IQ below 70 and majority below 90.

5. Occasional hypothalamic features, e.g. obesity, hypogonadism, premature puberty or diabetes insipidus.

Management
The diagnosis and often the cause of the hydrocephalus can be determined by a CAT scan. A Holter or Pudenz valve is often required.
   Complications of valve include: ventriculitis, *Staphylococcus albus* colonization of valve and septicaemia, acute and chronic obstruction of the valve, pulmonary embolization and superior vena caval obstruction.
   Revision of valve: replacement, change to opposite side, use of other types of valve, e.g. Pudenz, often required.

Chapter 97   *CEREBRAL PALSY*

Cerebral palsy occurs in 2·5 per 1000 of population. The term is given to any non-progressive brain lesion, manifested by disturbance of motor function. Following features may be more or less prominent: spasticity, athetoid movements, ataxia, tremor, rigidity, mental deficiency and epilepsy.
   The terminology is confused. Terms such as diplegia, quadriplegia, tetraplegia and double hemiplegia are used to describe the same condition by different authors. Word di (from Greek) means two or twice, tetra (from Greek) and quad (from Latin) mean four, plegia (from Greek) means a stroke; hemi (from Greek) means one-half. Para (from Greek) means near, or alongside of, and consequently can mean a hemiplegia but commonly is used to describe involvement of both legs and lower trunk.

Classification

Clinical
1. Diplegia or tetraplegia. The limbs are usually spastic but may be hypotonic.
2. Dyskinesia. Types: athetoid: choreoid; dystonic; tension; tremor.
3. Ataxia, simple or diplegic.
4. Hemiplegia, single or bilateral.
5. Mixed varieties.

Aetiological
Prenatal causes are rare. Spastic paraplegia and athetosis may be inherited. Different children in same family may have similar or different types of cerebral palsy.
Perinatal causes. Hypoxia is probably of aetiological importance but the exact role is difficult to determine. The following are noted more frequently in children with cerebral palsy than in normal children: history of prematurity (high incidence with paraplegia and quadriplegia, low incidence with hemiplegia), multiple pregnancies, maternal haemorrhage. Cerebral haemorrhage, especially intraventricular in preterm babies.
Postnatal causes. Infection, trauma, drugs or venous thrombosis.

Diplegia (*Spastic Cerebral Palsy; Little's Disease*)

'Spastic' is the commonest variety of cerebral palsy affecting the limbs symmetrically, the lower more than the upper. Bulbar palsy, fits, squints and mental retardation often occur. In 60% of cases there is a history of abnormal birth or prematurity.

History
The disorder takes some time to develop. The diagnosis is often made at routine follow-up clinic, either of an expectedly normal child, or one known to be at risk, e.g. pre-term. The baby may appear lethargic or irritable, or present because of delay in passing the normal milestones.

Significance of developmental delay—delay in motor development *alone* indicates motor disability, but with normal intelligence. Delay in non-motor development indicates mental deficiency. In severe mental deficiency without cerebral palsy all development is delayed.

Clinical Features
The signs and symptoms given here refer to spastic quadriplegia. In paraplegia and hemiplegia similar features are found in the affected limbs only.

On examination of the young child, the limbs are hypotonic in the early stages. Later there is poor head control and spasticity of varying degree. Held upright there is scissoring of the legs which are held stiff. When the baby is brought to the sitting position, there is spasm of the hamstrings and adductor spasm. Placed supine the infant may lie with an extended back. The knee jerks are brisk, and may even be obtained by tapping the dorsum of the foot. Sustained ankle clonus is often present. The primitive reflexes (Moro, grasp and tonic neck reflex) may persist (they normally disappear around 12 weeks). The hands should be loosely open; if tightly closed suspect spasticity. If an older baby with spastic upper limbs is offered an object he will take it with a characteristic grasp; the hand approaches the object slowly, flexed at the wrist, with excessive pronation and the fingers are splayed and bent before closing on the subject.

In older children the legs are held rigid, feet in plantar flexion, knees extended, hips adducted. Child walks with 'scissors' gait, due to spasm of adductors, and on toes, due to spasm of calf muscles. Muscle stretch reflex present (i.e. if muscle put on a stretch it contracts). Plantar reflexes extensor (only of value over 2 years old). Abdominal reflexes present if spasticity dates from birth. Arms held flexed. Tendon reflexes brisk. Dysarthria and drooling common in severe cases.

Hemiplegia

May be unilateral or bilateral. It accounts for 30% of cerebral pasly. Twice as common in boys—about half congenital, half acquired in early life, e.g. birth injury; may be preterm or large for dates. Arm always more affected than leg.

Clinical Features
There is poverty of movement of affected side, including face, limbs initially hypotonic, later spastic and reflexes increase. Can be recognized in newborn period by different intensity of movement on two sides, diminished movement and neonatal reflexes on affected side. Arm may be held at side, fist clenched over thumb.

Associated problems include:

1. Cortical sensory loss with absence of sense of position, two-point discrimination and homonymous hemianopia. Child may ignore affected side when sensory loss marked.

2. Vasomotor tone is poor and chilblains may develop in cold weather. Limb growth poor.

3. Convulsions occur in half the affected children.

Bilateral Hemiplegia
This is a term used when all four limbs are affected by paresis and spasticity (upper more than lower). Bulbar palsy also present, with early feeding problems and later speech difficulties. Epilepsy and mental retardation common. Often due to malformation of brain. Malformations may also occur elsewhere.

Acute Infantile Hemiplegia
Uncommon condition occurring in previously healthy baby, manifested by convulsion which may last for several hours and result in hemiplegia. Usually followed by further fits and mental retardation. Onset may be preceded by fever and vomiting.

The cause of the condition is unknown—thrombosis, dehydration, trauma or encephalopathy, after infectious disease or immunization have been suggested. May also follow hypoglycaemia or hypernatraemia.

Ataxic Cerebral Palsy

May present as a floppy baby with hypotonia, weakness, diminished movements and tendon reflexes. In ataxic diplegia, spasticity and increased jerks appear in the legs plus or minus the arms. Later children show delayed milestones. When walking may hold out arms to aid balance; gait wide-based. Examination shows weakness of voluntary movements, hypotonia, intention tremor, tendon reflexes depressed or sometimes increased; absence of nystagmus and Romberg's sign.

Dyskinesia

Initial hypotonia is followed by impaired voluntary movement due to unwanted involuntary movements and changes in tone. This occurs in all limbs, trunk and bulbar musculature. Speech is often badly affected.

Types

Athetosis
Slow, writhing movements of distal parts of limbs accompany voluntary movements. Less common now that haemolytic disease of the newborn can be adequately treated or prevented. May also be caused by neonatal hypoxia.

Dystonic Movements
Slow, involuntary movements of trunk and proximal part of limbs. Very rare, a genetic disorder.

Tremor
Rare, regular, alternating movements, tend to be rapid and rhythmic.

Complications of Cerebral Palsy

Frequent and cause severe disablement.

1. Mental Retardation
Occurs frequently. IQ often below 50. The more severe the motor defect, the lower the intelligence. Children with added fits have low intelligence. Often very difficult to assess intelligence of severely affected child, especially if two handicaps present, e.g. spasticity and deafness. Most intelligence tests demand either mechanical dexterity (e.g. building tower of bricks) or educational knowledge (e.g. naming picture). Former may not be possible because of spasticity and latter because of deafness, yet mentality normal.

2. Convulsions
Almost one-third of children with cerebral palsy have fits. Most common in quadriplegia and hemiplegia (50%). Attacks usually grand mal but 'salaam' spasms occur in infants.

3. Dislocation of Hips
Common in severely affected quadriplegics and paraplegics.

4. Sensory Loss
Almost one-half children with hemiplegia have sensory loss. Mainly astereognosis and decreased two-point discrimination. Visuospatial disorders occur. Sensory loss bears little relationship to severity of hemiplegia.

5. Hearing Loss
Hearing loss is common in athetosis but not in spastic children.

6. Visual Impairment
Squints, especially in quadriplegics and children pre-term, refractive errors and partial blindness common.

7. Speech Difficulties
Occur in 50%. Due to: dysarthria, mental retardation, hearing loss, cortical aphasia, emotional upset, possibly laterality in hemiplegic children (*see below*).

8. Laterality
If the child's normally dominant side is affected by late-onset hemiplegia, may have difficulty in changing speech centre to other side.

9. Incontinence
Due mainly to associated mental retardation and difficulty in training.

10. Drooling
From bulbar involvement. Common in severely affected children.

11. Behaviour Disorders
Antisocial, distractable, poor attention span. More important as child grows older.

Management

In any child with cerebral palsy there should be a full assessment of all skills and disabilities, social and educational factors. Important to assess vision, hearing and intelligence early. Team work by paediatrician, physiotherapist, occupational therapist, speech therapist, play therapist and social worker are important from the start. Parents must be fully acquainted with the results of the assessment and given advice as to their role in encouraging child to reach his full potential. Drugs rarely used (apart from control of epilepsy) but occasionally Diazepam of value. Baclofen may help spasticity. Orthopaedic surgeon's help needed for tendon elongations and treatment of dislocated hips.

Chapter 98   *EPILEPSY AND CONVULSIONS*

For International nomenclature, *see* Appendix 7, p. 518.

Convulsions, seizures and fits are synonymous terms and are often used interchangably although by common usage term 'convulsions' is applied to fits in infants. Epilepsy is the condition of recurrent convulsions. The word should be used with restraint in paediatrics because of its emotional overtones. It tends (quite wrongly) to conjure up vision of long-term physical, mental and social disability.

Convulsions are common, the cause may or may not be known in a particular case. Characterized physiologically by paroxysmal cerebral dysrhythmia and clinically by varying combinations of involuntary generalized or focal muscular movements, stereotyped sensory stimuli, behavioural change, loss of consciousness.

Status epilepticus is the term used for a single fit lasting more than 30 min, or a series of fits with failure to gain consciousness between attacks.

The incidence of convulsions is 6–7 % of all children under age of 5 years. Over 50 % of all fits in children occur in age group 6 months to 3 years.

Family History in Children with Convulsions

History of fits is often obtained from other members of family. Negative history may be inaccurate as parents may not know that they had fits in infancy. Electro-encephalogram performed on apparently normal relations of epileptics, often found to be abnormal. *Theory*: The predisposition to respond to certain stimuli by convulsions can be inherited. But the threshold above which stimulus produces fit varies from person to person. In particular individual, stimulus may never be strong enough throughout life to precipitate fit.

Clinical Classification

A. Clinical Manifestation Closely Related to Cerebral Maturity

Neonatal convulsions, myoclonic seizures, convulsions with fever and petit mal.

B. Convulsions not Necessarily Related to Cerebral Maturity

Major attacks, grand mal, akinetic fits, focal attacks, motor, sensory, psychomotor (temporal lobe), and Jacksonian.

Convulsions with Manifestations Related to Maturity

Neonatal Convulsions

Generalized tonic/clonic attacks rarely occur in infancy. Seizures in an infant are manifested by clonus, apnoeic spells, or cyanotic attacks. Sometimes rhythmic sucking, eye blinking, eyes rolling up or brief nystagmoid jerks occur. At the age 0–3 days the cause is usually structural brain damage, e.g. congenital malformations, or perinatal trauma. It may also be metabolic, e.g. hypoglycaemia, hypoxia, or vitamin B_6 dependency.

At the age 4–10 days metabolic disorders such as hypocalcaemia with hyperphosphataemia (especially in babies fed with full cream cow's milk), hypomagnesaemia, and electrolyte disturbances occur.

Throughout the neonatal period and early infancy causes are:

1. Infection, e.g. bacterial meningitis (especially gram-negative bacilli) with or without septicaemia, encephalitis (especially herpes simplex).

2. Inborn errors of metabolism e.g. hypoglycaemia, from leucine sensitivity, galactosaemia: pyridoxine dependency, phenylketonuria, hyperammonaemia.

3. Withdrawal symptoms. Mother addicted to heroin, morphine, barbiturates, alcohol.

EEG Findings

Normal records in the neonatal period are closely related to gestational age, and state of alertness. Abnormalities are not specific of any particular type of epilepsy.

Prognosis
That of underlying condition. Poor if fits occur in full-term baby in first 2–3 days, good for hypoglycaemic or hypocalcaemic fits occurring towards end of first week. Overall incidence for subsequent fits in next year—12%.

Myoclonic Seizures
These are manifested by sudden flexion of head and trunk with extension of arms forwards and thigh flexion, or sudden extension of head and trunk with abduction and extension of the arms. Usually associated with gross generalized cerebral disorder.

Types

1. Infantile Spasms (Hypsarrhythmia*)
Age at onset 3–12 months. The cause is often unknown, but it may be associated with congenital or perinatal brain damage of any sort, pertussis immunization, metabolic abnormalities, e.g. phenylketonuria, or tuberous sclerosis (with leaf-shaped areas of skin depigmentation).
EEG findings. Gross generalized disturbance with high-voltage slow waves and scattered spikes—so-called 'hypsarrhythmia'.
Prognosis. Poor. Spasms become less frequent with age but later onset of grand mal usual; 77% children with hypsarrhythmic EEG pattern are later mentally retarded. Normality more likely in cryptogenic and post-immunization groups.
Treatment. Is that of the underlying metabolic disorder if present. Seizure control is often difficult and has little effect on the long-term intelligence. Corticotrophin or steroids often helpful in reducing number of fits and aiding recovery.

2. Myoclonic Epilepsy in Childhood
Age at onset 18 months–4 years. Aetiology: Usually unknown. Can be associated with progressive cerebral degeneration of infective or metabolic origin.
Prognosis. Control of fits difficult. Myoclonic attacks tend to regress and grand mal fits may appear. Intelligence likely to be high-grade defective.

Convulsions with Fever
May be tonic or tonic/clonic. Often start focally and become generalized. Three per cent of all children are said to have convulsions with fever, commoner in males then females. Age of onset 6 months–3 years.

Predisposing Factors
1. Family history is positive for convulsive disorders in up to 60%. Dominant inheritance with incomplete expression.
2. Increased incidence of prenatal and perinatal abnormalities.
3. Preceding developmental histories suggest incidence of minor neurological deficits is high, but gross neurological disorder uncommon.

---

*Term 'hypsarrhythmia' should refer to EEG pattern only. However, by common usage the condition of infantile spasms often (wrongly) called hypsarrhythmia.

Precipitating Factors
Tend to occur in first 24 h of feverish illness or during rapid rise of temperature. Upper respiratory tract infection commonest clinical diagnosis with viral rather than bacterial aetiology.

Management
1. Convulsion should be controlled in the shortest possible time.
2. Investigate cause of fever, especially exclude bacterial meningitis by doing lumbar puncture.
3. Examine carefully for signs suggestive of symptomatic grand mal (*see* p. 326) and investigate accordingly.

Prognosis
Recurrence of convulsions with subsequent febrile illness. Overall risk 40–50%. Significantly increased risk if age at onset less than 19 months, family history positive for any convulsive disorder, neurological abnormality (however trivial) persists, initial convulsion has unilateral features, lasts more than 30 min or is repeated within same illness.
Later convulsions when afebrile
1. Grand mal. Overall risk 10–20%. The question the parents really want answered is, 'Will my child be an epileptic in later life?' This is improbable if the age of the child at the time of the first fit was over 9 months and under 3 years, there were no preceding or subsequent CNS abnormalities, the fit lasted less than 15 min and was generalized throughout, there is a family history of infantile febrile fits, but not of adult epilepsy, and the EEG is normal 2 weeks after the seizure. These are the criteria of true febrile convulsions.
2. Psychomotor fits (*see* p. 327). Overall risk 6%. Significantly follow prolonged unilateral convulsions.

Intelligence
Incidence of mental retardation 9%. Most of these probably subnormal before first convulsion, but prolonged fits in first year significantly related to reduced IQ. Uneven scoring on subtests common in those with full-scale IQ within average range.

Prophylaxis
Antipyretics and tepid sponging at onset of fever, and continuous anticonvulsants are indicated in cases with a significant risk of recurrence and after the second fit in all cases.

Petit Mal
In this condition there is a sudden momentary loss of consciousness without movement or loss or posture. The child is able to continue with his preceding activity immediately after the attack. Age of onset 3–10 years.
EEG findings are diagnostic. Normal background activity with sudden onset of synchronous 3 cycles/sec spikes and waves.

Prognosis
Usually good. Attacks rarely persist beyond puberty. Sometimes associated with

grand mal when prognosis for persisting epilepsy less good. Intelligence usually within average range, but very frequent attacks interfere with concentration and acquisition of knowledge.

Convulsions not Necessarily Related to Cerebral Maturity

Major Attacks (*Grand Mal Epilepsy*)
The appearance of the fits varies with age. In older children they resemble typical adult epilepsy with tonic and clonic phases. Under the age of 1 year the sequence of events tends to be less obvious with transient unconsciousness and some jerky movements. The aetiology of the attacks may be known (symptomatic seizures) or unknown (idiopathic or cryptogenic epilepsy), but in practice the distinction is seldom clear-cut as further investigations may reveal an unsuspected cause.

Idiopathic Epilepsy
No apparent cause found. There may be a positive family history of epilepsy. Intelligence is usually normal. EEG may or may not be completely normal between fits.

Prognosis is good if the fits can be controlled. The child may have only one or two fits in a lifetime.

Symptomatic Seizures
Here the fit is often an unpleasant incident in the life of a damaged child. They may be frequent in number, bordering on status epilepticus, or only occasional. Some causes of symptomatic seizures are:

1. Structural Cerebral Disorder
   1.1 Congenital malformation of brain, e.g. agenesis, cysts, hydrocephalus.
   1.2 Following trauma of any kind.
   1.3 Acute infections, e.g. meningitis, encephalitis.
   1.4 Acquired space-occupying lesions, e.g. tumour, abscess, haematoma, haemangioma.
   1.5 Circulatory or vascular changes, e.g. thrombosis, embolus, haemorrhage.
   1.6 Chronic or previous infections, e.g. toxoplasmosis, cytomegalovirus, toxocariasis, cysticercosis, measles (leading to subacute sclerosing panencephalitis).
2. Metabolic
   2.1 Temporary, e.g. hypoglycaemia, hyponatraemia, hypernatraemia, hypoxia, uraemia, hypocalcaemia, hypomagnesaemia, pyridoxine deficiency.
   2.2 Inborn errors of metabolism, e.g. hypoglycaemia, galactosaemia, phenylketonuria, hyperglycinaemia, hyperammonaemia, pyridoxine dependency.
   2.3 Degenerative brain disorder (*see* p. 329).
3. Others
   3.1 Hypertensive encephalopathy.
   3.2 Poisons: lead, analeptics.

3.3 Attacks precipitated by flashing lights, e.g. in discotheques, etc.; music or noise; a tap on the head; breath-holding etc.

Focal Attacks

Focal motor attacks are not such good indicators of localized cerebral disorder in children as in adults. Only part of the body is involved in the tonic or clonic movements. Adult-type Jacksonian fits are rare in childhood. Aetiology, management and prognosis are as for grand mal with structural cerebral disorder. The cause is not always identifiable.

Psychomotor (Temporal Lobe) Epilepsy

This condition accounts for up to 25% of the epilepsies of childhood. It is often associated with other types of fits, especially grand mal. In the attack there are behavioural or sensory disturbances, e.g. automatisms, lip smacking, repeated swallowing, olfactory, visual or auditory hallucinations. The attack is frequently preceded by an aura. Classically, the child complains of an unpleasant sensation or taste 'coming up from the stomach' into his mouth moments before some stereotyped movement or behaviour occurs.

Aetiology is usually unknown but may be subsequent to prolonged unilateral convulsions with fever (mesial temporal sclerosis).

EEG typically shows spikes in the temporal regions, but these may not always be seen.

The prognosis depends on the presence or absence of other types of convulsions, underlying cerebral disorder and behavioural accompaniments.

Investigation of Convulsions

The diagnosis idiopathic epilepsy is made by a process of exclusion. It is important to investigate carefully any child with fits in case there is some underlying treatable lesion and in order to establish the prognosis for further fits, intelligence and extension of the underlying cause. Some pointers to underlying causes are:

1. A fit in an older child without any obvious cause (e.g. no infection) and a negative family history.

2. A child with a prejudicial birth history or any CNS abnormality.

3. A child with below-average intelligence, particularly if there is any deterioration.

4. A child who fails to thrive (this may indicate a metabolic disorder or non-accidental injury).

5. A child with an unusual skin lesion (e.g. tuberous sclerosis or café-au-lait spots).

Electro-encephalographs (EEG) in Convulsions

Basic rhythms alter with brain maturation and state of alertness.

1. Records in newborns. Most information if baby sleeping. Basic rhythms up to 36 weeks' gestation similar in eye movement and non-eye-movement sleep and consist of low-voltage activity of 2–3 Hz with episodes of high-voltage slow activity (<1 Hz) with superadded fast (10–15 Hz). From 36 to 44 weeks' gestation marked difference between records in eye movement and non-eye-movement sleep. Non-eye-movement sleep—record similar to baby of <36 weeks. Eye movement sleep—basic rhythm continuous low-voltage 3–4 Hz activity. EEG abnormalities in newborns (*see* p. 323).

2. Waking records in older infants and children. Normal basic rhythms—age 1–3 yr, 3–4 Hz; age 3–7 yr, 5–7 Hz; age 8–12 yr, 8–12 Hz.

3. Abnormalities—of importance

>3.1 Asymmetry of basic rhythm—minor degrees allowable.
>
>3.2 Episodes of slower or faster frequencies (especially slower when not hyperventilating)—can be generalized or focal.
>
>3.3 Sharp waves.
>
>3.4 Spikes.
>
>3.5 Paroxysmal spikes or spikes and waves.

Significance of abnormalities—in absence of any other signs suggesting focal brain damage, focal slow waves are of doubtful significance, but may indicate space-occupying lesion. Focal spikes often seen in middle childhood and disappear at puberty in children who never have clinical fits. Paroxysmal spikes and waves are indicative of epileptic activity but may be seen in children without clinical fits. Diagnostic records found only in petit mal and in subacute sclerosing panencephalitis.

4. Activation of potential abnormalities

>4.1 Hyperventilation. Used for 3 min. Produces reduction of frequency and increased amplitude, especially in younger children, and may produce spike and wave complexes. Particularly useful for activation of 3 Hz spike and wave seen in classic petit mal.
>
>4.2 Photic stimulation. Stroboscope with variable frequency flashes of light. Precipitates spikes or spikes and waves in susceptible subjects.
>
>4.3 Drug influence, e.g. accentuation of irregularities by chlorpromazine; failure of appearance of fast activity with barbiturates (usually damaged areas).
>
>4.4 Sleep. Abnormalities may only occur in light sleep or on awakening.

Management of Convulsion

The choice of therapy for long-term drug prophylaxis depends on the type of seizure. The lowest dose possible should be given which controls the fits adequately, but if a breakthrough fit occurs, the dosage should be increased or other drugs added until control is achieved.

Therapeutic Level of Drug in Serum

For use as guide only. Many children are fit-free at levels well below that considered therapeutic.

1. Phenobarbitone. In single or 2 equal doses. *Serum levels*: therapeutic >15 μg/ml, toxic >40 μg/ml. *Toxic effects*: hyperactivity, irritability, short attention span especially in younger children, drowsiness, confusion and ataxia, rash, rickets, megaloblastic anaemia.

2. Primidone (Mysoline). In 3 doses. *Serum levels*: therapeutic >5 μg/ml, toxic >12 μg/ml. *Toxic effects*: as for phenobarbitone, with drowsiness, ataxia

and confusion presenting much more commonly. Diluted solution for small children unstable over more than 2 weeks.

3. Phenytoin (Epanutin). In 1 or 2 doses. *Serum levels*: therapeutic >10 μg/ml. *Toxic effects*: drowsiness, confusion, ataxia, nystagmus, gum hypertrophy, rash, blood dyscrasias.

4. Carbamazepine (Tegretol). In 2–3 doses. *Serum levels*: therapeutic >4 μg/ml, toxic >8 μg/ml. *Toxic effects*: aplastic anaemia, leucopenia, dizziness, jaundice, gastrointestinal upsets.

5. Ethosuximide (Zarontin). In 2–3 doses. *Serum levels*: therapeutic >40 μg/ml, toxic >100 μg/ml. *Toxic effects*: drowsiness, dizziness, headache, ataxia, blood dyscrasias, systemic lupus erythematosus (very rare), albuminuria.

6. Sodium valproate (Epilim). Dose 2–3 doses. *Serum levels*: therapeutic 50–100 μg/ml. *Other effects*: causes rise in serum barbiturate levels if given concurrently, occasional alopecia, nausea, drowsiness, changes in appetite, behaviour disorder, hyperammonaemia, liver failure.

7. Clonazepam (Rivotril). Dose in 3 divided doses. *Toxic effects*: drowsiness, ataxia, confusion, vertigo, appetite changes.

8. Nitrazepam (Mogadon). *Starting dose*: 0·25 mg/kg body weight/day in 2 doses. *Toxic effects*: drowsiness, ataxia, confusion.

Social Implications of Convulsions

1. Parental anxiety. The parents may over-indulge, over-protect, or reject the child. They may fear the child will die in a fit. They are also afraid of the fits continuing into adult life with deleterious implications for employment, marriage, or recreation.

2. Restriction of activities should be minimal and depend on the degree of control of fits, i.e. if the control is good, no restrictions required. However, it is wise always to have an adult in the water if a child is swimming. The child should be made to feel as normal as is compatible with his disability.

3. Young children are surprisingly unaffected by other members of the school class having fits and ostracization by peers is unusual unless reinforced by adults, or behaviour disorders coexist.

Educational Implications of Convulsions

Ideally educated in school most appropriate for intellectual abilities. Poor progress for intelligence likely if: convulsions very frequent (interfering with concentration), drug regimes lead to drowsiness or behaviour disturbance, underlying brain disorder causes uneven abilities or child feels rejected by peers and emotional factors contribute.

Chapter 99   *DEGENERATIVE BRAIN DISEASES*

A wide spectrum of diseases characterized by progressive loss of motor intellectual or sensory skills. Usually autosomal recessive, occasionally dominant—enzyme defects are becoming identified in many and some diseases can be diagnosed in utero.

Table 99.1.   Central nervous system storage diseases (All autosomal recessive except where * which are X-linked)

Type	Substance	Defect	Features
1. *Lipid*			
Ganglioside storage Tay–Sachs' disease (GM$_2$ gangliosidosis, Type 1)		Hexosaminidase A	Dementia, fits, blindness, hyperacusis, cherry red spot on macula, starting in early months
Sandhoff disease (GM$_2$ gangliosidosis Type 2)		Hexosaminidase A and B	Dementia, fits, blindness, hyperacusis, cherry red spot on macula, starting in early months
Juvenile GM$_2$ gangliosidosis, Type 3		Partial absence of hexosaminidase A	Dementia, fits, ataxia, spasticity
Generalized gangliosidosis GM$_1$ gangliosidosis		β galactosidase A, B and C	Retarded psychomotor development, hepatosplenomegaly, face like Hunter's syndrome, bones involved
Juvenile GM$_1$ gangliosidosis, Type 2		β galactosidase B and C	Dementia, ataxia, spasticity
Gaucher's disease	Glucocerebroside	Glucocerebrosidase	Acute infantile form affects CNS with swallowing difficulty, cyanotic attacks, rigidity. Abnormal cells obtained from marrow. Serum acid phosphatase raised. Hepatosplenomegaly
Niemann–Pick disease	Sphingomyelin	Sphingomyelinase	Fits, blindness, quadriplegia. Failure to thrive, hepatomegaly, foamy lymphocytes. Raised serum lipids and GOT
Fabry's disease (Angiokeratoma corporis diffusa)*	Cerebroside trihexoside (may be found in urine)	Ceramide trihexosidase	Burning feet sensation, severe limb pains, macular or nodular rash. Cerebrovascular accidents and thromboses of myocardium and kidney. Lung deposits. Tend to die in middle age
Metachromatic leucodystropy	Sulphatide	Aryl sulphatase	Dementia, fits, spastic quadriplegia, bulbar palsy. Urine deposit metachromatic and white cell aryl sulphatase low
Refsum's disease	Phytanic acid	Defect in oxygenation of phytanic acid	Peripheral neuropathy, retinitis pigmentosa, ataxia, ichthyosis, serum phytanic acid and caeruloplasmin raised, CSF protein raised

Disease	Stored substance	Enzyme deficiency	Clinical features
Wolman's disease	Cholesterol triglycerides	Acid lipase	Retarded development, vomiting, diarrhoea and abdominal distension, acanthocytosis, calcified adrenals
Lipoprotein deficiency β lipoprotein deficiency			Peripheral neuropathy. Ataxia posterior column loss, retinitis pigmentosa, low cholesterol, malabsorption, acanthocytosis
α lipoprotein deficiency			Peripheral neuropathy, recurrent weak legs, ptosis, diplopia, colitis, low cholesterol
Ceroid lipofuscinosis	Lipopigments		Clinical features like Tay–Sachs' but presents over age 3 years
Fucosidosis	Fucose containing glycolipids	α-fucosidase	Progressive dementia and quadriplegia, cardiomegaly, myocarditis, thickened skin, high sweat sodium
2. Carbohydrates			
Glycogenosis Type I (von Gierke)	Glycogen	Glucose-6-phosphatase	Hypotonia, fits, mental retardation, recurrent hypoglycaemia, xanthomata occasionally
Glycogenosis Type II (Pompe)	Glycogen	Acid maltase	Floppy infant, mental retardation, big tongue, big heart, may look hypothyroid. Poor outlook
Type III (limit dextrinosis)	Abnormal glycogen	Amylo 1,6-glycosidase	Floppy, myopathy, recurrent infections, failure to thrive
Type V (McArdle)	Glycogen	Muscle phosphorylase, phosphofructokinase, phosphoglucomutase	Muscle pains on exercise, odd gait, occasional myoglobinuria, dyspnoea, absence of rise in venous lactate on exercise
Mannose storage	Mannose glucosamine		Floppy, psychomotor retardation, hepatosplenomegaly, face like Hurler's syndrome, lens opacities, acidosis, hypogammaglobulinaemia
3. Protein			
Amyloidosis	Polypeptide. Hexosamine and sialic acid		Occasionally occurs in childhood. Can present with peripheral neuropathy and systemic features of nephrotic syndrome
4. Metals			
Wilson's disease	Copper		Involuntary movements, emotional lability, rigidity, dysarthria, dysphagia. KF ring, amino-aciduria, low caeruloplasmin

Type	Substance	Defect	Features
Juvenile haemochromatosis	Iron		Presents with diabetes or liver failure, suntanned skin, **raised serum iron**
Hallervorden–Spatz syndrome	Iron		Athetosis, rigidity, dementia, onset late childhood
Fohr's disease	Calcium		Hypoparathyroidism with symptoms from calcification of basal ganglia and hypocalcaemia—cataracts, monilia, etc.
4. Mucopolysaccharidoses affecting brain			
Type I (Hurler)	Dermatan sulphate, Heparan sulphate	β-galactosidase	Mental deficiency, characteristic face, hepatosplenomegaly, cloudy cornea, bone changes
Type II (Hunter)*	Dermatan sulphate, Heparan sulphate	β-galactosidase	Coarse features, limited extension of joints, deaf, dwarf, hepatosplenomegaly, bone changes
Type III (Sanfilippo)	Heparan sulphate		Severe mental retardation, deaf, joint deformity, retinitis pigmentosa
Type V (Scheie)	Dermatan sulphate		Mental retardation, retinitis pigmentosa, hand deformities
Lafora body (progressive myoclonic encephalopathy)	Mucopolysaccharides		Progressive dementia, myoclonic fits and abnormal eye movements; occurring late childhood

Classification
1. Degeneration of Cerebral White Matter

Usually present with abnormalities of motor function, spasticity or hypotonia sometimes with ataxia.

1.1 Leucodystrophies
Metachromatic leucodystrophy.
Krabbe's disease.
Pelizaeus—Merzbacher disease.
Canavan's disease.
Dawson's encephalitis.
1.2 Demyelinating diseases
Schilder's disease.
Multiple sclerosis.
Neuromyelitis optica.

2. Degenerations of Cerebral Grey Matter
Often present with fits and loss of intellectual function.

2.1 Neuronal storage diseases
2.1.1 Gangliosides.
2.1.2 Other sphingolipids.
2.1.3 Other substance, e.g. glycogen.
2.2 Degenerations without neuronal storage
Alper's, Leigh's, Menkes' diseases, subacute sclerosing panencephalitis.

3. System Diseases

3.1 Spinocerebellar degenerations
Ataxia-telangiectasia.
A-beta-lipoproteinaemia.
Refsum's disease.
3.2 Basal ganglia degenerations
Wilson's disease.
Torsion spasms.
Huntington's chorea.

Chapter 100

DISORDERS OF MYELINATION OF CENTRAL NERVOUS SYSTEM

---

*Metachromatic Leucodystrophy**
(Greenfield's Disease)

Rare autosomal recessive condition with accumulation in various organs of lipid metachromatic substances (sulphatides) due to absence of enzyme, aryl sulphatase.

*Metachromatic leucodystrophy. A review of 38 cases. MacFaal R., Cavanagh N., Lake B.D. et al. (1982) *Arch. Dis. Childh.* **57**, 168–75.

Clinical Features

Symptoms start at age of about 1–2 years:

Stage I. Hypotonia; unsteady gait; power of walking lost.

Stage II. Spasticity, hyper-reflexia and extensor plantar responses. Later flaccid weakness, atrophy distal muscles when peripheral nerves involved.

Stage III. Ataxia, dysarthria, nystagmus, optic atrophy, mental regression, fits and non-functioning gallbladder (because of sulphatide in wall).

Terminally: variable rigidity; bulbar palsy; decerebrate rigidity.

Investigations

   1. Urine shows metachromatic granules. Chromatography: sulphatides.

   2. CSF: Protein high; cells normal.

   3. Cholecystography: non-functioning gallbladder.

   4. Biopsy may show metachromatic substance. This can be found in pulp of a tooth, rectal mucosa.

   5. Nerve conduction velocity decreased.

Other members of group of neurolipidoses are:

   Niemann–Pick disease—sphingomyelin.

   Gaucher's disease—cerebroside.

   Tay–Sachs' disease—ganglioside.

Krabbe's Disease
(Globoid-cell Leucodystrophy)

Very rare fatal form of leucodystrophy. Manifested in first 4 months of life with failure to thrive, fretfulness, apathy, dysphagia, spasticity, fits, and blindness.

Canavan's Disease
(Spongy Degeneration of White Matter)

Autosomal recessive. Commoner in Jews. Develops in early infancy, poor head control, optic atrophy, rigidity and hyper-reflexia. Head becomes enlarged. Death before sixth birthday.

Subacute Sclerosing Panencephalitis (SSPE)
(Dawson's Encephalitis)

Very rare condition occurring between ages 2 and 20 years. Maximal incidence 8–14 years. Clinical Course. Slowly progressive. Progressive intellectual failure, personality changes, emotional lability. Later, regularly recurring myoclonic jerks of increasing amplitude appear, later still child becomes demented, bedridden and has major fits and spasticity. Has akinetic mutism and echo-phenomenon.

Investigations

   1. CSF. Gammaglobulin raised, measles titre raised and first zone colloidal gold curve present.

   2. Blood measles titre very high.

   3. Measles virus may be cultured from brain biopsy.

4. EEG usually relatively flat with periodic bursts simultaneous with myoclonic jerks.

Treatment
Not effective. Antiviral agents and interferon tried unsuccessfully. Relationship to measles immunization not established.

Chapter 101   *THE ATAXIAS*

Friedreich's Ataxia

Inherited as Mendelian dominant or recessive. Sporadic cases also occur. Age of onset of neurological symptoms 5–15 years. Pes cavus may occur earlier.

Clinical Features
1. Ataxia. First symptom, especially lower limbs. Occurs at age of about 5 years and may be history that child was slow in starting to walk. Later ataxia of upper limbs, head and trunk occurs with nystagmus, dysarthria and grimacing. Choreic movements may occur. Nystagmus present.
2. Weakness. Upper motor neurone lesion modified by associated sensory loss. Thus: ankle- and knee-jerks absent due to loss of deep sensation breaking reflex arc. Plantar responses always extensor in established cases.
3. Loss of proprioceptive and joint sense. Due to posterior column degeneration.
Associated lesions
   1. *Pes cavus and kyphoscoliosis.* Almost invariable. Due either to weakness of muscles from nervous lesion or to congenital bony abnormality.
   2. *Optic atrophy.* Uncommon. Retinitis pigmentosa very rare.
   3. *Mentality.* Child often facile and progressive loss of intellect.
   4. *Cardiac enlargement.* Rare. May lead to heart failure.

Ataxia-telangiectasia (*Louis–Bar syndrome*)

Very rare autosomal recessive disease manifested clinically by:
1. Ataxia. Cerebellar in type. Later in the disease athetoid movements, nystagmus, inability to fix eyes on object voluntarily and dysarthria develop. Tendon reflexes absent.
2. Telangiectasia. On bulbar conjunctivae and cheeks.
3. Infections. Especially of ears and chest, associated with absence of IgA and IgE and reduced T- and B-cell function. Alpha-fetoprotein raised.
4. Progressive mental deterioration.

Chapter 102   *MENINGITIS*

Meningitis is a very important disease in childhood. Diagnosed early and treated correctly the child will probably be cured with no sequelae. Poor treatment will result in death or a mentally retarded child with neurological impairment and often deafness.

Clinical Features

The meningeal involvement is usually preceded by 1–7 days of mild respiratory infection, and malaise with persisting fever. Instead of recovering as expected, the fever increases with vomiting and increasing lethargy and loss of consciousness. Often a fit ushers in the acute meningeal phase of the disease. Dehydration occurs rapidly.

Findings on examination will depend on the age of the child, the acuteness of onset and the type of organism.

Under about 1 year of age: bulging of the fontanelle, separation of the sutures and a cracked-pot sign on percussion of the skull are valuable signs. It may be difficult to be certain of neck stiffness under the age of six months, but this sign becomes increasingly valuable thereafter. The tendon reflexes becomes brisk and ankle clonus may occur. Later other neurological signs such as a squint and hemiplegia may develop. Other evidence of meningeal irritation such as Kernig and Brudzinski's signs, are of little value in young children. Any of the following organisms may cause meningitis:

Meningococcus, *Haemophilus influenzae*, pneumococcus, streptococcus (often secondary to injury), staphylococcus, *E. coli* (mainly in the neonatal period), *Bacillus proteus*, and *Listeria monocyytogenes*.

Management

Meningitis is the most urgent condition in paediatric practice. The diagnosis should be suspected and confirmed by lumbar puncture within half an hour of the child entering hospital. An intravenous line with appropriate fluid and broad-spectrum antibiotics should be running by one hour. An accurate bacterial diagnosis should be available within 12 h and the antibiotics changed appropriately. Blood culture taken at the time of lumbar puncture may give confirmatory evidence of the type of organism involved.

Note: Because of the real risk of missing a case of meningitis, a lumbar puncture should be seriously considered in every child with a fit and fever, and certainly if there is any suspicion of meningeal irritation.

Complications

1. Those common to any seriously ill, septicaemic child: skin rashes, mouth ulcers, conjunctivitis, etc. Less commonly disseminated intravascular coagulation (DIC) (*see* p. 423) causes bleeding and haemolytic anaemia, infarction, gangrene and shock.

2. Inappropriate ADH (antidiuretic hormone) secretion. The degree and duration of hyponatraemia correlates with complications of meningitis. Therefore, early diagnosis important. Body weight, serum electrolytes, urine volume and specific gravity and serum and urine osmolality should be measured on admission and several times in the first 48 h. If retention of fluid occurs fluid administration should be restricted to 800–1000 ml/m^2/day.

3. Local intracranial lesions: nerve palsies may be caused either by raised intracranial pressure and are then only temporary, or by thrombosis and infarction of the brain giving rise to, e.g. hemiplegia which may be permanent.

4. Subdural fluid collection. May occur with any organism, but most commonly with *H. influenzae* infection.

5. Later and more permanent complications include: progressive hydrocephalus, mental retardation. Nerve deafness is probably caused through infection of the perilymph via its connection with the subarachnoid space. It may not be noticed during the acute stage of the illness and is discovered during convalescence.

Prognosis
Prognosis is determined by the type of organism, age of child, speed with which effective treatment is commenced and efficiency of treatment. Mortality varies in different series. If recovery occurs it is usually complete but sequelae such as those mentioned above may occur.

Special features associated with particular organism:

Meningococcal Meningitis
Clinical features depend on the presence or absence of coincidental septicaemia. The child is often desperately sick and may die, but with adequate therapy improves within a few days and makes a complete recovery. Deafness is the commonest permanent complication.

Haemophilus Influenzae Meningitis
It is particularly in this condition that subdural collections of fluid may develop. They should be suspected if there is any deterioration of the child's condition, particularly if the fever which has gradually fallen to normal for about 4–5 days starts to rise again. Diagnosis by a CAT scan. If a large collection of fluid is present careful needling of the subdural space may be required.

Pneumococcal Meningitis
Is not common in older children. The main danger is a development of progressive hydrocephalus from blockage of the CSF pathways by exudate.

Streptococcal Meningitis
Is rare and occurs mainly in infants. May be secondary to a ruptured spina bifida or dermoid sinus.

E. Coli, B. Proteus, Pseudomonas Aeruginosa Meningitis
These types of meningitis usually occur below 3 months of age; more commonly in babies with meningocele or hydrocephalus, but may occur for no obvious reason. The onset is often insidious with failure to thrive, mild pyrexia and a bulging fontanelle. The first manifestation may be a fit. The outcome is usually poor, despite the use of the newer antibiotics. Cases which survive may develop hydrocephalus.

Listerial Meningitis
Rare meningitis caused by *Listeria monocytogenes* which morphologically resembles diphtheroids. May occur in infants. Usually responds to broad-spectrum antibiotics.

Treatment of Meningitis
Different antibiotic schedules are used in different centres. Some principles include:

1. Two or more broad-spectrum antibiotics (often ampicillin and chloramphenicol) should be used in the first instance until the type of organism and its drug sensitivity profile have been established. Antibiotics given for at least 14 days.

2. Antibiotics should always be given intravenously. It is better to be on the side of underhydration owing to the possibility of oedema of the brain from inappropriate ADH secretion.

3. Mannitol is of value if there is evidence of persistent raised intracranial pressure.

4. Anticonvulsants should be given as prophylactic.

Aseptic (Virus) Meningitis

Not uncommon, benign disease of multiple aetiology, manifested clinically by the abrupt onset of fever, vague muscle pains, headache which is often severe, nausea and vomiting, stiff neck and positive Kernig sign. A macular rash occurs with ECHO infections. The CSF contains a number of lymphocytes. Several different viruses have been incriminated in cases showing very similar clinical pictures:

Mumps Virus
Common especially during mumps epidemic.

Echo Viruses (*Enteric cytopathogenic human orphan*)
Many distinct serotypes. Types 4, 6 and 9 especially liable to cause aseptic meningitis.

Coxsackie Viruses
Two main groups: Groups A and B; organisms from both groups cause meningitis.
A similar picture may be caused by:
Other infections such as toxoplasmosis, leptospirosis or tuberculosis in the initial stages.
Non-infectious agents such as lead poisoning.
Virus meningitis merges into virus encephalitis (*see below*).

Management
The problem is to distinguish between bacterial meningitis which requires active antibiotic therapy, and virus meningitis which does not. This can be particularly difficult if an antibiotic has been given to child before lumbar puncture performed. If in doubt an antibiotic course must be commenced and clinical condition and laboratory findings reviewed after a few days with a view to ceasing treatment.

Chapter 103   **ENCEPHALITIS**

Encephalitis means inflammation of brain tissue, often due to infection with a virus, but the aetiological agent is not discovered in one-third of cases. It overlaps somewhat with viral meningitis.

Encephalopathy is clinically often similar to encephalitis, but due to non-infectious agents such as poisons. It may be very difficult to distinguish the two clinically or even pathologically.

Aetiology
Some causes of encephalitis include:
RNA viruses. Mumps commonest cause (usually mild); measles; rubella in newborn; enteroviruses.
DNA viruses. Herpesvirus hominis; varicella zoster; cytomegalovirus–congenital or acquired; Epstein–Barr virus; variola.
Note: RNA and DNA viruses spread from man to man.
Arthropod-borne agents. Rare in UK, e.g. Eastern and Western equine; St. Louis: Murray Valley.
Mammal-borne viruses. Rabies from saliva of many animals; Herpes virus simiae from monkeys' saliva; lymphocytic choriomeningitis from rodents' excreta.
Non-viral. Mycoplasma; toxoplasmosis; TB; syphilis; fungi, e.g. cryptococcosis; trichinosis and echinococcus.
(*a*) Para- and post-infectious, e.g. with specific diseases—measles; rubella; influenza; hepatitis; pertussis; (*b*) With vaccines—pertussis; rabies; measles; influenza vaccine.
Slow viral infections, e.g. SSPE (*see* p. 334).

Clinical Features
Vary somewhat with the causative organism. In general they resemble those of bacterial meningitis with fever, headache, neck stiffness, screaming spells, fits, stupor and coma.

Progress
Progress is very variable and according to aetiology, e.g. with mumps encephalitis there are mild constitutional symptoms only; neck stiffness lasts a few days. With Murray Valley encephalitis there is an acute onset with fits and coma and severe CNS signs. Cranial nerve lesions and decerebrate rigidity. If the child survives he usually has residual mental retardation and CNS involvement. This condition occurs in widespread epidemics based many years apart following severe flooding in the area.

Chapter 104   *REYE'S SYNDROME*
(Acute toxic encephalopathy with fatty degeneration of the viscera)

An uncommon disease of childhood, of unknown aetiology, characterized by acute encephalitis with deposition of fat in the liver, renal tubules and myocardium. Viral infections such as chickenpox or influenza usually precede the disorder, and salicylate administration has also been suggested as a predisposing factor.

Clinical Features
1. Onset insidious with upper respiratory tract infection; cough, sore throat, earache, etc. Not ill, apparently recovering.
2. Latent period of 1–3 days (occasionally up to 2–3 weeks).
3. Abrupt deterioration:
> 3.1 Persistent severe vomiting for a short time.
> 3.2 CNS signs: stupor, coma, intense irritability with wild delirium, violent flapping movements. Often convulsions. Hyperpnoea prominent.
> 3.3 Examination
> 3.3.1 Sometimes opisthotonos or lying on back with elbows flexed, hands clenched, legs extended.
> 3.3.2 Pupils dilated. Muscle tone and tendon reflexes increased.
> 3.3.3 Decerebrate rigidity, tentorial herniation, IIIrd nerve paralysis and respiratory arrest in some.
> 3.3.6 Liver enlarged and enlarging, firm. No jaundice. Occasional rash.

Autopsy Findings
Brain swollen. Liver: cut surface bright yellow, fatty degeneration. Kidney: fatty degeneration.

Laboratory Investigations
1. Blood ammonia levels and liver enzymes are increased but serum bilirubin is normal or only slightly raised.
2. Hypoglycaemia is usual, and in young children may be profound and resistant to treatment.
3. Blood films show a marked polymorphonuclear leucocytosis.

Management
1. Intravenous 10% dextrose.
2. Control of raised intracranial pressure by bolus injections of intravenous 20% mannitol as required. Dexamethasone may help.
3. Monitoring of intracranial pressure by insertion of a subdural or intraventricular transducer is valuable in severe cases. Aim to keep below 50% of mean arterial pressure. Peritoneal dialysis for hyperammonaemia.

Prognosis
Mortality is high (75%) in severe cases usually under 2 years, but milder cases are being increasingly recognized and the true figure may be much lower. Survivors make complete recovery.

Chapter 105   *SPACE-OCCUPYING LESIONS OF SKULL*

The manifestations of raised intracranial pressure in the child differ from those in the adult, because the adult skull is a rigid box whereas the child's sutures can widen. Thus, signs of raised intracranial pressure appear late and are less conspicuous in the child than in the adult.

Rising intracranial pressure compresses the thin-walled veins resulting in oedema of the brain and poor absorption of CSF. These cause further increase of pressure and a vicious circle is established. Sometimes the lesion itself may obstruct the CSF channels directly, especially if it is subtentorial in position. The falx cerebri and tentorium cerebelli tend to limit pressure changes to separate compartments.

The clinical features of raised intracranial pressure depend mainly on the rapidity with which the lesion expands and the site of the lesion. If rapidly enlarging (e.g. malignant tumour or brain abscess) symptoms and signs may be gross. If slowly enlarging clinical features are minimal or absent, they include:

1. *Headache.* At first paroxysmal, worse on lying down, therefore more prominent at night and early morning.

Aggravated by straining or coughing.

2. *Vomiting.*

3. *Papilloedema* is usually bilateral, more marked in subtentorial lesions. If fundi difficult to examine, general anaesthetic may be required. Diminution of vision may not appear till late.

4. *False localizing signs.* These are signs which appear to indicate direct involvement by lesion, but are merely manifestations of raised intracranial pressure. For instance:

>4.1 Sixth nerve involvement leading to lateral rectus palsy. Nerve most commonly disturbed owing to long, vulnerable intracranial course. Less commonly VIIth nerve.
>
>4.2 Extensor plantar responses from pressure on pyramidal tracts.

5. *Hydrocephalus.* Occurs commonly in small children with open sutures.

6. *Convulsions.* Surprisingly rare, as lesion seldom involves motor cortex. Chronic subdural haematoma may give rise to convulsions.

7. *Bradycardia.* Occurs only with rapidly growing lesions.

8. *Mental changes.* Not common in children except for terminal coma.

Investigations
A CAT scan is a most valuable investigation in the diagnosis of a space-occupying lesion.

Lumbar puncture should only be performed if there is a likelihood that the child may have meningitis. It is potentially dangerous owing to the risk of 'coning' of the medulla. This danger is less in small infants with separated sutures. Papilloedema is always a warning sign and should be looked for prior to any lumbar puncture. If necessary a neurosurgeon should be consulted first. In practice examination of the CSF yields very little information in space-occupying lesions. Very occasionally malignant cells may be found.

Brain Abscess

This condition is very rare in children, apart from post-trauma or in a child with right-to-left shunt from congenital heart disease.

Intracranial Tumours

Intracranial tumours are not uncommon in children under 8 years of age, but they are rare in infancy. Two-thirds are subtentorial, the commonest being midline cerebellar tumours. One-third are supratentorial, mainly around the third ventricle.

In any child with headache and vomiting the possibility of a cerebral tumour, or possibly other space-occupying or vascular lesion should be considered first. Such conditions as school phobia (*see* p. 352), migraine, encephalopathy (*see* p. 339) must also be thought of. The prognosis for cerebral tumours has improved recently with better surgical techniques, radiotherapy and cytotoxic drugs.

Pathology of Various Types of Tumour

Gliomas
Comprise about 75% of tumours in children. Derived from supporting tissue cells of brain.
Medulloblastoma. Macroscopically: rapidly growing, infiltrating tumour usually of cerebellum. Arises from region of floor of 4th ventricle. Rarely disseminated throughout subarachnoid space and outside CNS. Microscopically: composed of rounded undifferentiated cells. Duration of life from first symptoms to death: about 9 months.
Astrocytoma. Macroscopically: white, infiltrating benign tumour, normally of cerebellum. Frequently becomes cystic. Microscopically: composed of astrocytes—dark-staining cells with fibrillary network. Duration of life from first symptom to death may be several years.

Craniopharyngiomas
These are rare tumours of craniopharyngeal or Rathke's pouch; hypophysial epidermoid tumours. The onset may be insidious over a period of years. Sometimes presents as an endocrine disorder with involvement of the pituitary or hypothalamus. Local pressure on the optic nerve may result in bitemporal hemianopia, partial blindness and optic atrophy.

Radiography of the skull will show evidence of raised intracranial pressure and sometimes calcification of the cyst.

Clinical Features of Particular Tumours
Note: Most tumours present with symptoms of raised intracranial pressure.

Cerebellar Tumours
Signs. Vary according to whether tumour is midline or lateral. Most pronounced with rapidly growing lateral tumour.

1. Onset: Medulloblastoma—onset rapid with signs of raised pressure appearing first. Pituitary hypofunction common. Astrocytoma—onset gradual.

2. Ataxia: Unilateral lesions: incoordination on same side as lesion. Midline lesions: incoordination on both sides. Upper limbs more obviously affected than lower.

Signs of Ataxia: coarse tremor, dysdiadokokinesis, staggering gait, hypotonia and nystagmus, etc., are typical of cerebellar lesions in adults.

Chapter 106   *MIGRAINE*

Not uncommon in childhood. Unilateral headache caused by vasodilatation of cranial arteries, often preceded by vasoconstriction.

Clinical Features
Classical adult migraine with 'aura'—visual disturbances, sometimes limb paralysis—followed by throbbing unilateral headache, nausea and vomiting, is sometimes seen in children. Headache alone or headache and vomiting without an aura are more common. The symptoms are relieved by sleep. A family history of migraine is usual. Recurrent abdominal pain (*see* p. 204) is probably a migraine equivalent in some young children.

Treatment
Aspirin. A metered-dose ergotamine inhaler can be useful in older children. Frequent attacks may be treated prophylactically with pizotifen 1 mg at night in children aged over 5 years.

14

Chapter 107

PSYCHOPATHOLOGY

Incidence

Studies in primary school children show that about 5% are regarded as maladjusted. The figure increases in adolescence and more boys than girls are referred for psychiatric help.

It is difficult to define frequency of abnormal behaviour in children because criteria are socially and age dependent. For example:

1. Behaviour which is acceptable in a city ghetto, or a Third World village, may be quite unacceptable in a suburb.

2. Behaviour which is normal in a 2-year-old is not in a 12-year-old.

3. Some parents are very lenient with their children and uncomplaining while others are hypercritical and may seek help for a child with similar behaviour.

Some factors which control behaviour:

1. Genetically inherited personality factors.

2. Intelligence.

3. Parents' or surrogate parents' attitudes.

      3.1 The child's requirement is for a constant parent figure who supplies emotional stimulation and love. If the child is rejected, he may be stunted intellectually, socially and/or physically and develop a cold, affectionless, psychopathic personality.

Parental rejecting behaviour may show itself by:

      3.1.1 Neglect—where the mother does not establish a loving relationship with the child, e.g. she may favour a sibling. *Reaction*: The child often develops attention-seeking behaviour.

      3.1.2 Perfectionism. *Reaction*: The child is rebellious.

      3.1.3 Compensatory over-protection (smother love)—here the mother gives the child everything except love. *Reaction*: The child becomes over-dependent.

      3.2. Paternal. Absence of a father figure. Result:

      3.2.1 On boys—it has been shown that there is a relationship between delinquency and the lack of a stable father figure.

      3.2.2 Girls require a stable, loving father on whom to model their ideal of male behaviour.

345

*Childhood Psychiatric Disorders**

No classification is entirely satisfactory. The classification below has overlaps.

1. Adaptation reactions (reactive disorders). Caused by transient and reversible conditions related to stress, e.g. the precipitating factor may be the loss of a parent. There is no significant distortion of general development. The child may react by compulsive habits (*see* Chapter 109); enuresis, soiling, etc.

2. Specific developmental disorders. Related to biological maturation. These include:

> 2.1 Speech and language disorders.
> 2.2 Stammering (stuttering).
> 2.3 Enuresis.
> 2.4 Encopresis (*see* Chapter 109).
> 2.5 Also included is a heterogeneous group of disorders variously known as the hyperkinetic syndrome, minimal brain dysfunction, the clumsy child or specific learning disorders.

3. Conduct disorders. This group of disorders includes juvenile deliquency, which is often contributed to by mild mental retardation. It will not be considered further.

4. Neurotic disorders. The difference between a neurotic disorder and a psychosis is that the neurotic child has no loss of reality. Neurotic disorders are common in children and include: acute anxiety attacks, phobic reactions, depression and obsessive/compulsive behaviour. These conditions must always be considered in any child who is abnormally anxious or depressed. Such children usually require skilled treatment by a child psychiatrist. Some common conditions are: school phobia or abdominal pain.

5. Psychoses. These are major mental disorders in which behaviour is bizarre and unpredictable. They include:

> 5.1 Infantile autism (infantile psychosis) which commences before the third year of life (*see* Chapter 112).
> 5.2 Late-onset psychosis which occurs after 4 years of age. This resembles adult type psychosis and will not be considered further.

6. Psychosomatic disorders. These can be regarded as a spectrum ranging from:

> 6.1 The child's normal and understandable action to any physical illness, often made worse by his dislike of the sights, smells and noise of the hospital, the temporary separation from his mother, and particularly, his terror of needles, through.
> 6.2 Latent, such as some cases of asthma, ulcerative colitis, peptic ulceration or dermatitis which are brought to light by psychological stress, to
> 6.3 Bizarre hysterical conversion reactions resulting from stress, such as sudden non-organic blindness or paralysis.

---

*Modelled on Rutter N., Shaffer D. and Shepherd M. (1975). *A Multi-axial Classification of Child Psychiatric Disorders*. World Health Organization.

Chapter 108 **PSYCHOLOGICAL ASSESSMENT**

A battery of tests is often performed in children with suspected mental or psychiatric problems to assess:
1. Intelligence—Cognitive function.
2. Personality—Projective testing.
3. Educational achievement.
4. Motor and perceptual development.

The result of an intelligence test is given as the mental age which, when compared with the chronological age, gives the intelligence quotient (IQ) as follows:

$$IQ = \frac{\text{mental age} \times 100}{\text{chronological age}}.$$

For children below about 2 years of age, the less accurate Developmental Age is calculated from which a Developmental Quotient (DQ) can be derived.

For measuring intelligence, many different tests are available. For details *see* textbooks of psychology.

One of the most useful screening lists for younger children's development is the Denver Developmental Screening Test (DDST) (*see* Appendix 3).

Grading of Intelligence Scores

IQ	Designation
Below 69	Mentally subnormal
70–79	Borderline mental handicap
80–89	Dull normal
90–109	Normal intelligence
110–119	Bright normal
120–129	Superior
130+	Very superior

Value of IQ Testing
Intelligence quotient ascribes to mental ability a convenient number which can be easily recorded and, as tests are standardized, used for comparison.

If child's mental health and environmental situation do not greatly alter, IQ usually remains approximately the same throughout life. Serial IQs can be used to determine progress, for instance, in a progressive mental disease or after treatment for hypothyroidism.

It must be remembered that intelligence is not the all-important factor for future achievement and happiness. Many other factors such as religion, home environment, education, opportunity, physical health, perseverance and motivation all help to determine a person's future role in life.

Chapter 109

COMPULSIVE HABITS

This group of conditions is characterized by repetitive actions which appear to give pleasure to the child and are used as an emotional outlet for stress or boredom. Of little significance unless excessive or of prolonged duration, when they may be due to mental retardation or emotional distress.

Masturbation

Most children masturbate at some time, condition of no importance, unless indulged in to excess. Should then be regarded as symptom of some underlying emotional disturbance.

Treatment
Parents should be reassured that condition is both normal and harmless. Any sources of irritation should be removed and genitalia kept clean. Child should be encouraged to find interest in other activities.

Rocking, Head-banging, Head-rolling

Common in normal children and also in mentally defective or emotionally disturbed children. Common ages, 6 months to 4 years.

Thumb-sucking

Common habit in young babies which may persist for first few years of life. Often associated with some movement such as rubbing ear or grasping clothing.

Results
Physical. Usually nil. In a very few persistent cases forward displacement of front upper teeth may occur. Callosities, ulcers or rotation of thumb may develop.

Treatment
Usually none required. Restraints, strapping or painting thumb with bitter aloes, very rarely effective.

Nail-biting

Very common. Sometimes symptom of emotional disturbances such as school difficulties.

Treatment
Wearing gloves or appeals to pride of appearance may be effective in older children.

ENURESIS

Very common condition. Involuntary wetting occurs beyond age when child should have gained control—usually 18 months for day and 4 years for night control.

Causes
1. *Organic.* Rare.
       1.1 Urinary infection.
       1.2 Developmental abnormality of urinary tract.
       1.3 Diabetes mellitus or insipidus.
       1.4 Chronic renal failure.
       1.5 Neurological lesions.
       1.6 Mental deficiency.
2. *Psychological.*

Differentiation between Organic and Psychological Types
Following findings indicate possibility of organic cause and warrant full urinary investigations:
1. History
       1.1 If child wet all the time both day and night.
       1.2 If there have been recurrent attacks of urinary infection.
       1.3 Other urinary symptoms, e.g. dysuria or precipitancy.
2. On examination
       2.1 If other congenital abnormalities present.
       2.2 If child has repeatedly palpable bladder.
       2.3 If child has growth failure.
       2.4 If child has any neurological abnormality.
       2.5 If there is a poor stream of urine, or if child dribbles urine.
Following investigations should be made:
   1. Blood pressure. Blood urea.
   2. Biochemical and microscopic examination of urine.
   3. Intravenous pyelogram. If necessary retrograde pyelography should be performed.
   4. Micturating cystogram.

Psychological Enuresis

Clinical Features
Three main types of enuresis occur:
   1. Very common. Children wet from birth. Some of these children sleep very deeply. Probably delayed maturation. Merges into group (2) because child has emotional stress due to his wetness; develops a conditioned reflex to wet.
   2. Less common. Children who had achieved control but who relapse. Common story is that child was dry at night until age of about 3–5 years old and then, perhaps following some upsetting circumstance, such as a new baby, or attack of whooping cough, he suddenly started to wet at night. Usually child not wet every night, whether he is wet or not often depends on circumstances, e.g. child may always be dry when staying with grandmother or in hospital. Uncommonly obvious emotional stress present. Often history that one or both parents were enuretic.
   3. Children dry by night but wet by day (rare). May be associated with organic or psychological disorders.

Prognosis

Majority of children improve as they grow older with or without treatment. Said that 10% of untreated children with enuresis improve per year, i.e. of 100 5-year-old children 90 will still wet at 6 years, 82 at 7 years, approximately 73 at 8 years, etc. Thus a small number will persist into adult life. In addition, enuresis is not an all-or-none phenomenon; many children are mostly dry with occasional wet nights.

Treatment

Unsatisfactory. Three main methods attempted:

1. Mechanical prevention

> 1.1 Limiting fluids in the evening. This merely limits quantity of urine passed. May make matters worse if concentrated urine irritating to bladder.
>
> 1.2 Lifting at intervals.
>
> 1.3 Bladder training. Child taught to hold water for gradually increasing lengths of time during day. Theory is that bladder thus becomes accustomed to holding large quantities of urine.
>
> 1.4 Electric alarm which wakes child as soon as he is wet. Results in cure in about 80% of cases. Should be reserved for older child.

2. Drugs, e.g. Imipramine

Mode of action uncertain. Note risk of unpleasant side-effects and danger of introducing dangerous drug into household which may contain young children.

3. Psychological

> 3.1 Parents told to encourage rather than punish child. If each wet bed magnified to a major issue, child becomes tense and anxious and enuresis persists.
>
> 3.2 Child should be told not to worry, that many children do it, that he will grow out of it. Placebo drugs often given.
>
> 3.3 Reward for bladder control e.g. by using a star chart with star awarded for each dry night. May be used in conjunction with antidepressant drugs but these measures alone or in combination are unlikely to succeed unless child is motivated to become dry.

4. Summary

Best therapy is combination of psychological help and electric alarm.

Encopresis

Far less common than enuresis. Characterized by repeated passing of faeces at inappropriate places and times. To be differentiated from **overflow incontinence**, where child's abdomen is loaded with faecal masses, which child voluntarily retains. In overflow incontinence some stools become fluid and pass anus to give faecal soiling; examination of abdomen and rectum discloses masses of faeces. Illness may follow a fissure-in-ano or fear of toilet or be a reaction against parental attitudes, especially inappropriate toilet training. Child strongly resists enemas, suppositories and rectal examinations. Enuresis present in a third of cases.

True encopresis child passes regular and formed motions—often achieves control of faeces at appropriate age but relapses. Mothers may be overdemanding and meticulous; often neurotic and require psychotherapy.

Management
1. True encopresis: refer to child psychiatrist.
2. Overflow incontinence: combination of stool-softening agent, mild laxative and 'informal psychotherapy'. Ultimate prognosis good but symptom may persist for several years. Social worker may be helpful if domestic or school problem.

Hair Pulling, Scratching

Rare in normal, but may occur in sick children, e.g. picking lip or scar. May swallow hair causing hair ball in stomach.

Tics (*Habit Spasms*)

Repetitive, quasi-purposeful movements. Age: later childhood.

Character of Movements
Usually involve face, shoulders or upper extremities. Sinking, shoulder shrugging, etc. common. Becomes more frequent when child obviously watched, but can be temporarily stopped on command. Child can demonstrate movement if asked to do so. Cease with sleep.

Differential Diagnosis
Chorea: movements non-repetitive, incoordinate and purposeless; become worse if child told to stop; limbs more affected than trunk in early stages; individual movements cannot be demonstrated. Other signs of rheumatic activity may be present, such as carditis.

Treatment
Most important that parents should be reassured as to benign nature of condition. Tic should be ignored. If cause can be discovered, e.g. emotional tension while working for examination, correction should be attempted.

Breath-holding Attacks

Common, very alarming habit. Occurs in children between ages of 6 months and about 5 years. May be precipitated by anger, thwarting, fear (e.g. of a dog) or pain (e.g. a fall).

Sequence of Events
Child cries, holds breath in expiration, goes blue in face, falls to ground and, in severe cases, may have convulsion. At last he takes sudden breath. Never fatal except in association with cyanotic congenital heart disease.

Treatment
Essential that child should learn that he cannot have his own way by indulging in these methods. Ignoring attack may be effective.

Pica

Habit of dirt eating. Most children pass through stage of eating coal, feathers, paper, hair or chewing paint. Occasionally habit persists and is severe.

Chapter 110   ## SCHOOL REFUSAL (*School stress syndrome: School phobia: Truancy*)

These three conditions are linked by the common factor that the child manages to avoid school. All commoner in boys.

School Stress Syndrome

Aetiology
A child may not function well at school because of:
 1. Specific learning disability.
    1.1 Dyslexia (specific reading disability).
    Example: Child of 11 years with mental age of 11 (excluding reading) but reading age of 8 years. Often thought to be 'dull' or 'not trying'.
    1.2 Dyscalculia (difficulty with mathematics).
    1.3 Dysgraphia (difficulty with writing).
 2. A degree of mental retardation sufficient to prevent him from succeeding well at school but too slight to have been noticed before he entered school, e.g. IQ around 85.
 3. Poor teaching, especially in big class.
 4. Unrecognized physical handicap, e.g. marked myopia, unilateral deafness; chronic urinary tract infection giving rise to perpetual ill health.
 5. Known physical handicap, full effects of which are not appreciated.

Clinical Features
Child becomes psychologically stressed under pressure, especially at examination times. Avoids school by:
 1. Psychosomatic disorder. Commonest are: abdominal pain; nausea; vomiting; headache. Thus symptoms may mimic cerebral tumour or renal infection, etc.
 2. School phobia.
 3. Rarely, malingering.
 N.B. Important to make correct diagnosis between psychological or organically-based symptoms rapidly and certainly. Remember that absence of organic evidence does not mean that trouble is necessarily psychological. To diagnose psychological problem, must have positive evidence of psychological difficulties as well as negative evidence of organic.

Management
 1. Rapid work-up for organic disease once and for all—in order:

1.1 To make sure nothing important is missed.
1.2 To reassure parents and child.
1.3 To reassure doctor so that it need never be repeated (continual uncertainty on part of doctor reinforces psychological problem).
2. Full psychological testing, discussion with teacher.
3. Explanation to child, parents and teachers that child is not sick. Correction of disability as far as possible.

School Phobia

Child refuses to go to school because:
1. Does not want to leave home (commonest cause).
    1.1 Mother may not want him to go to school, and may obstruct him.
    1.2 Child may be afraid mother will become ill or desert home.
2. Fear of school, e.g. bullying.

Management
A psychological emergency. The longer the child remains away from school the harder it is to get him back. Discover cause and have full discussion with child, parents and teachers.

Truancy

Child goes off to school but fails to arrive. Factors include mild to moderate mental retardation; home with little academic interest, mother may keep him (or her) at home to look after other children. Some bright pupils may develop such severe hatred of school that they opt out. Modern classes are big and weeks may go by before child's absence is noted by teacher. Even professional parents may be deceived. Condition requires considerable discussion between teacher, parents and child.

Chapter 111   # SPEECH DEFECTS

Classification
1. *Disorders of voicing (dysphonia).* Loss of volume and tone of voice. May be due to laryngitis, nodules, papilloma.
2. *Disorders of rhythm (dysrhythmia).* Manifested by hesitation, repetition of syllables, stammer or prolongation of syllables, slurring. Made worse by excitement or stress.
3. *Disorders of articulation with dysfunction of articulatory apparatus (dysarthria)*
    3.1 Due to Neurological Abnormalities
    3.1.1 Cerebral palsy: Especially diplegia, athetosis, severe ataxia.

3.1.2 Suprabulbar paresis: Facial diplegia (Moebius' syndrome).

3.1.1 Myopathies.

3.2 Due to Local Abnormalities

3.2.1 Cleft palate or submucous cleft palate.

3.2.2 Adenoid or tonsillar enlargement.

3.2.3 Palatal disproportion—nasopharynx unduly big—allows air to escape giving nasal speech, often history of milk coming down nose during feeding. Can be successfully treated by pharyngoplasty.

3.2.4 Malocclusion of jaw, e.g. Pierre Robin syndrome.

4. Disorders of articulation due to secondary causes

4.1 Developmental Speech Disorder Syndrome, e.g. no words by age of 2 years; affects boys more than girls; family history often positive. May have history of birth difficulties and presence of 'soft' neurological signs. In severe varieties children appear not to understand spoken comments and rely on lip reading—auditory imperception. Outlook for severe varieties poor but good for milder groups.

4.2 Developmental articulatory dyspraxia—where voluntary control of muscles of speech is defective but involuntary movements are normal. Often drool. Require teaching about correct positioning of muscles.

Stammer (Stutter)

Definition
Stammer (or stutter) is involuntary repetition of a sound during speech, with inability to continue beyond it.

Aetiology
Age of onset: 2–4 years. Sex: more common in boys than girls. Familial incidence: not marked but condition may be acquired by imitation.

Causes. Unknown.

1. Emotional disturbance common but may be result of anxiety over stammer rather than cause.

2. Problems with right/left handedness have been incriminated but no firm evidence.

Clinical Features
1. Very common as temporary phenomenon during development of speech.

2. Persistent stammering. Either:

2.1 Child stops at difficult consonant, then suddenly brings it and rest of sentence out with a rush. During silent period associated activity such as grimacing or hand movements.

2.2 Rapid repetition of particular consonant occurs especially 'p' or 'b'. Eventually offending consonant and rest of word is said. Sentence continues until another difficult consonant is reached. Two types (*a*) and (*b*) usually occur together.

3. Secondary emotional disturbance common. Child may shun company and avoid speech. Can usually sing without difficulty.

Treatment
Speech therapy required.

Faulty Articulation

Lisping (Sigmatismus)
Difficulty in pronouncing certain consonants, for instance:
'th' pronounced 'f', e.g. 'thumb' becomes 'fumb'.
's' pronounced 'th', e.g. 'spoon' becomes 'thpoon'.
'r' pronounced 'w', e.g. 'rabbit' becomes 'wabbit'.

Causes
1. Almost universal when child learns to talk.
2. Malocclusion of teeth, etc. in later childhood.
3. Functional: sometimes from copying other child who lisps.
4. Familial.
5. Mental deficiency.

Lalling
Substitution of wrong consonants for ones with which difficulty is experienced. More severe defect. May be life-long.

Idoglossia
Development of individual language understood by child alone. Normal in young children for a short time.

Echolalia

Parrot-like repetition of words without understanding their meaning. Normal in young children, but only as passing phase. May persist in mental defectives and autism.

Chapter 112   *INFANTILE AUTISM*

A rare syndrome in which the child withdraws from people but relates to inanimate objects. Often misdiagnosed as mental retardation which is often present. Boys: girls, 4 : 1.

The following types may be recognized:

1. True infantile autism (Kanner syndrome). Commences before age of 3 years. Very often retrospective evidence that it commenced before age of 12 months, or even in neonatal period. May occur in more than one member of the family, occasionally in identical twins.

2. Secondary to brain damage. Child apparently normal until some damaging episode occurs, e.g. meningitis, measles, encephalitis, etc.

3. Secondary to severe emotional deprivation.

4. Pseudo-psychotic reaction to acute stress, physical or emotional.

Note:

1. (1) and (2) above permanent. (3) and (4) above perhaps reversible.

2. Psychoses of later childhood and adolescence are probably different conditions more akin to adult psychoses and will not be considered here.

Clinical Features

Early history. Difficult baby, unresponsive and implacable sometimes from birth. At about 6 months does not make usual anticipatory movements to being picked up; does not mould to the body of the person carrying him. Head-banging and rocking may commence.

Late history. *Note*: Normal children occasionally do some of the things listed here, but autistic children do them all day, every day.

1. Gross and sustained impairment of emotional relationships with people:
> 1.1 Aloof and distant manner as though other human beings did not exist.
> 1.2 Turning away from or looking past people.
> 1.3 Difficulty in playing with other children.

2. Self-examination. Studies parts of body.

3. Preoccupation with particular objects. Collects things, anger if lost.

4. Sustained resistance to change in environment or routine.

5. Apparent abnormality of special senses. Child considered to be deaf or blind. Later proved false. Lack of sensation of pain, hot or cold.

6. Abnormalities of mood. Temper tantrums; irrational fears; periods of laughing for no apparent reason; lack of fear of real danger.

7. Speech disturbances. May speak late (after 4 years) or never. *Note*: Prognosis is particularly bad in those who never speak. May have odd parrot-like repetition of phrases, sentences or even whole poems without apparent understanding or meaning. Often substitutes 'he' or own name for 'I'. Love of music.

8. Disturbances of movement. Often overactive, especially by night, often walks on tip-toe. Flapping movements. Extreme pleasure in bodily movements. Head-banging, rocking, etc.

9. Islets of normal or even above-normal skill may appear against a background of serious retardation, e.g. proficient at jigsaws and puzzles; other mechanical skills; reading; memorizing, etc.

Note: Very difficult to assess level of intelligence; usually low.

Chapter 113   # *MENTAL RETARDATION*

The term 'mental retardation' is given to a heterogeneous group of conditions occurring before the completion of growth and development and characterized by reduced intellectual capacity to the point of impaired learning ability and social inadequacy. It comprises a spectrum of intelligence from mild retardation to the completely incapacitated, bedridden ament; the aetiology may or may not be known (*see below*).

Retardation may be discovered:

1. At birth, e.g. Down's syndrome, microcephaly, or during a screening programme.

2. By the parents who suspect there is something wrong in the first year or so of life.

At Birth

The parents should be informed as soon as possible after the diagnosis has been made. Both father and mother are seen together if possible in the initial interview. The parents are naturally shocked and take in very little of the initial interview except that the child is mentally retarded. Subsequent interviews should therefore be arranged soon afterward to discuss the parents' feelings and reassure them that guilt feelings are inappropriate. They should be told the probable prognosis for life, and for education, and informed about the remedial programmes available. The family attitude to the child should be assessed. Early liaison with the general practitioner, health visitor and social services is important.

Parental Diagnosis

When the child is brought to the doctor because of the parents' anxiety, initial discussion with the mother will reveal her estimate of the child's developmental progress and she will probably be right, although she may have unrealistically high hopes. The child should have a full medical investigation to determine the cause if possible, so that treatment, if any, and informed genetic counselling may be given. Full investigation is also essential in order that the parents may realize that everything possible is being done. Assessment will include paediatric, neurological, psychological, hearing, speech, vision, physiotherapeutic and social evaluations.

Parental Reactions

Parents go through different stages after receiving bad news. These are:

1. Shock and denial.
2. Adjustment and sorrowing.
3. Later, realistic acceptance.

These reactions are compounded by guilt, remorse, anger, worry, fear of the future, secret desire to maim or kill the child (which may occur), blaming of the spouse or of doctors. Some accept with grace and equanimity. The parents may:

1. Refuse to accept the diagnosis.
2. Overprotect the child.
3. Reject and demand care in an institution.

The strain on the family of a child with mental retardation can be very great for all concerned, including the siblings. Positive benefits can include greater family cohesion, a greater understanding and empathy for others with problems and motivation for life of service for others.

Aetiology

Congenital Abnormalities acquired before or at birth:

1. Genetic

        1.1 Static, i.e. the pathology is present at birth and does not progress. Comprises 50% of all mental retards. Cause usually not found but includes certain specific syndromes, e.g. Cockayne's syndrome, DeLange's syndrome and numerous others.

1.2 Progressive unless given treatment where possible, cerebromacular degeneration; Huntington's chorea; the leucoencephalopathies; some of the neurocutaneous syndromes, e.g. tuberous sclerosis.

1.3 Chromosomal abnormality, e.g. Down's syndrome, other trisomies, Klinefelter's syndrome. (*See* Chapter 5.)

2. Acquired in utero

2.1 Maternal infections, e.g. rubella, toxoplasmosis, cytomegalovirus.

2.2 Maternal alcohol, phenytoin or drug ingestion.

2.3 Hypoxia from any cause.

3. Perinatal

3.1 Hypoxia. May be due to many causes, e.g. accidents to the placenta; oversedation of mother by drugs or anaesthetic; difficulty with delivery.

3.2 Obstetric damage; cerebral haemorrhage.

3.3 Prematurity, probably through intraventricular haemorrhage.

3.4 Severe rhesus incompatibility or other condition giving rise to kernicterus.

3.5 Metabolic inborn errors of metabolism, e.g. amino acidopathy, hypoglycaemia, etc. *see* Chapters 50, 51.

Acquired Abnormalities

1. Infections: meningitis and encephalitis, septicaemia and intravascular coagulations.
2. Encephalopathies, e.g. postvaccination.
3. Injury, including non-accidental injury.
4. Poisoning, e.g. lead.
5. Cerebrovascular accident.

Investigation of Mental Retardation

Some causes are obvious, e.g. Down's, Turner's or rubella syndromes. Some are detected by routine biochemical population screening, e.g. homocystinuria.

History

1. Pregnancy (infections, bleeding).
2. Birth (*a*) asphyxia, gestation and development; (*b*) neonatal abnormalities.
3. Infantile illnesses, e.g. hyperosmolar dehydration, meningitis.
4. Family history, e.g. neurocutaneous syndromes, Tay–Sachs' disease.

The Stigmata of Mental Retardation

It is often possible to guess that a child is mentally retarded by his physical appearance because he has some of the stigmata of mental retardation. These include:

Skull is usually smaller than normal.

High palate.
Jaw protrusion or recession
Pinna deformed and low-set.
Eyes abnormal; marked epigastric folds frequently occur.
Nose often flat.

If his intelligence is very low, the child may make ceaseless, strange and poorly co-ordinated gestures; may struggle. Often physically well developed so that control is difficult. Older children may rush around the room touching and moving objects (so-called 'hyperkinetic mental deficiency') and make odd noises.

The child may lie listless and apathetic. Saliva dribbles from the mouth; teeth grinding, masturbation, head banging, etc. may continue for hours on end. The circulation is often poor, resulting in cyanosis of the extremities. Puberty may be delayed, but reproduction is usually possible. Convulsions are common.

Clinical
Neurological examination, note ?cerebral palsy. Head size—too big or too small. Eyes—cataracts, e.g. rubella, Lowe's syndrome, galactosaemia, hypoparathyroidism. Retinopathy, e.g. rubella, CMV, toxoplasmosis. Retinitis pigmentosa—in various syndromes. Dislocated lens (homocystinuria), cloudy cornea (mucopolysaccharidoses). Transillumination of skull—hydranencephaly.
Laboratory tests. Include, where relevant, chromosome analysis, urine and blood amino acids, urine mucopolysaccharides, reducing substances, serology for infections. White cell enzymes.

Blood lead and calcium and thyroid tests. X-ray skull for calcification (toxoplasmosis, CMV and epiloia). CAT scan for brain morphology.

Differential Diagnosis
1. Blindness. Difficulty only arises in first few months of life. Mentally retarded child may take no interest in surroundings, and be thought to be blind.
2. Deafness. May be difficult to diagnose (*see* Chapter 59).
3. Language and *speech disorders.* Child may hear and see but not understand meaning or symbolism of words.
4. Organic nervous disease, e.g. in cerebral palsy the child is often mentally defective but not always so. Intelligent children must be distinguished as they can benefit from training and education.
5. Epileptic states, e.g. psychomotor epilepsy, may give rise to confusional states. In addition, child may be on anti-epileptic drugs which make him sleepy.
6. Autism (*see* Chapter 112).
7. Environmental deprivation, e.g. lack of social stimulation and educational opportunity, inadequacy at home.

Management
Management includes prolonged support by paediatrician and family doctor and genetic counselling service, support by community services, e.g. pre-school play group, physiotherapy, speech therapy, occupational therapy (to advise and provide appropriate aids) some advice over educational placing and prospects. Often helpful to introduce family to parents' association concerned with the particular child's disability, e.g. Spastics Society. Psychologists can help by providing graded limited goals for parents to aim at.

Some doctors give fluoride tablets where water not already treated to prevent dental caries. Drugs have little part to play—hyperkinesia can be treated by methylphenidate, amphetamines or chlordiazepoxide; haloperidol useful for severe behaviour abnormalities, e.g. rage reactions. Epilepsy if present, must be treated.

Mental Retardation without known cause ('Simple' or Primary Amentia)

Varies in severity from slight backwardness to child who is unable to do anything. Probably this group contains many subgroups not yet recognized.

Pathology
Brain sometimes appears normal macroscopically and microscopically. Sometimes nerve cells are deficient in number and lack orderly arrangements. Associated congenital abnormalities or stigmata of mental deficiency are often found in severe cases.

X-Linked Mental Retardation

There is a 25% excess of males in the population of retarded individuals. This suggests that there are some X-linked causes of mental retardation. These include:

1. Renpenning's Syndrome. These children are usually severely retarded with small heads, short stature, but no other physical abnormalities. In particular, their facial appearances are unremarkable and the testes are of normal size.

2. The macro-orchidism–marker X syndrome (MOMX) (fragile X-linked mental retardation syndrome). This syndrome has the following characteristics:

> 2.1 Birthweight may be increased, although the adult height is normal.
> 2.2 The head circumference may be slightly increased with a prominent forehead and the mid-face is hypoplastic. The mandible is frequently prominent and prognathic.
> 2.3 The ears are larger than normal.
> 2.4 Macro-orchidism is present from birth. It is occasionally unilateral. Penis normal.
> 2.5 The speech is 'narrative and compulsive'.
> 2.6 Retardation ranges from profound to mild. Most cases are moderately severe.
> 2.7 Chromosome analysis shows a fragile site on the long arm of the X chromosome.

Chapter 114   # MINIMAL BRAIN DYSFUNCTION (MBD)

This unsatisfactory term describes a not uncommon heterogeneous group of conditions which often go under such names as the hyperactive child; the clumsy child; specific learning difficulties, etc. They are more common in boys than girls and are particularized by a variety of behavioural abnormalities. Not every manifestation is present in every case and the severity varies considerably. Principal manifestations include one or more of the following:

1. Hyperactivity. Difficult to define because:

    1.1 A child may be described by one adult as hyperactive whereas another will consider his behaviour to be within normal limits.

    1.2 Some children are constantly hyperactive, whereas others are calm unless stimulated.

    1.3 The cause of the hyperactivity may be largely environmental, e.g. the child in ghetto situation.

However, the hyperactive child is restless, does not stay still for long, cannot concentrate effectively and is consequently slow in learning, difficult to discipline and annoys parents and sibs.

2. Impulsiveness, low frustration tolerance, distractability, aggression, clumsiness.

3. Learning problems; these may be specific, e.g. dyslexia (difficulty in reading), or dyscalculia (difficulty with maths).

4. Secondary behavioural problems are common, e.g. temper tantrum because of frustration, or showing-off behaviour to hide the very real physiological deficits.

On Examination

Conventional CNS examination often reveals little, but 'soft' neurological signs may be present.

1. Hyper- or hypotonia.
2. Depressed gross motor skills.
3. Poor eye/hand coordination, e.g. inability to tie shoelaces.
4. Poor perceptual function, e.g. child cannot copy simple shapes.
5. Vestibular or proprioceptive dysfunction, e.g.

    5.1 Absent or abnormal postrotatory nystagmus.

    5.2 Abrupt loss of tone when vision is occluded, by supporting the child in the horizontal position and asking him to close his eyes. If he is relying on vision to determine where his body is in space, he will lose tone and flop dramatically.

6. Crossed laterality is present in some children.
7. Any of the above may occur in conjunction with mild cerebral palsy, mental retardation or epilepsy.

Management

Despite the normal appearance and paucity of convincing CNS and other signs, the child has a genuine physical handicap. It is of the greatest importance that the parents learn to distinguish between 'can't' and 'won't'. Sometimes the child says he is unable, e.g. to dress himself. This may be true—'he can't'. But it may be that he does not want to—'he won't'. The key is observance. If he can dress himself on one occasion, then he can on another. To try to force a child to do something he is genuinely unable to accomplish, is merely to increase frustration and secondary behavioural problems.

Behaviour management programmes administered by skilled psychologists can prove very helpful and benefits are found after even a few weeks. Child's ability to concentrate improves coincidentally and so rate of learning increases.

The child's environment should be unstimulating but he should be allowed adequate exercise. A trampoline is helpful.

A small number of children may benefit from a Feingold diet, the most important element of which seems to be the absence of artificial colouring matter.

Some children seem to be helped by psychic stimulant drugs. Most often used are methylphenidate (Ritalin) or dextro-amphetamine. Medication should be given early in the day as both of these drugs causes sleep disturbance.

Chapter 115   ANATOMY AND PHYSIOLOGY

Embryonic Development and Prenatal Maturation of the Kidney

By 16 weeks of fetal life the kidney is formed and urine production starts although further branching of tubules and nephron formation occurs until 36 weeks. At that time there are approximately one million nephrons per kidney. At birth the glomerular diameter is approximately half that of the adult size. The juxtamedullary nephrons are formed first. The outer cortical nephrons continue to be formed up to the 36th week. By the 6th week of intrauterine life the cloaca has differentiated into the urogenital sinus and rectum. The gonads and reproductive organs start to appear at 8 weeks and are fully formed by 3 months. Developmental anomalies of the genitalia are sometimes associated with anomalies of the renal tract.

Anatomy (Fig. 115.1)

The kidney weighs 13 g at birth, 47 g at 2 years and 100 g at teenage. The adult kidney measures approximately 15 cm. The mean glomerular diameter at birth is 0·115 mm and 0·28 mm in adults. The juxtamedullary glomeruli are relatively larger at birth than the outer and more recently formed glomeruli. The loops of Henle and the proximal convoluted tubules of the juxtamedullary nephrons are longer and more developed. The renal tubules are, however, less well developed at birth than the glomeruli.

The capsular blood supply provides a network of capillaries over the surface of the kidney and a small amount to the collecting system. When the main renal artery is occluded the kidney may receive sufficient blood by the alternative supply. The venous system is in parallel with the arterial supply to the kidney. It receives venous blood from the capillaries supplied by the efferent arterioles.

On cross section the renal cortex and medulla are clearly differentiated, the cortex being lighter in colour. The cortex is the outer part of the kidney and it surrounds the medulla which has papillae with the papillary ducts opening at the tips. The papillae are the cause of the normal cupping of the minor calyces recognized radiologically. These drain into the major calyces, renal pelvis and ureters. After passing through the muscular wall of the bladder the ureter has a submucosal segment which acts as a flap valve and prevents vesico-ureteric reflux. The very small size of the pelvis in infants allows the bladder to be easily felt in the abdomen. The female urethra is much shorter than the male urethra, facilitating

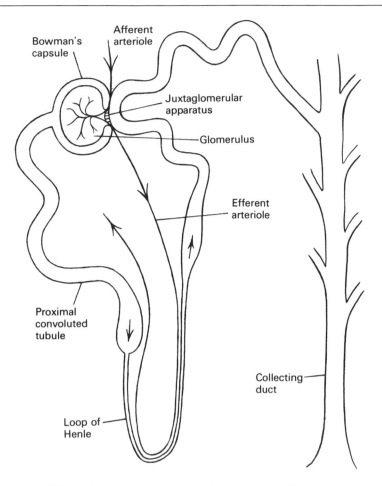

Fig. 115.1. Schematic representation of a glomerulus with blood supply.

the entry of bacteria into the bladder. Obstructive lesions are relatively rare in the female urethra.

Physiology

Blood Flow

Renal blood flow comprises 20–25% of the cardiac output; 93% of which goes to the cortex (500 ml/min/100 g kidney tissue). Renal blood flow is influenced by neurogenic stimuli acting on alpha receptors. There is also an autoregulatory system involving the juxtaglomerular apparatus and prostaglandins. In utero homeostasis is accomplished via the placenta and mother's kidneys. Renal blood flow is approximately one-third that of the adult and renal vascular resistance is very high. At birth there is an immediate fall in renal vascular resistance and an increase in renal blood flow. A further fall in renal vascular resistance occurs during infancy and childhood and renal blood flow increases to take a greater proportion of total cardiac output. In early infancy there is relatively more blood flow to the juxtamedullary glomeruli than to the other cortical nephrons.

Glomerular Filtration
The glomerular filtrate is formed from water and solutes which are filtered through the endothelial lining of the glomerular capillaries, the basement membrane and the epithelium of Bowman's space. The glomerular filtration rate is influenced by the renal blood flow, the surface area of the glomeruli, the hydrostatic pressure in the glomerular capillaries and Bowman's capsule and the oncotic pressure. The glomerular basement membrane is a semipermeable membrane and the oncotic pressure will be the same on both sides, except for the component due to colloid osmotic pressure, since colloids are not filtered. Glomerular filtration occurs in the human fetus at 9–12 weeks but this is not necessary for intrauterine growth. At birth there is a sudden increase in glomerular filtration rate mainly due to an increase in blood supply to the juxtamedullary nephrons. An increase in blood flow to the superficial cortical nephrons continues during the first 2 years of life. Thereafter glomerular filtration rate is proportional to surface area. Because of the large volume of fluid filtered, 99 % is usually reabsorbed in the tubules.

Tubular Function
Whilst glomerular filtration is a passive process depending on blood flow and the filtering characteristics of the glomerular basement membrane the tubular functions involve active and passive transport mechanisms and therefore involve energy consumption. The main source of energy is glucose, but free fatty acids, citrate and lactate are also utilized. Of the 180 litres filtered by the mature kidneys every day, 179 litres are reabsorbed by the tubules. Similarly, huge quantities of sodium, potassium, glucose and bicarbonate are reabsorbed by an active process. Tubular function is summarized in *Fig.* 115.2.

Sodium Balance
Excess interstitial fluid resulting in generalized oedema is always accompanied by an increase in total body sodium. In the healthy adult increased sodium intake results in fluid retention and an increase in weight. This is followed by an increased sodium excretion to restore balance. Aldosterone which stimulates sodium and water retention is secreted in response to volume depletion via volume receptors in the heart and arteries or to a fall in osmolality or serum sodium detected by osmoreceptors within the central nervous system.

Renin
Renin is produced in the juxtaglomerular apparatus which is situated in the media of the afferent arteriole just before it reaches the glomeruli. The portion of the distal convoluted tubule in close proximity to the juxtaglomerular cells is called the macula densa. Renin release increases in response to a fall either of blood pressure or extracellular fluid volume whilst an increase in pressure or volume decreases renin release. Renin release is stimulated by the sympathetic nerves, and is influenced by the amount of sodium reaching the distal tubule. Renin release is decreased by a potassium load and increased with potassium depletion. Renin is an enzyme synthesized in the kidney and reacts with angiotensin to form angiotensin 1 which is changed by a converting enzyme to angiotensin II, the

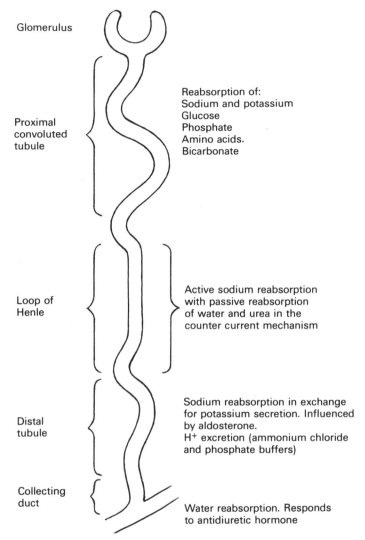

Fig. 115.2. Diagram of a tubule showing function of different parts.

active form. Angiotensin II has a direct action on arteries causing constriction and stimulating aldosterone secretion. It also has a central action on the brainstem.

Erythropoietin
This hormone, responsible for erythropoiesis, is produced in the kidney and is reduced in renal failure, causing anaemia.

The Counter Current Mechanism
The arterial supply to the loop of Henle comes from the capillary arteriolar loops descending from the cortex with the blood flow in the opposite direction to that of the tubular fluid. Sodium is actively transported from the tubular lumen as it leaves the medulla into interstitium and may enter the vascular space only to be

carried back into the medulla again. This counter current multiplier system makes a very high osmolar concentration in the renal medulla. Chloride ions and urea also contribute by diffusing from the tubules passively. Thus the fluid reaching the distal convoluted tubule is hypotonic.

Antidiuretic Hormone (ADH)
Antidiuretic hormone is secreted by the posterior pituitary gland and acts on the distal tubule and collecting ducts, making them permeable to water, thus enabling fluids to be removed from the tubules by osmosis into the hyperosmolar renal medulla. Endorgan unresponsiveness occurs in nephrogenic diabetes insipidus.

Tubular Secretion
Some waste products are actively secreted by the tubules, e.g. uric acid and some drugs.

Chapter 116	ASSESSMENT OF RENAL FUNCTION

Examination of the Urine

Colour
The urine is normally yellow, the shade depending on the concentration of the urine. Cloudy urine is usually due to crystalline deposits of phosphates but increased numbers of white or red cells or heavy bacteriuria cause some cloudiness. Very dilute urine such as occurs in chronic renal failure (particularly dialysed patients) or nephrogenic diabetes insipidus is very pale or colourless. Other causes of coloured urine are summarized in *Table* 116.1.

Milky coloured urine is sometimes seen in the nephrotic syndrome and is occasionally due to chyluria.

Table 116.1.   Causes of abnormal colour in the urine

Red	Brown/black	Green/blue
Haematuria*	Azodies	Obstructive jaundice
Haemoglobinuria*		
Myoglobinuria*	Alkaptonuria	Blue diaper syndrome
Porphyria	Methaemoglobinaemia	Hepatitis
Serratia marcescens	Melanin	Phenol poisoning
Urates	Tyrosinosis	Methylene blue
Anthrocyanine	Phenol poisoning	Indigo carmine
Rhodamine B	Aniline	Resorcinol
(food colouring)		
	Cascara	Tetrahydronaphthalene
Blackberries	Resorcinol	Methocarbamol
Phenolphthalein	Senna	Carotene
Pyridium	Thymol	Riboflavin
Aminopyrine	Hydroxyquinone	
Phenytoin		

*Positive test with haemastix.

Odour
Fresh urine has a distinctive smell. Infected urine may have a fishy odour. An ammoniacal smell is due to urea breakdown and may occur within the urinary tract if the urine is infected with proteus and some of the coliform organisms. However, an ammoniacal smell in infants is usually caused by splitting after the urine has been passed into the napkin. Some inborn errors of metabolism may give rise to unusual odours, for example maple syrup urine disease.

pH
Urine pH is usually measured with paper impregnated with chemicals which change colour in direct relationship to hydrogen ion concentration. A pH meter should be used for accurate measurement. pH must be measured on freshly voided urine or, alternatively, the urine can be kept under liquid paraffin whilst transported to the laboratory. If bacteriuria is present it is essential that the urinary pH is measured as soon as possible after voiding, since bacteria may metabolize the normal urinary constituents, thus affecting pH. The normal range is from pH 4·5 to pH 7·5 and a pH of greater than 7·5 suggests the presence of urea-splitting organisms and ammonia. Interpretation of the urinary pH is more meaningful if the metabolic state of the patient is known (e.g. inappropriately neutral in the presence of a metabolic acidosis). In the presence of normal renal function and a metabolic acidosis the urine pH should be less than 5·3. Less acid urine suggests a urinary acidification defect. It is particularly useful to document urinary pH during an acute illness and the observation of a normally acidified urine in the presence of a metabolic acidosis obviates the need for a formal urine acidification test.

Osmolality
With widespread availability of techniques measuring the depression of freezing point, osmolality has superseded specific gravity as a means of assessing the concentration of the urine. Only very small quantities of urine are required for this technique and it is less affected by the presence of urinary proteins than specific gravity measurements. The osmolar concentration of the urine depends upon the sum of all the electrolytes and other solutes such as urea, creatinine and glucose. Proteins present in the urine will contribute only slightly to the osmolality because of their large molecular size. Osmolality is best interpreted in the context of the clinical state of the patient (e.g. concentrated urine with a high osmolality in the presence of shock and oliguria suggests a prerenal cause for oliguria).

Urine Testing on the Ward
Urine testing strips are prepared commercially and are widely available so that the presence of blood, protein, glucose can be detected readily by this very simple procedure. It is possible to test specifically for the presence of albumin in the urine. The test is very sensitive, and from time to time insignificant amounts of albumin may be detected. It is possible to test for the presence of haemoglobin: myoglobin and whole red cells also give a positive result. The glucose oxidase method is used for detecting the presence of urinary glucose but if other reducing substances are suspected, use Clinitest which depends upon the colour change associated with the reduction of Fehling's solution. Urine testing strips for the presence of bacteriuria depend on the reduction of nitrites

to nitrates by bacteria, but unfortunately these tests give too high an incidence of false negative results to be of much clinical value.

Microscopy of Urine
Microscopy of fresh urine is best done on an uncentrifuged sample since centrifugation may damage casts. The freshly obtained urine is placed in a Fuchs–Rosenthal counting chamber using a pipette. Observations on the numbers of red cells and white cells/mm^3 as well as the presence of bacteria, casts, crystals and epithelial cells can be made. Delay in examination of urine by this technique will result in failure to detect red cells or casts which may be damaged or lysed during the interval between urine formation and examination.

Proteinuria
The presence of persistent proteinuria is strongly suggestive of significant renal disease. In adults there is generally less than 200 mg of protein/24 h. However, benign postural proteinuria may result in up to 1 g/day. The collection of a timed overnight urine sample will exclude proteinuria produced in the erect position and in children the amount of protein excreted is generally less than 4 mg/m^2/h. The presence of excessive quantities of low molecular weight proteins in the urine such as β_2-microglobulin or lysozyme suggest tubular damage, whereas albumin originates from the glomeruli. Proteinuria of sufficient severity to lower the serum albumin results in the nephrotic syndrome.

Glycosuria
Glycosuria may be due to hyperglycaemia or a reduced renal threshold. It occurs in tubular disorders including interstitial nephritis and Fanconi syndrome from a failure of tubular reabsorption.

Amino Aciduria
Excessive quantities of amino acids in the urine may be due to high serum levels or, alternatively, because of specific tubular defects with failure to reabsorb these compounds, e.g. cystinuria when 4 amino acids, cystine, lysine, arginine and ornithine are in the urine. In cystinosis there is a generalized amino aciduria which is due to a more generalized tubular defect (Fanconi syndrome). In children with phenylketonuria raised blood levels of phenylalanine, phenylpyruvic and phenyl lactic acid result in amino aciduria.

Phosphaturia
Phosphate is normally filtered at the glomerulus and reabsorbed in the renal tubules; failure to reabsorb it lowers the serum phosphate. The normal serum phosphate is slightly higher in females than in males, and higher in infants than adults. Although the major fall occurs between birth and 20 years there is a small reduction during adult life.

Calciuria
The normal calcium excretion in a child is less than 4 mg/kg/day (0·1 mmol/kg/day). Hypercalciuria may predispose to renal stone formation.

Glomerular Filtration Rate (GFR)
Glomerular filtration rate is one of the standard means of assessing glomerular

function. It depends on the renal blood flow, the glomerular permeability and the pressure difference across the basement membrane. At birth the glomerular filtration rate is approximately $30\,ml/min/1{\cdot}73\,m^3$ or less in pre-term infants, but rises to the normal level of 120 ml/min/1·73 m² by the age of 2. Assessment of glomerular filtration rates can be made accurately by studying the clearance from the circulation of chelating agents such as ^{51}Cr-EDTA or ^{99}Tc DTPA.

Creatinine and Creatinine Clearance

Creatinine is a breakdown product of muscle. It is filtered by the glomerulus and very little is secreted in the renal tubules, thus the clearance of creatinine approximates to glomerular filtration rate. Because creatinine production is related to muscle bulk, levels of serum creatinine in healthy children are considerably lower than those observed in adults. An approximation of glomerular filtration rate can be obtained from the following formula:

$$\text{GFR (ml.min/}1{\cdot}73\,m^2\text{)} = 40 \times \frac{\text{Height in centimetres}}{\text{Creatinine in micromoles/l}}$$

There is a rapid increase in creatinine production during puberty and conversely with prolonged illness with muscle wasting there may be a reduction in creatinine production. These deviations are reflected in serum creatinine without indicating true alterations in glomerular function. Under these circumstances it may be helpful to undertake a formal creatinine clearance.

Urea

Urea is produced from dietary protein. Acutely ill patients in a catabolic state have increased urea production due to breakdown of body protein which in the presence of renal impairment causes a rapid rise in blood urea. Rapid changes in blood urea may occur as a result of altered dietary protein intake and do not necessarily indicate changes in renal function.

Electrolytes

Abnormalities of kidney function can significantly affect the serum electrolyte levels. Knowledge of the patient's sodium and potassium is of diagnostic and therapeutic value.

Physical Measurements

Parameters essential in management of a patient with renal disease include: height, weight, surface area, blood pressure and fluid balance. Careful and regular attention to these details is essential in the management of childhood renal disease.

Radiological and Other Diagnostic Investigations

Intravenous Urography

This investigation is one of the most useful investigations of the urinary tract. Before ordering such an investigation it is important to know the renal function. A higher dose of contrast medium is required with a reduced glomerular filtration rate. Infants, young children and those in chronic renal failure should not be dehydrated prior to an intravenous pyelogram as this investigation is potentially dangerous if carried out in pathologically dehydrated patients and is unlikely to yield a satisfactory result under these circumstances. If peritoneal dialysis is in progress this will have to be discontinued during the period of the pyelogram to prevent dialysis of the contrast media. The pyelogram gives information about the shape, size and position of the kidneys as well as the cortical mass, the shape of the calyces, the size of the ureters and bladder. It is helpful in excluding obstruction.

Micturating Cystourethrogram
This investigation is poorly tolerated by most children and is particularly difficult in toddlers. It is used to show vesico-ureteric reflux and if appropriate pictures are taken can demonstrate or exclude urethral valves. It requires an experienced radiologist. A combination of micturating cystourethrography with pressure measurements may help to differentiate obstructive from neurogenic bladder problems. Because of the risk of introducing bacterial infection, antibiotic cover is recommended.

Antegrade Pyelography
A nephrostomy tube is inserted after an IVP or under ultrasound into the renal pelvis. Contrast media is injected to outline the pelvis to demonstrate a block. The tube can be left in situ to permit drainage.

Ultrasound
This technique which is quick and non-invasive has widespread application in the investigation of childhood renal disease. It is possible to demonstrate the presence, size and texture of the kidneys as well as the presence of cysts and obstruction.

Isotopes and the Gamma Camera
The use of the gamma camera in conjunction with [99]technetium labelled diethylene-triamine-pentacetic acid (DTPA) enables dynamic studies of renal function to be undertaken. The relative function of each kidney can be obtained from the slope of the first two minutes of the renogram curve and if total GFR is measured subsequently then a precise GFR can be obtained for each kidney. In the presence of good renal function it is possible to differentiate between normal drainage and obstruction (*Fig.* 116.1), although with poor function these differences are less easy to detect. It has been possible to detect vesico-ureteric reflux indirectly by observing the radioactive counts over the bladder, ureters and kidneys before, during and after micturition. DMSA is a mercury-containing compound which is filtered and then fixed in the tubules. Filling defects such as tumours and cysts as well as renal scars can be clearly seen.

Renal Biopsy
This may be done as an open surgical procedure but more often a needle biopsy is undertaken. Histological examination by light microscopy after appropriate staining is combined with electron microscopy and immunofluorescent studies. Usually a needle biopsy is undertaken only if both kidneys have good or equal function and the renal size is normal. Mild sedation and local anaesthetic are usually satisfactory. Renal biopsy is particularly helpful in the management of

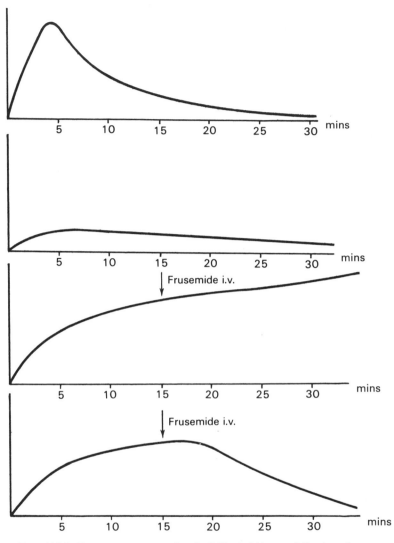

Fig. 116.1. Renogram curves for individual kidneys following the injection of ^{99}Tc DTPA. *a*, Normal; *b*, Poor renal function; *c*, Obstruction or acute tubular necrosis; *d*, Dilated collecting system.

glomerular disorders both in decisions about treatment and for prognosis. It is also helpful in cases of acute renal failure and in the management of renal transplants. Exclude coagulation disorders before undertaking a renal biopsy.

Chapter 117   ***URINARY TRACT INFECTION***

Definition

Urinary tract infection is present when organisms are multiplying in the urinary tract. The majority of infections recognized are bacterial although fungal, viral and parasitic infections also occur. To diagnose the condition with certainty bladder urine should be obtained by either suprapubic aspiration or urethral catheterization using an aseptic technique. Organisms obtained by either procedure originate in the urinary tract and are significant. These two techniques provide information which is more reliable and easier to interpret than midstream, 'clean catch' or bag urine samples which are prone to contamination. Unfortunately both suprapubic aspiration and urethral catheterization are invasive techniques and are not widely used for this reason. In practice, the first specimen of urine is obtained by bag and if infection is found, the urine is further examined after suprapubic or catheter aspiration. In the management of children with spina bifida where the abdomen is anaesthetic suprapubic aspiration of urine is usual.

Suprapubic Aspiration of Urine

After cleaning the skin of the lower abdomen with antiseptic solution a 20-ml syringe with a 19-gauge needle is advanced through the skin at right angles 1 cm above the symphysis pubis after ensuring that the child has a palpable bladder. If negative pressure is applied to the plunger of the syringe, urine enters the barrel as soon as the needle is in the bladder. The bladder should be emptied completely where possible. When such a sample is sent to the laboratory it should be clearly labelled as a suprapubic aspirate so that laboratory staff can interpret the result appropriately.

Midstream Urine Sample

This is obtained by catching the middle part of the urinary stream from a patient after cleansing with water or green soap the perineum in females and retracting the foreskin and cleansing the glans penis in males. This procedure is rarely carried out properly in children and the presence of organisms in such samples is frequently due to contamination.

'Clean Catch' Urine

It is often possible to catch the urine from an infant when the nappy has been removed during physical examination or routine nursing care. Doctors, nurses and parents are to be encouraged in the use of this non-invasive technique. Although it is easier to obtain good samples from male infants they can be obtained from female infants if the perineum is clean. The specimen can be sent immediately to the laboratory.

Bag Urine Collection

This technique is used when the child is not toilet trained, or does not co-operate with formal collection. It is adequate for chemical analysis but not reliable for obtaining timed samples since leakage is common. It is unreliable in the diagnosis of bacterial infections since contamination is very common. The risk of contamination is increased if the bag is not removed immediately the urine is passed. A small number of contaminating organisms will multiply rapidly in warm urine thus producing a heavy growth when the urine is plated out. If this type of urine sample is to be used for the diagnosis of urinary tract infection several samples must be sent and infection should only be assumed if a significant growth of the same organism can be reproduced on two or three occasions.

Asymptomatic Bacteriuria

Two percent of schoolgirls and 5% of young women have covert bacteriuria. Many of them have mild symptoms referable to the urinary tract. A third of schoolgirls with covert bacteriuria have vesico-ureteric reflux and a quarter have renal scarring. In some girls bacteriuria ceases spontaneously while in others it may persist for many years. This condition is much less common in boys.

Urinary Tract Infection in Infants

Urinary infection may be present in this age group with no symptoms or it may result in irritability, excessive crying, poor weight gain, vomiting, fever or severe illness with septicaemia or dehydration. Urinary tract infection in infants is more likely to cause renal damage than later in childhood. In the first month of life infection is more common in males than in females. This ratio is reversed thereafter.

Urinary Infection in Childhood

The presentation in toddlers is with a fever or febrile convulsion. Frequency and dysuria or a change in the normal voiding pattern may be noted. Although loin pain is rare, tenderness may be detected on physical examination in pyelonephritis. Urinary tract infections are often recurrent although the symptoms may not be so severe or may be absent.

Investigation of Child or Infant with Urinary Infection

Investigation should be directed to establishing the level of renal function, the exclusion of urinary tract obstruction and the localization of any pyelonephritic scarring (calyceal clubbing and loss of overlying cortex on intravenous urography). All children should have an IVP. This should be followed by a micturating cystogram in all children under 4 years, and in older children with scarring and/or frequent symptomatic infections. Any congenital renal anomalies should be noted (*Table* 117.1). These may require surgical treatment, e.g. relief of obstruction. There is evidence to suggest that vesico-ureteric reflux (usually demonstrated at cystography) may predispose to the development and progression of renal scarring, but no evidence that surgical correction of reflux alters the prognosis.

Management

Children with proven infection should have an appropriate antibiotic intravenously or orally, and intravenous fluids may be required, as infants may develop dehydration, electrolyte losses, uraemia and acidosis, which should be corrected in 24–48 h. Obstructive lesions should be sought (especially by ultrasound) and

Table 117.1.   Congenital renal anomalies

Primary renal problems	Obstructive lesions	Ureteric abnormalities
Renal agenesis	Pelvi-ureteric junction obstruction	Vesico-ureteric reflux
Dyplastic kidney	Vesico-ureteric junction obstruction	Duplex ureter
Hypoplastic kidney	Ureterocele	Ectopic ureter
Multicystic kidney	Outflow obstruction	Megacystis, megaureter
Horseshoe kidney	*a.* Valves	Prune belly syndrome
Malrotation of kidney	*b.* Other urethral problems	Ureterocele
Ectopic kidney	e.g. diverticula, stenosis	
Single kidney	*c.* Neurogenic bladder	
Duplex kidney		

relieved as soon as possible. The child should be investigated radiologically when better. Many children will have further urinary tract infections. In the majority of children further reinfection can be prevented by the use of long-term low-dose prophylaxis with trimethoprim or nitrofurantoin. Such measures may prevent progressive renal damage in infants and older children with gross vesico-uretic reflux. In some girls over 4 with normal radiology where the risk of renal damage is minimal long-term antibiotic therapy may be used to prevent frequent attacks associated with distressing symptoms. This risk of renal scarring is greatest in infancy so prophylactic antibiotics are indicated at this age. Surgery can correct vesico-ureteric reflux but not necessarily alter the course of the disease.

Chapter 118   # GLOMERULAR DISORDERS

There are a number of ways of classifying glomerular disorders. Three different aspects are:
1. Clinical syndromes.
2. Aetiology or underlying disease.
3. Histological appearance.

1. Clinical Syndromes Associated with Glomerular Diseases

Proteinuria
After exclusion of postural proteinuria, urological abnormalities and reflux nephropathy, then persistent proteinuria is likely to occur from glomerular disease. Proteinuria occurs in any progressive renal disease as end stage is approached but in the presence of glomerular disorders may occur with a normal GFR. Heavy proteinuria of sufficient severity to lower the serum albumin is known as the nephrotic syndrome. Children with mild proteinuria (less than 1 g/day or 40 mg/m^2/h) with normal renal function and a normal pyelogram

generally follow a benign course and renal biopsy does not usually contribute significantly to management.

A ratio of IgG: albumin (or transferrin) of $<0\cdot1$ is 'highly selective' and typical of idiopathic nephrotic syndrome with minimal histological changes.

Nephrotic Syndrome

Aetiology

In childhood 85–90% of cases of nephrotic syndrome are idiopathic and steroid-sensitive responding to prednisolone. Renal biopsy shows minimal histological changes. Other causes of nephrotic syndrome are shown in *Table* 118.1.

Table 118.1.   Causes of nephrotic syndrome in childhood

Primary Renal Lesions
   Minimal change (steroid-sensitive nephrotic syndrome)
   Mild mesangial proliferation
   Focal glomerulosclerosis
   Membranoproliferative glomerulonephritis
   Membranous nephropathy
   Proliferative glomerulonephritis
   Congenital nephrotic syndrome (Finnish type)

Secondary to Recognized Disease
   Henoch–Schönlein purpura
   Disseminated lupus erythematosus
   Acute post streptococcal glomerulonephirits
   Alport's syndrome
   Goodpasture's syndrome
   Diabetes—rare complication in children
   Syphilis
   Malaria
   Polyarteritis
   Neoplasia
   Sickle-cell anaemia
   Amyloid
   Hepatitis (Australia antigen positive)
   Nephrotoxins
   Other infections

Clinical Features

These children present with odema due to low serum albumin and usually normotensive. Boys are more often affected than girls. The peak age of onset is 6 years but it ranges from 6 months to adulthood. Proteinuria is usually highly selective, the glomeruli allow the passage of albumin in large quantities but not of larger molecules. Haematuria is occasionally present in small amounts during relapses but clears when the child is in remission. Occasionally, rapidly developing proteinuria results in a sudden fall in plasma oncotic pressure causing acute hypovolaemia, shock, oliguria, hypotension and tachycardia. Abdominal pain or vomiting may occur.

Treatment and Prognosis
Short term
1. Prednisolone 2 mg/kg/24 h or 60 mg/m^2/24 h for 4 weeks. Remission occurs when proteinuria ceases and the serum albumin rapidly returns to normal in a well nourished child. Steroids may then be stopped or reduced over a 6–8 week period. One-third of children have further isolated attacks of nephrotic syndrome and one-third will have frequent relapses. Alternate-day steroids up to 1 mg/kg may reduce the frequency of the attacks. The use of Albustix at home enables relapses to be detected before the child becomes symptomatic. With prompt treatment an attack may be aborted with minimal symptoms.
2. Acute hypovolaemic symptoms may be temporarily relieved by the infusion of salt-poor albumin in a dose of 1 g/kg but because of the continuing urinary protein leak it produces temporary benefit. If oedema and ascites are causing symptoms and are resistant to diuretic therapy they may respond to an infusion of salt-poor albumin given in conjunction with frusemide. Diuretics, fluid and sodium restriction should be used with caution in children since over-zealous use of these conventional forms of treatment for the management of nephrotic syndrome may precipitate hypovolaemia.
Long term
1. Cyclophosphamide 2·5–3 mg/kg/24 h for 6–8 weeks lengthens the period between relapses but does not necessarily reduce the total number. The relatively small benefit must be balanced against the potential dangers of cytotoxicity and marrow depression. Monitor WBC count and reduce dose if less than 4000 or polymorphs below 1000. Serious side effects are uncommon, although viral illness such as varicella and measles are hazardous. Higher doses, up to 5 mg/kg/24 h lower relapse rate but increase risk of unpleasant side effects such as alopecia, haemorrhagic cystisis and bone marrow suppression. May damage spermatozoa and result in infertility.
2. Chlorambucil is also effective in the management of frequently relapsing nephrotic syndrome but is a dangerous drug which should be used only after careful evaluation of the alternative and safer forms of therapy.

Haematuria
Isolated haematuria (without significant protein) may occur in a number of conditions (*see Table* 118.2) and can be distinguished from other causes of red or brown urine by the finding of a positive Haemastix test and the presence of red cells on microscopy of fresh urine. Red cells can be overlooked because of lysis in dilute urine. Red cell casts indicate a renal origin. An IVP should be carried out to exclude a tumour. The anomalies which give haematuria include horseshoe kidney, medullary sponge kidney, renal stones, reflux nephropathy, urinary tract infection, disorders of coagulation from anticoagulants and cyclophosphamide. Blood is often present in the urine sample during menstruation. Occasionally contamination with blood may be self induced as in some cases of the 'loin pain, haematuria syndrome' and in girls before the onset of periods presumably to simulate menstruation. After excluding these causes haematuria can be assumed to be of renal origin.

Recurrent Haematuria
In this condition haematuria is not associated with proteinuria. Recurrent attacks of macroscopic haematuria may be associated with loin pain, renal colic and

Table 118.2.   Isolated haematuria

Anatomical and Surgical Causes
  Wilms' tumour
  Trauma
  Urethral or bladder polyp
  Horseshoe kidney
  Pelviureteric junction obstruction

Inflammatory Causes
  Balanitis
  Urinary tract infection
  Cyclophosphamide therapy

Glomerulopathies
  Acute post-streptococcal nephritis
  Henoch–Schönlein nephritis
  Mesangiocapillary glomerulonephritis
  Focal proliferative glomerulonephritis
  (Mesangial IgA nephropathy)
  Alport's syndrome

bladder symptoms. It may be precipitated by intercurrent infection, particularly, of the upper respiratory tract. Red cells are sometimes present in the urine between attacks. There is normal renal function and radiology. Sometimes other members of the family are affected, suggesting a dominant inheritance. Renal biopsy may show mild focal proliferative changes and mesangial IgA and IgG deposits seen on immunofluorescence (Berger's disease). It is important to distinguish benign haematuria from Alport's syndrome, a familial condition which leads to renal failure and is associated with high tone deafness. Haematuria may be the presenting feature of mesangiocapillary disease, lupus nephritis or a rapidly progressive nephritis and often follows an attack of Henoch–Schönlein purpura. In these conditions it is usually associated with proteinuria. Proteinuria in conjunction with haematuria suggests a worse prognosis.

Nephritic Syndrome (Acute Nephritis)
This is characterized by haematuria, proteinuria, retention of salt and water resulting in weight gain, hypertension and oedema. The oedema is not due to hypoproteinaemia but sodium retention by the kidneys which may cause severe hypertension and/or pulmonary oedema. These problems can be avoided by careful restriction of salt and water and by the use of diuretics and antihypertensives. The cause is usually post-streptococcal nephritis but it may also occur with Henoch–Schönlein nephritis, systemic lupus erythematosus, rapidly progressive nephritis and membranoproliferative (mesangiocapillary) nephritis. An acute nephritic syndrome may go on to oliguria and acute renal failure. Dialysis may be needed.

Rapidly Progressive (Crescentic) Nephritis
Occasionally children may have a nephritis or nephrotic illness which progresses rapidly over a period of months to end-stage renal failure. During the early stages the renal biopsy usually shows a proliferative glomerulonephritis with numerous epithelial crescents. Cytotoxic drugs, steroids, anticoagulants, anti-

platelet agents and plasmaphoresis are used but benefit from these is unproven.

Chronic Renal Failure
Occasionally children with chronic glomerular disease may present with end-stage renal failure.

2. Aetiology

Many glomerular disorders are due to immune-mediated mechanisms. Circulating immune complexes have been demonstrated and in some the antigen has been identified, e.g. shunt nephritis (antigen *Staph. albus*). In lupus nephritis the antigen is the patient's own DNA. The cause in Goodpasture's syndrome is a circulating antibody to glomerular basement membrane. The appearance of granular deposits on the basement membrane or in the mesangium on immunofluorescent studies suggests immune complexes in the glomerulus. A linear appearance is found in antiglomerular basement membrane disease. The aetiology of steroid-sensitive nephrotic syndrome has not yet been established.

Acute Post-streptococcal Nephritis
This usually develops 2 weeks after a streptococcal throat infection with a group A beta-haemolytic streptococcus, Lancefield group 12. The child develops general malaise, cloudy urine and a puffy face. The diagnosis is confirmed by the presence of a raised ASO titre and a low serum complement (3rd component) which rises to normal in 1–8 weeks. Streptococci may be grown from the throat of the child and the relatives. Casts, red cells and white cells as well as proteinuria are usually present in the urine. Improvement is usual after 2 weeks but occasionally may be delayed.

Lupus Nephritis
Systemic lupus erythematosus is a systemic disease with joint swellings, rash, fever, arteritis, pericardial and pleural effusions. Renal involvement causes haematuria and/or proteinuria. The renal lesion may progress to a nephritic, nephrotic syndrome or progressive nephritis. Histology shows a variety of lesions from mild mesangial proliferation to diffuse proliferation, membranous nephropathy, mesangiocapillary changes or crescentic nephritis. The biopsy is rarely helpful in making the diagnosis but may be helpful in management. The renal lesion of lupus is steroid sensitive. Azathioprine or cyclophosphamide are used in addition to steroids in some cases. Treatment is usually required for life. Lupus in uncommon in childhood and occurs more often in girls than boys.

Henoch–Schönlein Purpura
A systemic disease with red macular rash, usually seen on the legs and buttocks, joint swellings, abdominal pain, intussusception and testicular involvement. Many children have microscopic haematuria and in the majority this disappears over a period of months. Some children develop proteinuria, nephrotic syndrome and rapidly progressive nephritis leading to end-stage renal failure. During the acute illness some children have acute nephritis and renal failure.

Goodpasture's Syndrome
This is an aggressive illness due to circulating antibodies to glomerular basement membrane which also react with the alveolar basement membrane causing pulmonary haemorrhage as well as acute nephritis. Plasmaphoresis and immuno-suppression may help before oliguria occurs.

Alport's Syndrome
This is a hereditary nephritis associated with deafness and ocular lesions. Males are more severely affected than females.

3. Histological Findings

The finding of normal glomeruli or very mild abnormalities is indicative of a mild disease process and generally a good prognosis. Irreversible damage is characterized by hyalinized or sclerosed glomeruli and tubular atrophy.

Membranous Nephropathy
A thickened basement membrane in the absence of other abnormalities indicates membranous nephropathy. This is usually associated with the nephrotic syndrome. The disease may slowly progress over 20 years to renal failure, but spontaneous improvement may occur. It is uncommon in children but may occur with lupus nephritis, tumours, drugs and infective agents.

Proliferative Glomerulonephirits
Proliferative lesions may be divided into:

a. Focal Proliferative Glomerulonephritis
The usual histological finding in children with recurrent haematuria. Mesangial IgA and IgG deposits often seen on immunofluorescence.

b. Diffuse Proliferative Glomerulonephritis
In acute post-streptococcal nephritis there is gross swelling of the glomeruli with obliteration of glomerular capillaries, exudation and inflammatory infiltrate. Acute and subacute nephritis (with or without nephrotic syndrome) due to other causes may also show proliferation. The presence of crescents indicates a worse prognosis. In rapidly progressive nephritis more than 50% of glomeruli show crescent formation.

c. Mesangiocapillary Glomerulonephritis
Histological appearance indicates a serious renal disease which may progress to renal failure in 3–10 years. It may present as recurrent haematuria, nephrotic syndrome, acute nephritis or chronic renal failure.

d. Minimal Change and Mild Mesangial Proliferation
Lesions are found in children with steroid-sensitive nephrotic syndrome and are associated with a good prognosis.

e. Focal Segmental Sclerosis
This lesion may be overlooked. Occurs in children with nephrotic syndrome but is often associated with resistance to steroids and a bad prognosis. Massive

proteinuria in infants with focal glomerulosclerosis may occur from birth and is difficult to manage. The disease progresses to renal failure. Focal glomerulosclerosis may occur in siblings. It is the second commonest cause of nephrotic syndrome in children.

Chapter 119   # TUBULAR DISORDERS

Tubular disorders may be a primary inherited disorder or secondary to generalized renal disease such as reflux nephropathy.

Nephrogenic Diabetes Insipidus

This condition occurs in males and is an X-linked recessive condition. Affected infants usually present in infancy with dehydration or pyrexia. Treatment is an adequate fluid intake. Thiazide diuretics are sometimes helpful in reducing the urine output.

Hypophosphataemic Rickets

This is an X-linked condition in which males are more severely affected than females. A defect in the tubular reabsorption of phosphate leads to hypophosphataemia and rickets which respond to very high doses of vitamin D or 1 α-hydroxycholecalciferol. Phosphate supplements are advisable. Serum calcium must be closely monitored to avoid hypercalcaemia and renal damage.

Renal Tubular Acidosis

Renal tubular acidosis may be due either to a proximal or a distal tubular abnormality. In proximal tubular acidosis a failure to reabsorb bicarbonate results in bicarbonate wasting in the urine. Distal tubular acidosis is due to inadequate hydrogen ion excretion. Failure to acidify the urine below pH 5·3 in the face of a metabolic acidosis suggests renal tubular acidosis. Infants may present with failure to thrive, vomiting, acidosis or hypotonia. Other electrolyte abnormalities may be present. Renal calcification and metabolic bone disease are recognized complications. Treatment with an adequate fluid and electrolyte intake and supplements of sodium or potassium bicarbonate are usually necessary.

Fanconi Syndrome

This is a proximal tubular defect of reabsorption of glucose, amino acids, phosphate and electrolytes. Patients present with acidosis, dehydration or rickets. This syndrome is associated with a number of inherited conditions causing widespread abnormalities in addition to the renal problems, e.g. Lowe's syndrome. It may also occur secondary to nephrotoxic agents, e.g. lead.

Cystinosis

This is an inherited disorder in which cystine accumulates within cells, particularly those of the reticulo-endothelial system. Accumulation in the renal tubules results in rickets, Fanconi's syndrome and later progresses to renal failure. Other tissues affected include the cornea, the thyroid gland and the brain. As the metabolic defect is intracellular, renal transplantation can be performed when end-stage renal failure occurs.

Chapter 120   CYSTIC CONDITIONS INVOLVING THE KIDNEY (*Table* 120.1)

Solitary Cysts of the Kidney

Solitary renal cysts are common coincidental findings e.g. during IVP, ultrasound or at operation. In adults they are differentiated from malignant tumours by the presence of fluid on aspiration and the absence of malignant cells. They are rare in children, tend to be small and should be differentiated from other renal cysts. No treatment is required.

Table 120.1.   Cystic conditions of the kidney

1. Simple renal cysts
2. Cystic renal dysplasia
3. Polycystic kidneys
   a. Adult type
   b. Infantile type
4. Medullary cysts
   a. Familial juvenile nephronophthisis
   b. Medullary cystic disease
5. Microcystic disease (Finnish type congenital nephrotic syndrome)
6. Congenital and inherited disorders associated with cystic kidneys e.g. tuberous sclerosis, Jeune's syndrome

Cystic Dysplasia

The kidneys are cystic and show dysplastic features, are usually non-functional and do not have an ipsilateral ureteric orifice. May be diagnosed in fetus by ultrasound. If both kidneys are involved the condition may present with oligohydramnios and Potter's syndrome or severe renal impairment. May occur with pelviureteric junction obstruction or urethral valves.

Medullary Sponge Kidney

In this condition there is cystic dilatation of the collecting ducts in the renal papilla. Histological changes are found in the medulla and renal impairment is rare. Usually first recognized in teenagers. It presents with renal calculi, haematuria or urinary tract infection and may be detected incidentally. Occasionally renal papillary calcification or stones may be detected on plain radiography but usually the abnormal papillae are seen during intravenous urography. Treatment is of renal calculi, infection and pain relief. Hypercalciuria which is often present will require treatment to reduce the risk of recurrent stone formation.

Calyceal Cysts

Calyceal cysts or diverticula are small cystic cavities which lie in the renal parenchyma peripheral to but communicating with the minor calyces. They are lined with transitional epithelium. They may be congenital or acquired and are usually found incidentally when excretion urography has been undertaken for some other reason. Occasionally infection or stone formation may give rise to symptoms and require treatment.

Infantile Polycystic Disease

This is an autosomal recessive condition in which affected infants have large cystic kidneys which are easily palpable at birth. Infants may be stillborn or gross abdominal distension may interfere with labour. Oligohydramnios may occur from poor urine formation and infants may have pulmonary hypoplasia and other features of Potter's syndrome. Those that survive may have impaired renal function with problems in sodium handling or hypertension but some thrive and survive for several years before developing renal impairment. Affected children have multiple hepatic cysts, hepatic fibrosis and impaired hepatic function. The intravenous urography shows opacified cortical cysts easily visualized throughout which may remain opacified for several days. A film should be taken 24–48h after injection of contrast media if this condition is suspected.

Adult Polycystic Disease of the Kidney

This condition in which cysts are distributed throughout the kidney is transmitted as an autosomal dominant. Renal failure may develop after the 3rd decade although renal enlargement is usually present some years before. Hypertension, recurrent haematuria and septicaemia occur. Renal enlargement may be present at birth but renal impairment is rare in infancy. Cystic enlargement is progressive. Polycystic kidneys may look normal on intravenous urography or ultrasound examination during childhood. No treatment prevents progress and little is gained from investigation before the late teens or early twenties, prior to marriage.

Familial Juvenile Nephronophthisis

This condition is clinically similar to medullary cystic disease. It is autosomal recessively inherited and is a progressive condition leading to renal failure after the 3rd year. Impaired tubular function causing thirst and salt wasting occurs early; proteinuria may be absent or minimal until end-stage renal failure is reached. In some families the condition is associated with tapetoretinal degeneration (retinal renal dysplasia). In contrast, medullary cystic disease—an autosomal dominant—usually presents with uraemia in the 3rd decade. The kidneys are of normal size and the cysts are smaller than those seen in infantile or adult polycystic kidney disease. They do not opacify with contrast media.

Renal Cortical Cysts

Diffuse renal cortical cysts are seen in the Finnish type of congenital nephrotic syndrome. This condition which presents with nephrotic syndrome during the first months of life progresses to renal failure.

Renal Cysts Associated with Syndromes

A number of congenital syndromes, most of which are thought to be transmitted by recessive inheritance are associated with renal cysts:

Tuberous sclerosis

von Hippel–Lindau syndrome

Zellweger cerebrohepatorenal syndrome

Jeune's disease (asphyxiating thoracic dystrophy)

Ehlers–Danlos syndrome.

In addition cortical microcysts may be associated with multiple congenital malformations and chromosome abnormalities.

Chapter 121   # ACUTE RENAL FAILURE

This is usually a reversible condition of sudden onset. Oliguria is usually present (<0.5 ml/kg/h). There is an accumulation of waste products, urea, creatinine, uric acid, and loss of normal homeostasis (sodium, potassium, bicarbonate, water).

Causes of Acute Renal Failure

1. Prerenal causes (*see Table* 121.1)
2. Renal causes:
   - 2.1 Acute tubular necrosis
   - 2.2 Glomerulonephritis
   - 2.3 Nephrotoxins
   - 2.4 Interstitial nephritis
   - 2.5 Vascular catastrophes
   - 2.6 Haemolytic uraemic syndrome
   - 2.7 Malignant hypertension
3. Obstruction

In infants with acute renal failure, renal venous thrombosis and renal medullary and cortical necrosis should also be considered. These usually give haematuria. Recovery of renal function is often incomplete giving chronic renal insufficiency and hypertension.

On occasions children with chronic renal disease may present acutely following an intercurrent illness.

Initial management consists of identifying and correcting the precipitating factors (e.g. correction of poor renal perfusion, removal of nephrotoxic drugs, relief of obstruction). Subsequently fluid and electrolyte balance must be maintained.

Table 121.1.   Prerenal causes of acute renal failure

1. Pump failure
   Congenital heart lesion
   Acquired
      myocarditis
      infarction
      pericarditis
      valve lesions
      cardiomyopathy
      cardiogenic shock

2. Loss of circulating blood volume
   Haemorrhage
   Dehydration
      diarrhoea
      vomiting
      renal concentrating problems
      diuretics
      inadequate fluid intake
   Hypoproteinaemia
      burns
      nephrotic syndrome

Prerenal Failure (*Table* 121.1)

Any condition resulting in poor cardiac output and/or poor peripheral circulation can give rise to poor renal blood flow which will reduce the glomerular filtration rate. There is a redistribution of renal blood flow with less blood going to the outer cortical nephrons. If the renal blood flow falls below a critical level insufficient clearance of waste products occurs. This may occur with acute blood loss, dehydration, acute protein loss (in the nephrotic syndrome), shock following burns, trauma or septicaemia and in any cardiac condition in which cardiac output is severely reduced.

Features of Poor Peripheral Circulation
1. Poor colour and poor skin perfusion
2. Cold extremities
3. Normal or low blood pressure
4. Large central/peripheral temperature gap

Features of Low Circulating Volume
1. Normal or raised pulse rate
2. Normal or low blood pressure
3. Low JVP or CVP
4. Small liver
5. Weight loss (in dehydration)
6. Features of dehydration
7. Large central/peripheral temperature gap ($>2\,°C$)

Features of Pump Failure
1. Poor peripheral circulation
2. Evidence of cardiac pathology

3. Elevated wedge pressure
4. Elevated JVP or CVP
5. Big liver

Careful biochemical analysis of blood and urine enables distinction between oliguria due to poor perfusion (prerenal causes) and established renal damage.

In prerenal oliguria and uraemia the urinary sodium is low due to avid tubular sodium reabsorption facilitated by the renin–angiotensin–aldosterone mechanism. The urine to plasma urea and creatinine ratio is greater than 5 : 1 (10 : 1 for adults) and the urine osmolality is greater than the plasma osmolality (*Table* 121.2). This is not so in children with dehydration secondary to impaired renal function or salt-wasting conditions or from diuretics, where a ratio of urine to plasma urea of greater than five may be associated with an inappropriately high urinary sodium.

Table 121.2.   Urine : plasma ratio in renal failure

	Acute Tubular Necrosis	Prerenal
Urea	<5 :1	>10:1
Creatinine	<15:1	>20:1
Sodium	>30:1	<20:1
Osmolality	≤1·1:1	>1·5:1

Management of Acute Renal Failure

1. Correct prerenal causes.
2. Observe bladder and urinary stream or catheterise.
3. Give frusemide, 1 mg/kg i.v. initially. If no response after 2 hours repeat with a larger dose. Maximum 10 mg/kg.
4. Give mannitol, 0·4 g/kg i.v.
5. Provide fluids to cover insensible loss and urinary output and other measured losses (if patient is overloaded reduce intake further).
6. Provide a high calorie diet with protein 1 g/kg/day. Reduce sodium content if patient is overloaded or hypertensive. Reduce potassium content if hyperkalaemic.
7. Treat hypertension by a reduction in sodium and water intake, frusemide and antihypertensive drugs.
8. Hyperkalaemia (K^+ > 6·0 mmol/l) should be treated by a reduction in potassium intake, calcium or sodium resonium (1 g/kg up to 15 g q.d.s.) and in emergencies by glucose and insulin, sodium bicarbonate and calcium gluconate infusions. Dialysis may be required.
9. Acidosis may require supplements of sodium bicarbonate. If severe and worsening, dialysis is indicated. Elevated serum phosphate may be treated with phosphate binders and severe hypocalcaemia should be treated with intravenous calcium gluconate.
10. Blood transfusion should be given with caution because of the risk of precipitating severe hypertension. Packed cells in a dose of 10 ml/kg are usually well tolerated and raise the haemoglobin by 2 g/dl.
11. Ultrasound and/or intravenous pyelography (using a high dose and tomograph) should be undertaken if the cause is not clear to exclude obstruction.

12. If normal-sized kidneys are present and the diagnosis in doubt renal biopsy may establish the aetiology and give the prognosis.

13. During the recovery phase there may be a brisk diuresis. It is important to ensure adequate fluid intake at this time.

14. Peritoneal or haemodialysis may be indicated if conservative measures fail to hold the patient in a stable condition. In children haemodialysis is only occasionally necessary in acute renal failure. The introduction of dialysis may produce a dramatic improvement in the patient's condition and will often enable a free diet with better calorie intake to be given.

15. During the management of a child with acute renal failure frequent observations should be made of weight and blood pressure, and electrolytes and urea. Haemoglobin and blood film should be undertaken to exclude haemolytic uraemic syndrome and a clotting screen should be undertaken for intravascular coagulation.

Indications for Dialysis
1. Urea > 40 mmol/l and rising
2. Potassium > 6·5 mmol/l
3. Severe acidosis
4. Severe fluid overload
5. Severe hypertension

After the initial management an attempt should be made to establish the cause if this is not apparent.

Postrenal or Obstructive Causes of Renal Failure

Clues about the presence of an obstructive lesion are often obtained from the history or examination. In childhood the majority of obstructive lesions leading to acute renal failure are in the urethra or bladder, e.g. urethral valves, diverticula, ureteroceles and neurogenic bladders. Less commonly, bilateral lesions involving the ureters may occur, such as pelviureteric junction obstruction, renal calculi, clot retention in relation to trauma or malignancy or obstruction by malignant glands or pelvic tumour. In children with single kidneys, unilateral ureteric obstruction presents early because of oliguria. If the problem is related to urinary outflow tract there will be a large palpable bladder and usually bilateral hydronephroses will be felt. The finding of neurological signs in the lower limbs or of spina bifida occulta on radiography suggests a neurogenic cause. Ultrasound is now the primary investigation of choice in an experienced unit to exclude obstructive lesions. If obstruction is present it should be relieved as soon as possible by bladder catheterization and continuous drainage or by the use of a nephrostomy tube if there is ureteric obstruction. Ureteroceles may be treated by surgical 'decapping'. Retrograde pyelography is useful for defining ureteric obstruction in adults but is technically difficult in small children and rarely used. Urethral valves are the commonest cause of obstructive uropathy in male infants.

Renal Causes of Acute Renal Failure

When pre- and postrenal causes have been excluded it is probable that intrinsic renal damage has occurred.

Acute Tubular Necrosis
This is a reversible condition of sudden onset, which follows an identifiable insult such as haemorrhage or shock, and may be due to prolonged interference with renal blood flow. After restoration of the circulation and good renal blood flow filtration occurs although oliguria and renal failure persist. On renal biopsy there is a characteristic appearance with evidence of damage to the cells lining the renal tubules. Tubular necrosis usually resolves spontaneously in less than 6 weeks with a dramatic diuresis provided the patient has been kept alive by conservative treatment or dialysis. Occasionally it may present with polyuria.

Chapter 122	*CHRONIC RENAL FAILURE*

The major causes are listed in *Table* 122.1. Chronic renal failure is suspected if biochemical evidence of renal failure is present and no evidence for reversible causes can be found. Features favouring chronic rather than acute renal failure include a long history of malaise, absence of acute illness, normochromic anaemia, pigmentation, evidence of rickets or hyperparathyroidism and short stature. Antegrade pyelography may be very helpful.

Table 122.1.   Causes of chronic renal failure in children

Congenital
  Hypoplastic kidneys
  Dysplastic kidneys
  Cystic dysplastic kidneys
  Infantile polycystic kidneys
  Obstructive lesions, e.g. urethral valves

Acquired
  Reflux nephropathy
  Glomerulonephritis
  Obstructive uropathy
  Neurogenic bladder
  Focal glomerulosclerosis
  Cystinosis
  Oxalosis
  Alport's syndrome
  Interstitial nephritis
  Other inherited conditions
  Cortical or medullary necrosis
  Renal vein thrombosis

Management

Conservative Treatment
First correct contributory pre- and postrenal factors. Look for and treat obstruction and infection. Hypertension which occurs in approximately one-third of children with chronic renal failure, is usually due to sodium retention and responds to reduction of total body sodium, e.g. by salt restriction and/or diuretics. Beta-blockers and peripheral vasodilators are helpful. Persistent

hypertension hastens renal failure. Occasionally hypertension from excessive renin output occurs and is more difficult to manage but angiotensin-blocking agents may be helpful. Children who are not hypertensive may be relatively sodium depleted due to the loss of normal tubular sodium reabsorption. Under these circumstances the circulating blood volume and therefore the GFR is reduced.

An increase in sodium and water improves renal function. Individuals with chronic renal failure lose renal concentrating ability and have obligatory polyuria. Failure to provide sufficient fluids causes dehydration. Potassium output cannot be adjusted by the failing kidney and the intake must be manipulated to keep the serum potassium within physiological limits. Inadequate calorie intake and poorly treated metabolic bone disease contribute to the growth failure often seen in children with chronic renal failure. Dialysis and transplantation should be considered for children with end-stage renal failure. For the very young and severely handicapped child decisions about whether to treat are extremely difficult. Adequate discussion with parents and child about the present and future problems is most important. Preparation of vascular access by the formation of an arteriovenous fistula in good time and judicious sparing of forearm veins will aid the smooth transition from chronic renal failure to haemodialysis.

Haemodialysis
Haemodialysis in children requires equipment appropriate for the size of the child. It is usually required three times weekly for 3–6 hours per session but more frequent dialyses may be required during intercurrent illness. Provided vascular access is good most children do well on haemodialysis. However, home-based haemodialysis poses great stress on the families. Continuation with normal activities should be encouraged and full-time school is advised for the majority of children.

Haemodialysis does not restore normality as the patient remains in mild renal failure. Anaemia and metabolic bone disease are frequent. Fluid and sodium restriction should be related to the urine output. Hypertension can usually be controlled by dialysis provided the sodium and water intake is not excessive. Dietary potassium restriction is often needed. Linear growth is sometimes severely retarded on dialysis. A good calorie intake may aid normal growth. Puberty is often delayed.

Continuous Ambulatory Peritoneal Dialysis (CAPD)
This new treatment depends upon insertion of a Tenckhoff peritoneal cannula, usually under general anaesthetic. A suitable bag of fluid (30–50 ml/kg) is connected to the cannula and allowed to run into the peritoneal cavity. The empty bag may then be rolled up until the bag is run out and changed for a fresh one 4–8 hours later. Most children require 4 or 5 bags daily for adequate dialysis. There is probably a better exchange of large diffusible molecules than with haemodialysis. Anaemia is less severe on CAPD than with haemodialysis. Growth may be better but metabolic bone disease remains a problem. Peritoneal infection is the main drawback. Children and families find CAPD less stressful than haemodialysis.

Renal Transplantation
Renal transplantation is the best treatment for most children, especially for growth and rehabilitation. Many parents want to donate kidneys to their children, however the failure of a live donor kidney has far-reaching consequences on the family. Azathioprine and steroids are given to prevent rejection. Prednisolone on alternate

days produces less adrenal suppression than daily steroids and hence better growth. Acute rejection is shown by a sudden decline in renal function, development of hypertension or oliguria and usually responds to a large dose of steroids either orally or intravenously. Antilymphocytic globulin is occasionally useful. Cyclosporin is a new drug which may prevent transplant rejection but one drawback is its nephrotoxicity.

Patients with renal transplants are susceptible to viral infections. Measles and chickenpox can both produce serious life-threatening illness. Where possible if the child has not had natural exposure to measles the immunization should be offered 2 months before transplantation. Children who have not had these exanthemas should receive the appropriate immunglobulin if a definite contact has occurred.

Metabolic Bone Disease

Children with any form of chronic renal failure develop radiological features of rickets and there may be evidence of hyperparathyroidism (subperiosteal erosions of middle phalanges). Treatment is by lowering the serum phosphate using phosphate binders, ensuring an adequate calcium intake, giving vitamin D analogues such as 1 α-hydroxycholecalciferol and regular monitoring of calcium, phosphate, alkaline phosphatase and wrist radiographs.

Hyperparathyroidism may cause hypercalcaemia which prevents proper dosage of 1 α-hydroxycholecalciferol so that parathyroidectomy may be necessary.

Chapter 123	*BLOOD PRESSURE AND HYPERTENSION*

Blood pressure rises with age in normal healthy children (*Table* 123.1). The blood pressure in preterm infants is lower than that in term infants. Blood pressure tends to be slightly higher in tall children and is often raised in association with obesity.

Table 123.1. 10th and 90th centiles for blood pressure during childhood

Age	Systolic		Diastolic	
	10th	90th	10th	90th
Newborn	72	88	38	54
1	82	103	41	70
5	83	116	43	75
10	86	128	50	79
16	94	134	54	75

Measurement of Blood Presssure

Direct arterial blood pressure is sometimes used in intensive care both of neonates and older children. Most observations of blood pressure are made by a sphygmomanometer. The bladder of the cuff chosen must have a width sufficient to cover two-thirds of the upper arm and be long enough to surround the arm and applied carefully so that alterations in pressure within the cuff are transmitted to the tissues in the arm. When auscultation is impossible in infants the radial pulse may be used to determine systolic blood pressure. The Doppler method is similar and reliable. A Doppler sensor is placed over the antecubital fossa. Changes in the tone of the emitted sound indicate systolic and diastolic blood pressure. Recently, equipment has become available for measuring blood pressure by the detection of oscillation. The equipment is expensive but simple to use and reliable, provided the machine is calibrated against a mercury manometer.

Hypertension

Hypertension is present if the blood pressure exceeds the 97th centile for the patient's age. Untreated hypertension predisposes to heart disease, strokes and renal impairment. Severe or malignant hypertension in childhood may result in cardiac failure with pulmonary oedema, hypertensive encephalopathy, cerebral haemorrhage and renal failure. Hypertension commonly accompanies a renal disease, and is usually related to sodium overload. Less commonly hypertension is due to excessive renin output. Hypertension may present with a facial palsy.

Causes of Hypertension
1. Essential hypertension
2. Renal hypertension
   - 2.1 With diffuse renal disease
   - 2.1.1 With renal impairment—acute or chronic renal failure
   - 2.1.2 With sodium retention—acute nephritis—nephrotic syndrome—interstitial nephritis
   - 2.1.3 Obstruction—acute or—chronic
   - 2.1.4 Renal transplant rejection
   - 2.2 Unilateral renal disease
   - 2.2.1 Pyelonephritis scarring (may be bilateral)
   - 2.2.2 Hydronephrosis
   - 2.2.3 Congenital renal hypoplasia/dysplasia
   - 2.2.4 Renal artery stenosis
   - 2.2.5 Renal tumour (Wilms' tumour)
   - 2.2.6 Post-traumatic
   - 2.2.7 Arteriovenous fistulae and aneurysms
3. Non-renal hypertension
   - 3.1 Endocrine
   - 3.2 Miscellaneous: Guillain–Barré Syndrome, Stevens–Johnson syndrome, leukaemia, bacterial endocarditis, hypernatraemia, poliomyelitis, familial dysautonomia, hypercalcaemia, mercury poisoning, raised intracranial pressure, steroid administration, amphetamines, paraplegia.

Investigation of Hypertension
The history, examination and investigations should seek a renal or endocrine cause. Proteinuria or haematuria suggests diffuse renal disease. Intravenous pyelography will demonstrate unilateral disease, e.g. renal artery stenosis. Early films show delayed excretion of contrast on the affected side. Later films show

increased density of contrast medium on the affected side. Other causes of a small kidney include congenital renal hypoplasia or dysplasia and reflux nephropathy. The diagnosis of renovascular hypertension is supported by a high resting renin level and if unilateral disease is suspected the renin values from the affected side are generally elevated. Renal arteriography is the definitive method for demonstrating renal artery stenosis. Stenosis may be present in the segmental renal arteries. Renal artery stenosis may be a congenital anomaly or associated with other vascular lesions such as fibromuscular dysplasia. Compression of the renal artery by malignant glands or tumour also occurs occasionally.

Treatment
Treatment aims are to stabilize with antihypertensive drugs, and relieve reversible causative factors. The drugs commonly used are beta-blockers, peripheral vasodilators and diuretics with a reduction in sodium intake. Patients with a high renin output are helped by angiotensin-blocking agents (captopril), using a small initial dose to avoid severe hypotension. Differential renal function studies should be undertaken with unilateral renal parenchymal disease before considering nephrectomy which is done only if the function of the affected side is very poor. Obstruction should be relieved. A severely scarred pyelonephritic kidney should be removed only if the opposite kidney is normal and shows compensatory hypertrophy. Renal artery stenosis may be corrected in older children but is difficult in infants. Dilatation of the artery using a balloon catheter at arteriography is sometimes successful. If renal disease is bilateral then unilateral nephrectomy may make the problem worse rather than better.

Malignant Hypertension

Malignant hypertension is associated with fundal haemorrhages, exudates and papilloedema. Renal damage secondary to hypertension, heart failure and pulmonary oedema usually occur when fundal changes are present, as may hypertensive encephalopathy. Urgent treatment to lower blood pressure is required but too rapid a fall can lead to brainstem or cerebral infarction. Methyldopa, hydrallazine, frusemide and beta-blockers are usually effective but intravenous diazoxide given slowly or an infusion of sodium nitroprusside may be required. In very difficult cases dialysis may be indicated, particularly if renal function is severely impaired.

Chapter 124	*CONGENITAL ANOMALIES OF THE RENAL TRACT*

These may arise from early fetal damage or from inherited disorders, and are especially serious when normal renal tissue is reduced or obstruction is present.

Low-set ears, abnormalities of the ear lobe and single umbilical artery are associated with renal anomalies. If these anomalies are not obvious at birth routine radiological investigations are of little value since obstructive lesions are uncommon and most of the anomalies detected are unlikely to have pathological significance.

Potter's Syndrome

Arises when any renal condition causes reduced amount of urine in utero, e.g. renal agenesis, severe hypoplasia, infantile polycystic kidneys or obstructive lesions. Oligohydramnios is often noted during pregnancy. The affected infant may have low-set ears, a small chin, a broad flat nose and marked epicanthic folds. Other features include pulmonary hypoplasia and flexion deformities of the limbs, abnormalities of the genitalia. The appearance of the infant is thought to be due to the mechanical effect of insufficient amniotic fluid.

Renal Duplication

This varies from a bifid renal pelvis to a completely duplicated renal system with two ureteric orifices. The upper moiety of the kidney is associated with the lower ureteric orifice because the ureters cross. The ureters are occasionally complicated by a ureterocele at the lower end, which can cause bladder outflow obstruction. Hydronephrosis or pyonephrosis may develop. Vesico-ureteric reflux more commonly occurs in the upper and outer ureteric orifice to the lower moiety of the kidney. The ureter may have an ectopic orifice in the urethra or vagina, giving rise to continual dribbling requiring surgical correction. Many individuals with renal duplication are fit and well and the abnormality may be detected incidentally.

Renal Ectopia

In this condition the kidney is in an abnormal position such as in the pelvis or the opposite side of the body, and may have vesico-ureteric reflux, poor function, and infection. A pelvic kidney can be missed at IVP but will be detected with a DMSA scan.

Horseshoe Kidney

In this condition the lower poles are fused or joined by a fibrous band. The kidneys are often rotated so that the calyces are viewed end on at pyelography. Occasionally the ureters may be compressed where they pass over the lower poles. Vesico-ureteric reflux and infection often occur. Needle biopsy of a horseshoe kidney is dangerous because of the unusual position of the hilar vessels and should not be undertaken.

Pelviureteric Junction Obstruction

This condition which may be unilateral or bilateral may present with pain, infection, a mass or renal impairment. The child has unilateral abdominal pain and swelling after a large drink or a diuretic. The symptoms may disappear for weeks or months. IVP shows distended pelvis and calyces but no ureter. Isotope studies are characteristic. Surgery is required.

Vesico-ureteric reflux is usually due to a short submucosal segment within the bladder. It predisposes to urinary tract infection and renal scarring, is familial, and improves with age.

Obstruction at the Lower End of the Ureter

This is an uncommon congenital anomaly and may be associated with poorly functioning kidneys.

Megaureter

Megaureters are very large ureters with abnormally thin walls and deficiency or absence of smooth muscle. They may be associated with an abnormal bladder, (megacystis megaureter syndrome). Renal function is often poor.

Prune Belly Syndrome (*Triad Syndrome*)

This is a rare anomaly in which there is megacystis megaureter, absence of abdominal wall musculature and bilateral undescended testes.

Ectopia Vesicae

Ectopia vesicae is obvious at birth. The ureters open into bladder mucosa on the anterior abdominal wall. The pelvis is abnormal with failure of fusion of the symphysis pubis. The bladder mucosa is usually removed to prevent malignancy. Ureters may be implanted into a conduit.

Urethral Valves

This may present at birth with a big bladder and loin masses. Occasionally urinary ascites is present. The child may present with infection or renal failure. Early surgical relief after correction of electrolyte disturbances and infection is essential. In infants not fit for surgery free drainage should be provided by urethral or suprapubic catheter. Many infants and children with urethral valves have impaired renal function.

Neurogenic Bladder

Occurs with spina bifida and is apparent at birth. In spina bifida occulta the neurogenic bladder may remain undetected until the child presents with difficulty in walking, enuresis or infection. Neurogenic bladder gives dilatation of the upper renal tracts and vesico-ureteric reflux. Deterioration of renal function is common but may be delayed or prevented by intermittent self-catheterization or internal sphincterotomy. Neurogenic bladder may present with urinary tract infection. This problem requires careful evaluation and management. The advent of bladder pressure studies and intermittent self-catheterization have significantly altered the management of this problem in children.

Hypospadias

In this condition the urethral orifice is on the underside of the shaft of the penis. Surgery may be indicated especially with chordee.

Epispadias

The urethral orifice is on the dorsum of the penis.

Undescended Testes

In infants and toddlers the testes easily retract from the scrotum towards the inguinal ring particularly if the child is apprehensive or the examiner's hand cold. Truly undescended testes are unlikely to descend spontaneously after the first year and need surgery. If the testes are undescended bilaterally it is wise to confirm the sex.

Ambiguous External Genitalia

The external genitalia of virilized female hermaphrodite and incompletely masculinized male may be very similar. There is usually a significant phallus and an opening on the ventral surface or perineum with rugose skin in the region of the scrotum. At birth such anomalies will require urgent and full evaluation so that the parents can be properly advised about the sex of rearing for such an infant.

Chapter 125   *INTERSTITIAL NEPHRITIS*

A condition in which there are inflammatory cells in the interstitium of the renal parenchyma. The tubules may show atrophy, dilatation or cellular damage. In chronic cases interstitial fibrosis and tubular atrophy are accompanied by sclerosed glomeruli whereas in the early or acute lesions the cellular infiltrate predominates; chronic interstitial nephritis is seen in children with chronic pyelonephritic scarring. Other causes are juvenile nephronophthisis, cystinosis, oxalosis and uric acid nephropathy. Acute interstital nephritis is an allergic reaction to drugs, e.g. methicillin and phenytoin, and usually presents with acute renal failure and a rash.

Chapter 126   *STONES*

Renal calculi are uncommon in childhood—frequency is less than 1% of adults. Stones are often associated with urinary infection and can be divided into those which arise secondary to infection often with *B. proteus* and/or stasis in the urinary tract, those due to metabolic disorders and those with no predisposing cause. In the latter group minor metabolic abnormalities including hypercalcaemia may play a part. Recognized causes of metabolic stones include cystinuria, hyperuricaemia, oxalosis, hyperparathyroidism, renal tubular acidosis and abnormalities of xanthine metabolism. The stones of cystinuria may be radiolucent. In this disorder there is a failure by the renal tubule to reabsorb cystine, lysine, arginine and ornithine. The condition is recessively inherited. An increased fluid intake, particularly at night will enable an increased load of solutes to be excreted and is recommended whatever the cause. Infection should be treated, although sterilization of the urine is impossible in the presence of a large stone. Large stones which cannot pass spontaneously and any causing obstruction should be removed surgically.

Alkalinization of the urine with oral sodium bicarbonate will increase the solubility of cystine and uric acid. Renal calculi cause renal damage as a result of obstruction and infection and may lead to renal failure.

Bladder calculi are now uncommon in western countries but still occur in the Middle and Far East, mainly in males under 5 years of age.

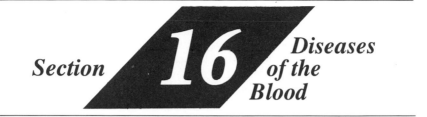

Section **16** *Diseases of the Blood*

Chapter 127

PHYSIOLOGY

Anatomy of Blood Formation

Normal blood values at birth, infancy and childhood, *see Table 127.1.*

Table 127.1. Mean red blood cell values at various ages

Age	Haemoglobin (g/dl)	Haematocrit (%)	Red Cell Count (10^{12}/litre)	MCV (fl)	MCH (pg)	MCHC (g/dl)
Cord blood	16·5	51	4·7	108	34	33
1 to 3 days (capillary)	18·5	56	5·3	108	34	33
2 weeks	16·5	51	4·9	105	34	33
1 month	14·0	43	4·2	104	34	33
3 to 6 months	11·5	35	3·8	91	30	33
6 months to 2 years	12·0	36	4·5	78	27	33
2 to 6 years	12·5	37	4·6	81	27	34
6 to 12 years	13·5	40	4·6	86	29	34

Biochemistry of Haemoglobin

Function of haemoglobin is to transport oxygen and carbon dioxide and help to buffer pH.

1. Normally composed of:

        1.1 Haem—an iron-containing porphyrin. Iron is in ferrous form (Fe^{2+}) and has bond available for loose union with oxygen.

        1.2 Globin—consisting of two alpha and two beta polypeptide chains of amino acids—total 574 per molecule.

        Varieties of haemoglobin all due to differences in globins. Substitution of but one amino acid is sufficient to alter the haemoglobin properties. Variants are best separated by electrophoresis. Two physiological types:

        1.2.1 Adult haemoglobin A. 2·5% is slow moving A_2 with a delta chain replacing a beta chain—denatured by alkali.

        1.2.2 Haemoglobin F. Both beta chains replaced by gamma chains. 60–90% of haemoglobin at birth in full-term babies consists of haemoglobin F, by 4–5 months less than 10% circulating haemoglobin is fetal haemoglobin, persists in

397

some anaemias, e.g. thalassaemia, and reappears in Fanconi's anaemia. Is resistant to alkali, takes up and releases oxygen at lower tensions than HbA—hence value to fetus.

2. Abnormal haemoglobins are associated with haemolytic anaemias designated by letters of alphabet, e.g. HbS found in sickle-cell anaemia is much less soluble in reduced state, incipient crystallization causes bizarre cell shape. Cells easily destroyed.

Cell Shape and Size

Anisocytosis and macrocytosis persist until about 12 weeks and then cells have approximately adult values but become slightly microcytic and hypochromic until puberty.

Blood Volume

Approximate values:

1. 3500 g (7 lb) baby at birth has blood volume of 300 ml. Can be increased by amounts of up to 100 ml if placenta allowed to empty into baby before cord is clamped.

2. Until 7000 g (15 lb) (6 months) figure can be calculated as 100 ml/kg body weight. After 1 year is approximately 80 ml/kg.

Chapter 128   *CLASSIFICATION OF ANAEMIAS*

Aetiological Classification
Inadequate production of haemoglobin or red cells
1. Deficiency of specific substances:
      1.1 Minerals—iron, copper.
      1.2 Vitamins—B_{12}; folic acid.
      1.3 Amino acids.
      1.4 Hormones—thyroid; adrenal; pituitary.
2. Marrow failure
      2.1 Congenital hypoplastic anaemia.
      2.2 Acquired aplastic anaemia due to drugs.
      2.3 Replacement: e.g. leukaemia and other malignancies.
      2.4 Erythropoietin deficiency due to renal failure.
Excessive loss of blood
1. Haemorrhage, acute or chronic.
2. Haemolysis.
      2.1 Intracorpuscular defect.
      2.1.1 Abnormal shape, e.g. spherocytosis.
      2.1.2 Abnormal haemoglobins, e.g. sickle-cell anaemia.
      2.1.3 Abnormal enzymes, e.g. glucose-6-phosphate dehydrogenase deficiency
      2.1.4 Parasitization, e.g. malaria.
      2.2 Extracorpuscular defects, e.g. immune reactions; haemolytic disease of newborn; toxins and burns.

Morphological Classification

Red-cell size
   1. Increased—macrocytic.
   2. Normal—normocytic.
   3. Decreased—microcytic.

Chapter 129   ***ANAEMIA IN THE NEONATAL PERIOD***

Cause
If severe, anaemia at birth is either due to haemorrhage or haemolysis. Loss of 50 ml blood may shock infant.

Cause of Haemorrhage in Newborn
   1. Prior to birth, e.g. twin to twin or feto-maternal transfusion, spontaneous or following version or amniocentesis.
   2. Occurring during birth
             2.1 External: placenta praevia, abruptio placentae, rupture of umbilical cord, incision of placenta during Caesarean section.
             2.2 Internal: ruptured liver or spleen, intracranial, subgaleal or cephalhaematoma.

Haemolytic Anaemia, *see* p. 402.

Impaired Blood Production
Congenital hypoplastic anaemia (Blackfan–Diamond syndrome), may present at birth. *See* Chapter 132.

Polycythaemia in the Neonatal Period
Diagnosis. Venous haematocrit greater than 65 %—or haemoglobin greater than 22·0 g/dl during first week of life.
   Note: Thrombocytopenia and reticulocytosis may occur.
Clinical features. Respiratory distress, cyanosis, convulsions, necrotizing enterocolitis, congestive heart failure, priapism, jaundice, renal vein thrombosis, tetany. More common in male. Most infants with polycythaemia have no symptoms.
Causes. Twin-to-twin transfusion, maternal→fetal transfusion, placental insufficiency and postmaturity, congenital adrenal hyperplasia, neonatal thyrotoxicosis, maternal diabetes, Down's and Beckwith's syndromes.
Treatment. If symptoms are present, a small exchange transfusion with fresh frozen plasma.

Chapter 130

IRON-DEFICIENCY ANAEMIA

Sources of Iron in Infancy
1. Two-thirds of iron present in infant at term acquired during last 3 months of intra-uterine life.
2. Breast milk contains small amount of iron which is highly bio-available.
3. Cow's and goat's milk do not contain sufficient iron.

Aetiology
Prenatal causes of iron lack
> *1. Premature birth*
>> 1.1 Fetus prevented from receiving iron which is normally obtained during last weeks of pregnancy and this leads to the late anaemia of prematurity.
>> 1.2 Investigational blood loss in sick pre-term infants leads later to iron-deficiency anaemia.

2. Twin birth. Fetus has to share available iron stores with twin. May also be born prematurely. Vascular anastomoses may allow one twin to bleed into the other (in monozygotic twins).
3. Maternal anaemia. Only when extreme is infant affected.
4. Intra-uterine haemorrhage: from fetal into maternal portions of the placenta; from premature placental separation; or ruptured fetal blood vessel.

Postnatal Causes of Iron Lack. Prolonged milk feeding without supplementation, e.g. over 1 year on breast or bottle.

Additional Factors. Constant gastrointestinal loss of small amount of blood (1–7 ml daily) associated with heat-labile protein in cow's milk, or protein containing iron (transferrin); malnutrition; chronic infection. In later childhood malabsorption syndromes, peptic ulcer, polyp or haemangioma.

Age Incidence
Usually develops by third to sixth month, especially after pre-term delivery.

Haematology
1. Peripheral blood: hypochromic and microcytic anaemia; *see Table* 127.1 for normal values.
2. Bone marrow: shows absence of stainable iron.

Clinical Features
Onset: insidious, child often noted to be pale at routine examination. Commonly brought to doctor because of some intercurrent infection, or child irritable, off food, may have pica. Early and developing iron deficiency is easily missed clinically. Splenomegaly in 10% of cases. Anaemic infants, particularly prone to infections: bronchitis, upper respiratory infections, etc. which in turn aggravate anaemia.

Prevention
1. Prenatal. Pregnant mothers usually given extra iron.

2. Postnatal

2.1 Premature and twin babies should be given iron from age of 4 weeks, e.g. ferrous sulphate.

2.2 Weaning on to adequate mixed diet at age 4 months. In practice in Western society most iron for infants is obtained by baby foods which have had iron added.

Treatment

1. Correct cause; educate mother about diet when necessary.
2. Any iron-deficient child should be given iron in adequate dosage which may need to be given systemically if oral route ineffective.

Sideroblastic Anaemias

Mixed group of hypochromic, microcytic anaemia due to abnormalities of haem or iron metabolism. Serum iron raised. Marrow contains nucleated red cells with a collar of haemosiderin granules—sideroblasts. One variety X-linked. May respond to vitamin B_6.

Other Deficiency Anaemias

1. Folic-acid Deficiency

Folic-acid deficiency occurs in malabsorption syndromes; in pre-term infants; in infants receiving goat's milk or diet for phenylketonuria unless correct supplements or intravenous nutrition given; in leukaemia and haemolytic anaemias. Certain anticonvulsants, e.g. primidone and sodium hydantoinate induce folic-acid deficiency. Methotrexate, pyrimethamine and pentamidine also cause folic-acid deficiency.

2. Vitamin B_{12} Deficiency (*Juvenile Pernicious Anaemia*), very rare, results from:

2.1 Genetically determined inability to secrete intrinsic factor, onset 7 months onwards.

2.2 Occurrence of intrinsic factor antibodies and gastric atrophy. May have abnormality of other exocrine glands.

2.3 Specific defect of vitamin B_{12} absorption associated with proteinuria.

2.4 Associated with resection of terminal ileum or infestation by *Diphyllobothrium latum*.

2.5 Vegetarian diets.

3. Vitamin E Deficiency

Vitamin E deficiency in very pre-term babies or with cystic fibrosis presents as haemolytic anaemia with acanthocytes, thrombocytosis, oedema and snuffles. May be precipitated by iron therapy if given very shortly after birth, worsened by formula feeds rich in polyunsaturated fatty acids.

4. Thyroid Deficiency

Anaemia of hypothyroidism cured largely by thyroid hormone.

5. Pyrimidine Deficiency
Occurs in a rare inborn error of metabolism—gives rise to combination of hypochromic anaemia, megaloblastic marrow and orotic aciduria.

Chapter 131   **THE HAEMOLYTIC ANAEMIAS**

Classification

1. Inherited haemolytic disorders

>1.1 *Defects in Red Cell Membrane.* Hereditary spherocytosis; elliptocytosis, stomatocytosis, etc.
>1.2 *Deficiency of Red Cell Glycolytic Enzymes.* Pyruvate kinase, hexokinase, phosphofructokinase; aldolase, etc.
>1.3 *Deficiency of Pentose Phosphate Pathway and Glutathione Metabolism.* Glucose-6-phosphate dehydrogenase deficiency (G-6-PD), glutathione reductase; glutathione peroxidase, etc.
>3.4 *Other Red Cell Enzyme Deficiencies*
>3.5 *Defects in Globin Structure and Synthesis.* Unstable haemoglobin disease, thalassaemia, sickle-cell disease, double and mixed heterozygous disorders.

2. Acquired haemolytic diseases

>2.1 *Immune Haemolytic Anaemias.* Haemolytic disease of newborn; with antibodies following mycoplasma and viral diseases, malignancies, systemic lupus erythematosus; drugs; with cold reactive antibodies.
>2.2 *Traumatic and Microangiopathic Haemolytic Anaemias.* Haemolytic uraemic syndrome, disseminated intravascular coagulation—prosthetic valves.
>2.3 *Infections.* Malaria, toxoplasmosis, clostridia, typhoid, cholera.
>2.4 *Chemicals.* Naphthalene, nitrofurantoin, sulphonamides, PAS, phenacetin, penicillin and methyldopa, etc.
>2.5 *Burns*
>2.6 *Liver Disease*
>2.7 *Paroxysmal Nocturnal Haemoglobinura*

Haemolytic Disease of Newborn

Definition
Not uncommon group of diseases in the newborn with the same aetiology, but showing different clinical manifestations, ranging from macerated fetus to mild anaemia. Disease nowadays commonly due to ABO incompatibility, less frequently Rh(D) and other blood group incompatibility, e.g. C, E, c, Kell, Lewis, M, Duffy or Kidd.
Racial incidence of Rh group
   1. Eighty-five% of Europeans and White Americans are Rh positive (38% homozygous positive, 47% heterozygous positive). Fifteen per cent Rh negative.

2. Percentage in other races varies, e.g. Chinese 100% Rh positive.

Subdivisions of Rh factor. Rh factor now known to be divisible into at least six subdivisions, known as Cc, Dd, Ee. Of these, D is most potent. So-called 'Rh positive' really means 'D positive' and 'Rh negative' means 'D negative'.

Immunization by Rh antigen can be caused in one of following ways:

1. By Intravenous Transfusion of Rh-positive blood into Rh-negative recipient. Result:

>1.1 If recipient has not been previously immunized, nothing happens clinically, but antibodies are formed. These can be detected by indirect Coombs' test.
>
>1.2 If few antibodies present, some transfused cells are haemolysed. More antibodies form.
>
>1.3 If many antibodies present, all transfused cells may be haemolysed, giving rise to dangerous or fatal reactions.

2. Rh-negative Mother Carrying Rh-positive Fetus. Following sequence of events occurs:

>2.1 Rh-negative mother reacts to presence of Rh-positive fetus as if she had transfusion. Fetal red blood corpuscles pass through placental barrier into maternal circulation during pregnancy and labour. Minimal amounts, less than 1·0ml, are sufficient to sensitize mother. Antibodies then appear in her plasma.
>
>2.2 Antibodies pass freely back through placenta to react with fetal corpuscles.

Note: Two-way passage across placental barrier required. Fetal red cells→maternal circulation; maternal antibodies→fetal circulation.

3. By Dilatation and Curettage following abortion of Rh-positive fetus.

4. Combination of Methods may occur, e.g. Rh-negative woman who has previously had Rh incompatible blood transfusion may carry Rh-positive fetus.

Note: Not every child of Rh-negative mother and Rh-positive father affected for following reasons:

1. Father may be heterozygous (Dd). One-half of children can then be Rh positive, one-half Rh negative.

2. Placental permeability may vary.

3. Several pregnancies may be required to raise titre of antibodies to required level. If family is small this may never be achieved.

4. ABO incompatibility of mother and fetus protects infant as fetal cells in mother's circulation are removed before sensitization can occur.

Clinical Classification

1. Haemolytic disease of fetus
>1.1 Macerated fetus.
>1.2 Hydrops fetalis.

2. Haemolytic disease of newborn
>2.1 Icterus gravis neonatorum.
>2.2 Congenital anaemia of newborn.

Pathology

1. Hydrops fetalis. Infant stillborn or dies within few hours. All organs grossly oedematous; serous cavities full of fluid; liver and spleen enlarged and site of active haemopoiesis; gross anaemia present. Placenta oedematous often with disseminated intravascular coagulation thrombocytopenia and hypoalbumin-aemia.

2. *Icterus gravis neonatorum*. Persistence of fetal erythropoiesis occurs. Liver may become necrotic with deposits of bile pigment and iron; plugged bile canaliculi. Brain: pathognomonic yellow staining of basal nuclei occurs, known as kernicterus (*see* p. 406).

Haematology
1. *Anaemia*. Varies in degree from extreme in hydrops fetalis to mild in congenital anaemia of newborn. Anaemia usually macrocytic with numerous normoblasts and reticulocytes present.
2. *Haemolysis*. Coombs' test positive. Antibody present in mother's serum detected by *indirect* Coombs' test but also coated to fetal red cells and detected by *direct* Coombs' test.
3. *Jaundice*. May be marked. Serum bilirubin level raised, unconjugated but can be conjugated if obstruction present; urine contains little urobilinogen.
4. *Disseminated intravascular coagulation (DIC)* can complicate the anaemia. The excessive haemolysis liberates thromboplastin which causes intravascular coagulation with deficiency of consumed factors and platelets. Liver damage can cause depletion of Factors II, VII, IX and X.

Clinical Features
1. *Onset*. All gradations occur from severe types in which vernix is golden yellow at birth and jaundice develops rapidly, to mild anaemia only, which commences at end of second week.
2. *Jaundice*. Commonly present within first 24 h after birth. (Physiological jaundice never seen within first 24 h.) May be severe, last several weeks and become obstructive in type.
3. *Anaemia*. Often clinically masked by degree of jaundice. Haemorrhage may occur from DIC and low prothrombin level.
4. *General condition*. Child tends to be lethargic and difficult to feed. Liver and spleen often palpable especially in severe cases with heart failure.
5. *Nervous lesions*. Acute kernicterus may occur if serum indirect bilirubin level over 340 µmol/l (20 mg/dl) in full term—but lower amounts in pre-term infants.

Differential Diagnosis
From other causes of neonatal jaundice (Chapter 14).

Prognosis
Depends upon:
1. *Degree of maturity*. Immature babies more likely to develop kernicterus than mature babies. Death rate higher.
2. *Severity of disease*. Best gauged by haemoglobin level of cord blood.
        2.1 If over 17·5 g/dl prognosis good in mature and immature.
        2.2 Below 8 g/dl prognosis poor.

Antenatal Detection

1. ABO and Rh blood grouping should be performed during early months of pregnancy on all pregnant women.

2. If mother Rh negative, Rh group of father should be determined.

3. Important to look for antibodies in every mother in every pregnancy at 12–16 weeks, at 32 and 36 weeks. If antibodies present repeat titre estimations weekly from 32nd week onwards. Antibody titre correlates poorly with severity of disease after first pregnancy.

4. Spectrophotometric examination of liquor amnii: test performed on high-risk mothers (i.e. if titre over 1 : 32 in first pregnancy and over 1 : 16 in subsequent pregnancies) from 20 weeks onwards. Blood contamination invalidates test for next 2 weeks. Also invalidated by meconium staining, exposure of fluid to light.

Postnatal Diagnosis

ABO and Rh grouping, Coombs' test, haemoglobin estimation and serum bilirubin should be performed on cord blood.

Postnatal Assessment of Severity.

Following methods of assessing severity and therefore of necessity for treatment have been suggested:

1. Haemoglobin of cord blood. Most valuable sign. Hb less then 15 g/dl—moderately severe. Hb less than 9 g/dl—severely ill.

2. Strength of Coombs' test. Course of disease usually indicated by severity of Coombs' test, e.g. a strongly positive result often means infant will require exchange transfusion.

3. Cord serum bilirubin. Of significance if over 50 μmol/l.

Treatment by Exchange Transfusion

To remove sensitized red blood cells antibody and bilirubin.

Indications for exchange transfusion

1. Any Coombs-positive baby irrespective of value of cord haemoglobin or bilirubin if:

> 1.1 There is history of previous baby being stillborn with haemolytic disease, or having hydrops or kernicterus.
> 1.2 The baby is very low birth weight.

2. Other affected babies if:

> 2.1 Cord haemoglobin less than 15 g/dl.
> 2.2 Cord haemoglobin over 15 g/dl but cord serum bilirubin over 50 μmol/l.
> 2.3 Serum bilirubin (indirect) rises above 340 μmol/l or at a rate greater than 10 μmol/l/h.
> 2.4 Clinical evidence of kernicterus.

3. Subsequent transfusion required if: serum indirect bilirubin rises above 340 μmol/l in first week of life. Direct bilirubin can be ignored. Take lower levels for pre-term or anoxic infants.

Note: Exchange transfusion performed far less commonly than in past owing to efficacy of: Prevention by anti-D gammaglobulin and phototherapy.

Technique of Exchange Transfusion
Time. At birth if infant severely affected. If cord Hb over 10·0g/dl can be left up to 6h, but the earlier the better.

Apparatus. Polyvinyl tube should be used. Via umbilical vein. This route can be used up to 5 days after birth.

Quantity. Attempt exchange of at least 170ml/kg body weight. Not more than 200–300ml/h in 10–20 ml amounts keeping accurate records.

Venous pressure. Should be measured as babies with severe anaemia are often in heart failure.

Drugs
    a. Vitamin K_1 i.m., 1mg at birth.

    b. Calcium gluconate may be reqiured to counteract the effect of citrate in donor blood. Check calcium after every 100ml exchanged.

    c. 1·0 mEq sodium bicarbonate for every 100 ml blood during first transfusion to counteract acid of donor blood.

Specimens. Last sample withdrawn from baby should be examined for haemoglobin, serum potassium and serum bilirubin.

Other treatment
    1. Transfusion of concentrated red cells. Blood given by slow drip if haemoglobin falls too low. Amount of concentrated red cells required in ml = (desired PCV—observed PCV) × body weight in kg.

    Note: Blood volume calculated as 85ml/kg (40ml/lb) body weight.

Indications for Induction of Labour
1. With previous stillbirth or hydrops fetalis.
        1.1 If father homozygous, induce at 35 weeks.
        1.2 If father heterozygous, do amniocentesis and spectroscopic examination of bilirubin in liquor amnii at 30 weeks.
2. If previous infant moderately affected and rising maternal titre (over 1 in 8), induce at 36 weeks.

Prevention
Anti-D gammaglobulin given to Rh-negative mothers imediately after delivery will destroy any fetal cells in mother and reduce degree of sensitization of mother.

Kernicterus
Very rare, serious result of hyperbilirubinaemia. Pre-term babies especially vulnerable. Preventable (*see above*) in all except Crigler–Najjar syndrome.

Causes
1. Haemolysis. Due to:
        1.1 Extracorpuscular defect—Rh or ABO incompatibility; excess vitamin K.
        1.2 Intracorpuscular defect such as pyruvate-kinase deficiency.
        1.3 Red cell membrane defects, e.g. hereditary spherocytosis.

2. *Liver enzyme deficiency*. Lack of or reduced glucuronyl-transferase—as in pre-term infants and Crigler–Najjar syndrome.

Pathology
Direct toxic action of indirect bilirubin on lenticular and caudate nuclei of brain.

Clinical Features
Onset—Haemolytic cases, within first 4 days; liver enzyme deficiency cases, 5th to 9th day. Baby ill, feeds poorly, markedly stiff or at times flaccid. Lies in position of opisthotonos with trismus and spasm of bulbar muscles. High-pitched cry, irritable. Moro reflex absent or may occur spontaneously. Fits common. Cyanotic attacks may occur.

Prognosis
Majority of severe cases die. If they survive they may develop athetosis, deafness and yellow teeth. Children with Crigler–Najjar syndrome survive intact with intensive continuous phototherapy initially and later nocturnal phototherapy.

Haemolytic Disease of the Newborn due to ABO Incompatibility

Should be suspected if baby develops jaundice within first 24 h of birth with no evidence of Rh incompatibility and negative Coombs' test. First-born affected as often as subsequent infants.

Diagnosis
Confirmed if mother Group O, baby Group A or B (more commonly A_1) and if mother's blood contains haemolytic antibody (immune antibody) to baby's AB group. Baby's blood shows microspherocytes and reticulocytes. Coombs' test often negative, may be weakly positive. Occasionally associated thrombocytopenia. Kernicterus rare except in pre-terms.
Note: ABO incompatibility seems to protect against Rh iso-immunization.

Other Haemolytic Disorders in Newborn
Besides rare blood group incompatibilities, congenital infection, e.g. rubella, syphilis, toxoplasmosis, cytomegalovirus, spherocytosis and red cell enzyme deficiencies also may cause haemolytic disease in newborn. Coombs' test negative in these diseases. Homozygous α-thalassaemia causes stillbirth due to hydrops fetalis. Coombs' test negative in these diseases.

Heinz-body Anaemia of the Newborn

Rare type of haemolytic anaemia caused by factors which lead to Heinz-body formation and disintegration of red cells. Heinz bodies are intracellular inclusions of precipitated haemoglobin seen in red cells after staining with supra-vital dyes. Heinz bodies usually removed quickly by spleen. Heinz bodies seen often in glucose-6-phosphate dehydrogenase deficiency, in very immature infants, in unstable haemoglobin disease, in thalassaemias and injury from chemicals, e.g. vitamin K in large doses, nitrofurantoin, sulphamethoxypyridine, *p*-aminosalicylic acid, naphthalene.

Clinical Features
Occurs in very premature babies. Child not anaemic at birth. Haemolytic anaemia and jaundice develop, in second or third week. Coombs' test negative; no immune bodies present in mother's serum. Heinz bodies present in increasing numbers during first few weeks of life and methaemalbuminaemia may occur. Death from anaemia may occur.

Acute Haemolytic Anaemia
(*Acquired Haemolytic Anaemia*)

Definition
Acute haemolytic anaemia very rare. Varied aetiology.

Aetiology
(*see* Classification, p. 402).
   1. Toxic: red cell damage—bacteria, burns, potassium chlorate, etc.
   2. Antibodies: induced in patient by autoimmune process.
   3. Genetic: potential weakness associated with enzyme deficiencies of red cell—haemolysis induced by contact with drugs or vegetable products.

Haematology
   1. Rapidly developing normocytic, normochromic anaemia with reticulocytosis. There may be erythrophagocytosis, Heinz bodies and fragmented red cells in peripheral blood.
   2. Leucocytosis common.
   3. Platelet count usually normal; low if immune thrombocytopenic purpura present (Evans syndrome).
   4. Coombs' test strongly positive and IgG specific antibodies (against red cell antigen) present in anaemias with warm antibodies. Cold antibodies of IgM type often with mycoplasma infection.

Clinical Features
Child acutely ill with rapidly developing pallor, jaundice, pyrexia, and often vomiting and diarrhoea, haematuria. Splenomegaly and lymphadenopathy may be present.

Treatment
Blood transfusion usually causes dramatic recovery. Steroids useful. Parents warned of possible precipitating causes.

Inherited Haemolytic Disorders

Hereditary Spherocytosis (*Congenital Haemolytic Jaundice; Acholuric Jaundice; Familial Spherocytosis*)

Definition
Not uncommon chronic familial disease characterized clinically by splenomegaly, mild jaundice and spherocytic anaemia which becomes more marked in periodical crises.

Aetiology
1. Pathophysiology. Red blood corpuscles are spheroidal with defective cell membrane. *Note*: Normal corpuscles are biconcave. Abnormal shaped red cells cannot traverse capillary slits in spleen, become sequestrated and removed. Occasionally a hypoplastic crisis follows infections. Disease may remain 'latent', however, and relations sometimes only discovered to be affected when specially examined.
2. Inheritance. Inherited as autosomal dominant but up to one-third have no family history.
3. Age. May be manifested in infancy by jaundice and/or anaemia. Usually first noticed in late childhood.

Investigations
1. Anaemia. Slight degree usually present, which becomes severe during crises.
2. Red blood cells. Mean corpuscular volume normal or above normal. Anisocytosis marked. Reticulocyte count usually over 10%.
3. Red cell fragility test. Normal red cells show median fragility at 0·445–0·45% saline. In hereditary spherocytosis increased osmotic fragility is found although detectable in some cases only after incubation for 24h at 37°C. (Test may be difficult to interpret in infants up to 3 months of age; family studies may help.)
4. Bilirubin level of blood increased
5. Coombs' test. Negative.
6. Urine. No bilirubin (hence name 'acholuric jaundice'). Urobilinogen increased.

Pathology
1. Spleen enlarged and engorged with blood.
2. Bone marrow hyperplastic.
3. Gallbladder may contain pigment stones.

Clinical Features
1. Presentation. May be in one of following ways:
> 1.1 Mild jaundice or anaemia. Jaundice may be present on first day of life and lead to kernicterus, although fragility test is not always positive.
> 1.2 Routine examination and discovery of enlarged spleen or on special examination if sibling known to have disease.
> 1.3 Aplastic crisis, rare.

2. Appearance during latent period. May have mild anaemia. On examination conjunctivae icteric. Spleen palpable and firm. Liver not usually enlarged, but biliary obstruction and colic may develop. Very rarely ulcers occur on shins; corneal opacities.
3. Appearance during crises. Medical emergency, often precipitated by infection, hence several members of family may be affected simultaneously. Anaemia and

jaundice become more marked and spleen may enlarge. Child often complains of abdominal pain. General condition deteriorates.

Diagnosis
Should always be considered in child with enlarged spleen, anaemia, jaundice or gallbladder disease. Family history often obtainable although examination of apparently normal individuals may be required. Blood should be examined for reticulocytes and increased fragility of red cells.

Prognosis
Condition not usually very severe, but crises may be dangerous to life.

Treatment
Splenectomy curtails the haemolysis and the anaemia although the red cells remain spherocytic. The later risks of biliary stones and aplastic crises are averted. Splenectomy should not be performed before 4 years of age. Splenectomy in young children predisposes to overwhelming septicaemia for several years and vaccination against pneumococci is advised. Folic acid supplements (0·5 mg/day) should be given for the increased folate demands because of the haemolysis.

Congenital Non-spherocytic Haemolytic Anaemias

Definition
A rare group of anaemias with clinical features similar to those found in congenital spherocytosis but associated with various inborn errors of red-cell metabolism, e.g. glycolytic enzymes, pentose phosphate pathway and glutathione metabolism. Main clinical entities: glucose-6-phosphate dehydrogenase deficiency including favism; pyruvate kinase deficiency.

Normal Metabolism
Relevant features:
    1. Red cell requires energy for maintaining biconcave shape and electrochemical gradients of sodium, potassium, etc.
    2. Haemoglobin is an unstable molecule undergoing spontaneous oxidation to methaemoglobin at rate of 2% per day. Normal cell has enzymes present to prevent this.
    Abnormal shapes, e.g. poikilocytes, or burr cells, always have short life.

Abnormal Metabolism
Two types:
1. Deficient energy potential. Red-cell energy derived from breakdown of glucose. Enzymes necesary for maintaining energy metabolism include pyruvate kinase and triose phosphate isomerase.
2. Reduction potential diminished. Cell unable to combat haemoglobin oxidation. The enzymes which are deficient are glutathione reductase or glucose-6-phosphate dehydrogenase. Disease is sex-linked dominant. Denatured haemoglobin appears in cell as inclusion bodies. Occurs in varying degree in different races. Some may have complete deficiency with severe haemolytic anaemia. In other cases episodes of haemolysis occur in presence of various drugs, e.g.

certain antimalarials, sulphonamides, sulphones, nitrofurans, antipyretics, ascorbic acid, Fava bean.

Clinical Features
May present in neonatal period with marked haemolytic crisis. Increased tendency to haemolysis persists. Crises are precipitated by infection or drugs. Splenectomy and steroids are not indicated. Blood transfusion often necessary; phototherapy, exchange transfusion may be required in infancy.

Defects in Haemoglobin Structure and Synthesis

Thalassaemia

Definition
Syndromes found in Mediterranean, Indian and Chinese races. A heterogeneous group of chronic anaemias which are partly haemolytic but the main defect is decreased production of haemoglobin polypeptide chains. Defect is decreased production of haemoglobin polypeptide chains (α, β, γ or δ). Homozygotes have thalassaemia major but heterozygotes have thalassaemia minor and few or no symptoms. Most common varieties are associated with defect in β chain synthesis, called β-thalassaemia.

β-Thalassaemia
May be minor (heterozygous) or major (homozygous). Occurs in Mediterranean races. There is decreased production of normal β chain with:
1. Reduced HbA production.
2. Normal or increased HbF production.
3. Relative increase in percent of HbA_2.

Thalassaemia Minor
Heterozygous β-thalassaemia, associated with mild anaemia, hypochromia, microcytosis, poikilocytosis, low MCV (about 70 fl) target cells. HbA_2 levels from 3 to 7%. Fifty per cent cases have HbF of 2–6%.

Thalassaemia Major (*Cooley's Anaemia; Homozygous Thalassaemia*)

Pathological Features
Severe microcytic, hypochromic anaemia, with poikilocytosis, target cells and bizarre shaped cells present, red-cell count may be raised, moderate reticulocytosis, nucleated red cells, stippling, inclusion bodies. Typical target cells seen in blood smear. Leucocytosis present. Haemoglobin electrophoresis demonstrates haemoglobin abnormality. Anaemia severe (5 g/dl), high serum iron. HbF often >5%. HbA_2 less than 3% but HbA_2 : HbA increased.

Clinical Features
1. Peculiar pigmentation—partly due to transfusion haemosiderosis and jaundice.
2. 'Mongolian' facial expression caused by thickening of cranial and malar bones due in part to marrow hyperplasia.
3. Enlarged liver, spleen and often heart. Leg ulcers. May be retarded.

4. Growth impaired, puberty delayed or absent, diabetes secondary to pancreatic siderosis.

Radiological Changes
Very characteristic, consequent upon hypertrophy of erythropoietic tissue. Vertical striations of skull bones occur, 'hair-on-end' appearance. Long bones become thin and fractures frequent.

Prognosis
Thalassaemia major almost invariably fatal in second or third decade.

Treatment
Keep haemoglobin above 9–10 g/dl by repeated small transfusions at 4–6 weeks intervals. Use fresh packed red cells. Cross-matching must be meticulous to prevent iso-immunization. Splenectomy may be necessary because of huge size of spleen or secondary hypersplenism. Followed by severe infection in one-third of cases. Delay as long as possible until over 8 years. Use of desferrioxamine and ascorbic acid to minimize haemosiderosis by increasing iron excretion is useful.

Other Thalassaemic Syndromes
A group of diseases found in South-East Asia and China, characterized by decreased production of α chain causing:
    a. Less HbA, HbA_2, HbF.
    b. Formation of haemoglobins rarely found normally: HbH ($\beta 4$), Bart's haemoglobin Hb Barts ($\gamma 4$).
    In homozygous state α-thalassaemia causes hydrops fetalis with Hb Barts. HbH syndromes resemble Cooley's anaemia.
    Other thalassaemic syndromes include haemoglobin S-thalassaemia, haemoglobin C-thalassaemia, haemoglobin D-thalassaemia.
    HbF can persist in high levels as a genetic defect with levels of up to 30% in blood. Little anaemia or illness results. If combined with sickle gene, protects against sickling.

Sickle-cell Anaemia
Common disease in Negro races. Caused by mutant autosomal gene which substitutes valine for glutamic acid on β polypeptide chain ($\alpha_2\ \beta_2^{6val}$). Result: deoxygenated molecule has altered physical properties and stacks into monofilaments forming crystals which deform cell.

Aetiology
Gentically inherited disease.
1. Heterozygous children have sickle-cell 'trait'. No symptoms, except occasionally infarction from hypoxaemia at high altitude. Erythrocytes appear normal *in vivo* but can be induced to sickle *in vitro*. Protects against malaria. Both HbA and HbS present.
2. Homozygous children have sickle-cell anaemia. Disease severe. Erythrocytes show sickling *in vivo*. HbS and a little HbF present. No HbA.
    Sickle-cell anaemia and thalassaemia not infrequently occur in same patient.

Clinical Features

Symptoms appear towards end of first year when HbF level decreased.

Note: Sickle-cell anaemia may mimic any disease. In any ill Negro child, blood should be examined for sickling. If the test is positive this may be heterozygous (trait) or homozygous sickle-cell disease.

1. The anaemia. Children show evidence of haemolytic anaemia with pallor and enlarged spleen which atrophies after age of 6 years because of recurrent infarction and fibrosis. Low haemoglobin (6–8g/dl) and reticulocytosis; bilirubinaemia. Target cells, hypochromia, Howell–Jolly bodies, leucocytosis and thrombocytosis.

2. The crises. Following types may occur:

2.1 Vaso-occlusive. Common. Due to capillary obstruction by abnormal shape of erythrocytes. Results in infarcts which may occur in any organ in body. Common symptoms; pain in abdomen or extremities, haematuria, fits, coma, hemiplegia. Hands and feet may be swollen in young; and bigger joints in older children. Characteristic X-ray of bone destruction and periosteal reactions.

2.2 Haemolytic. Rare. Symptoms as above, also sudden fall in haemoglobin and rise in bilirubin. Patient usually has G-6-PD deficiency as well.

2.3 Aplastic. Rare. Occurs especially in association with infection.

2.4 Sequestration Crisis. Blood pools in liver and spleen causing hypotension.

Note: Although sickle-cell disease patients are susceptible to salmonella osteomyelitis in Great Britain, *Staphylococcus aureus* is the commonest cause of osteomyelitis worldwide.

Tests for Sickling

1. During crisis peripheral blood often contains sickle cells.

2. If drop of blood placed on slide, sealed from oxygen by cover slip and petroleum jelly, and incubated from 1 to 24h, erythrocytes will develop characteristic sickle shape. Reducing substances, e.g. sodium metabisulphite, act similarly.

Note: This test does not distinguish sickle-cell anaemia from the sickle-cell trait.

3. Quantitative electrophoresis shows more than 90 % HbS in sickle-cell disease and less than 40 % HbS in the trait.

Treatment of Crises

1. Hydration therapy. Child given fluid by mouth and if necessary intravenously. Dextran and glucose intravenously of some value.

2. Blood transfusions. Required if anaemia severe, but avoid unless symptoms of hypoxaemia marked.

3. Antibiotics. Should be given for infection.

4. Analgesics

5. Oxygen

Haemolytic Uraemic Syndrome

Definition

Rare acute haemolytic disease associated with thrombocytopenia and uraemia.

Occurs mainly in infants under 1 year old. Cause unknown, may be related to infection, e.g. gastro-enteritis or immunizations.

Features
Onset often with diarrhoea. Rapid development of pallor, drowsiness and stupor. May have coma and convulsions. Scanty dark or black urine. Blood shows evidence of haemolysis, severe anaemia, reticulocytosis and abnormally shaped red cells—burr cells. Hypertension occurs. Blood shows severe anaemia, fragmented, distorted red cells, reticulocytosis, leucocytosis and sometimes thrombocytopenia. Plasma contains haemoglobin, little or no haptoglobin, urea and bilirubin raised.

Prognosis
Prognosis guarded. Many die from intracranial complications or uraemia. Mortality c. 25%.
   Autopsy shows intravascular thrombi in brain and kidneys.

Treatment
Blood transfusion; heparin sometimes dramatic; vitamin E or steroids may help. May benefit from peritoneal or haemodialysis.

Further Reading

Modell B. and Petrou M. (1983) Management of Thalassaemia major. *Arch. Dis. Childh.* **58**, 1026–30.

Chapter 132   APLASIA AND HYPOPLASIA
                 OF BONE MARROW

Marrow Failure

Causes

Hypoplasia
   1. Genetic. Fanconi syndrome (*see below*).
   2. Drugs, e.g. sulphonamides, chloramphenicol, chlorpromazine, meprobamate, benzene compounds, nitrogen mustard, 6 MP and methotrexate.
   3. Severe infection, e.g. herpes simplex, infective hepatitis and mononucleosis (in neonatal period, toxoplasmosis, torulosis, herpes simplex, cytomegalic inclusion disease may cause hypoplasia).
   4. Irradiation with radium, other radioactive material or X-rays.

Marrow infiltration
   1. Infiltration with malignant growth, e.g. leukaemia, neuroblastoma. Infiltration with lipid in lipid storage disease. Encroachment on marrow by bone disease, e.g. osteopetrosis or myelofibrosis.

2. Preleukaemic state.

Pathology and Haematology
1. Red marrow in bones replaced by yellow marrow or by the infiltrating substance, e.g. malignant growth. Replacement rarely complete; islands of normal tissue remain.
2. Peripheral blood: Usually is normochromic, normocytic anaemia with reduced reticulocyte count but may be leucoerythroblastic; usually neutropenia and thrombocytopenia.

Special Features of Fanconi Syndrome
Autosomal recessive. Half children have absence of radii and thumbs, microcephaly and microphthalmos, also abnormalities of heart and kidneys. Children often short, pigmented with café-au-lait spots. Anaemia develops by age 3–12 years. Blood and marrow show pancytopenia. HbF level of 5–15%. Chromatid breaks common.

Diagnosis
Essential feature is progressive anaemia with:
1. No haemolysis—serum bilirubin normal and Coombs' test negative.
2. No blood regeneration—reticulocyte count normal.
3. No blood loss.
Bone-marrow biopsy shows aplasia.

Treatment
Treatment by blood transfusion; androgens, e.g. testosterone propionate or oxymetholone together with prednisone. Drugs should be gradually withdrawn after remission. Prolonged androgen therapy causes haemorrhagic cysts of the liver and malignant hepatoma. Leukaemia commoner in relatives. Bone-marrow transplantation under review. Acyclovir can sometimes cure.

Neutropenia

Definition
Neutropenia is a reduction in the numbers of circulating neutrophils below $2 \cdot 0 \times 10^9$ cells/l. Commonly associated with some viral infections, typhoid and brucellosis.

Aetiology
1. *Drugs and X-ray therapy.* Following may cause neutropenia: some antimitotic drugs; various sulphonamides, analgesics, e.g. phenacetin, indomethacin, anticonvulsants, e.g. carbamazepine, phenytoin, troxidone; phenothiazines; antithyroid drugs and antibiotics, e.g. chloramphenicol, ampicillin, PAS and INAH.
2. Neutropenia may also occur in leukaemia or malignant disease.
3. Familial cases may be associated with hypogammaglobulinaemia.
4. In newborn: (i) transient leucopenia caused by maternal leucoagglutinins, severe infections—viral and bacterial; (ii) severe lethal familial variety occurs.

5. Periodic (cyclic) neutropenia, with recurrent skin or mucus membrane infections and fever. May be associated with hypo- or hypergammaglobulinaemia. Granulocytes may drop to very low levels but return to normal after 10 days.

6. Chronic neutropenia—mild illness recovering at adolescence—with recurrent pneumonia, pyoderma and mouth ulcers. Usually sporadic. Associated with hypergammaglobulinaemia.

7. Associated with hypoplasia of exocrine pancreas (Shwachman's syndrome).

Clinical Features
Infection usually takes form of necrotic ulceration of pharynx and mouth, which is often first manifestation of disease. Ulceration may also occur elsewhere.

Treatment
Remove offending agent, if known, and prohibit its future use. Warn parents of possible significance of adverse reactions if patient given potentially noxious drug. Strenuous efforts to stop infection until white cells return. Prophylactic antibiotics should not be given but every effort made to identify and treat organism at first suspicion of infection. White-cell transfusion may help but can lead to antibody formation.

Erythrogenesis Imperfecta
(Congenital Hypoplastic Anaemia; Pure Red-cell Aplasia; Blackfan–Diamond Syndrome)

Very rare condition manifested within few weeks of birth by progressive anaemia. Peripheral blood shows low red-cell count, haemoglobin and reticulocyte count, but normal white cells, platelets may be raised. Failure of red-cell formation possibly due to inborn error of metabolism affecting erythrocyte maturation. Tryptophan metabolism may be abnormal. High levels of erythropoietin in blood and urine. Patients may have Turner's syndrome appearance but with normal karyotype. May be associated with prematurity or abnormalities of pregnancy.

Treatment
1. Blood transfusion until steroids have controlled anaemia. May need repeated transfusion with danger of siderosis.

2. Steroid therapy may affect remission. Should be given intermittently. Prognosis better if steroids started early.

Anaemias Secondary to Disease

Following conditions often cause anaemia. Exact mechanism unknown:

1. Acute rheumatism. Anaemia common during acute stages of disease, especially if pericarditis present. May be due to fluid retention.

2. Acute nephritis and nephrotic syndrome. Usually have associated anaemia. This may appear greater than is actually the case owing to oedema.

Chapter 133

PURPURA

Classification and Causes

Platelet Deficiency
1. Congenital

1.1 Rubella embryopathy at any time in pregnancy. Other intra-uterine infections may cause hepatosplenomegaly with haemolysis.

1.2 Associated with maternal thrombocytopenia.

1.3 From transplacental passage of maternal platelet antibodies.

1.4 Maternal thiazide treatment.

1.5 Thrombocytopenia with absent radii (TAR syndrome). Haemorrhage may occur in early weeks. Autosomal recessive.

2. Immunologically-mediated thrombocytopenic purpura

3. Secondary (symptomatic) thrombocytopenic purpura

3.1 Leukaemia.

3.2 Drugs, e.g. quinine and sedormid.

3.3 Malignant disease.

3.4 Severe infections.

3.5 Exanthemata, e.g. rubella.

3.6 Marrow failure.

3.7 Gaucher's disease.

3.8 Associated with large haemangioma.

3.9 Thrombotic thrombocytopenic purpura.

3.10 Wiskott–Aldrich syndrome.

Diseases due to Capillary Damage
1. Henoch–Schönlein purpura

2. Secondary (symptomatic) purpura

2.1 Meningococcal septicaemia (meningococcaemia).

2.2 Scurvy.

2.3 Mechanical causes, e.g. following severe bout of coughing in pertussis; vomiting; stomach wash-out; lumbar puncture. Petechiae on front of chest seen with wearing of cellular vests.

2.4 Congenital weakness: cutis laxa, haemorrhagic telangiectasia.

Idiopathic Thrombocytopenic Purpura

Definition
Disease of unknown aetiology manifested haematologically by reduction in number of platelets and prolonged bleeding time; clinically by bruises and frequent haemorrhages especially of skin and mucus membranes.

Aetiology
Unknown. Most probably immune mechanism destroys platelets. Role of platelet agglutinins at present uncertain. Some cases follow viral infection, e.g. rubella. There is usually an associated weakness of endothelium.

Haematology
1. Anaemia may be present owing to recurrent haemorrhages.
2. Platelet count less than $40 \times 10^9/l$ (normal $>100 \times 10^9/l$). Purpura does not usually occur until count falls below $25 \times 10^9/l$.
3. Bleeding time prolonged.
4. Coagulation time normal.
5. Clot retraction and formation poor.
6. Hess test positive.

Types
1. Acute—commoner, 90% self-limiting disease by 1 year.
2. Chronic—10%. Case can be regarded as chronic if thrombocytopenia persists for more than 100 days.

Clinical Features of Chronic Type
Condition proceeds by alternate remissions and relapses. During relapses bruises are seen which may be large, and haemorrhages from nose, mouth, uterus or urinary tract may occur. Spleen palpable in less than one-third of cases. Relapse may last for about 1 month.

Differential Diagnosis
1. From haemophilia, *see* p. 421.
2. From other causes of thrombocytopenic purpura, e.g. leukaemia. Diagnosis of 'idiopathic' purpura should never be made until all forms of symptomatic purpura have been eliminated.

Treatment
Majority recover spontaneously, but treatment may be needed when there is severe thrombocytopenia (below $20 \times 10^9/l$) or with bleeding.
1. Blood or platelet transfusion of little benefit as transfused platelets rapidly disappear.
2. Steroids. Of especial value in acute cases if bleeding severe. Maintenance therapy may be required for about 4 weeks to raise platelets to $50 \times 10^9/l$. As greatest change is in first few weeks of the disease, steroids (if justified) should be given then or probably not at all.
3. Splenectomy. Dangerous and unnecessary in acute cases. About 60–70% cure in chronic cases, but note:

> 3.1 Only required if bleeding tendency not controlled by steroids. (Actual level of platelets less important.)
> 3.2 May lead to subsequent infections.

Syndrome of Thrombocytopenia, Eczema and Infection

(Wiskott–Aldrich Syndrome)

Very rare sex-linked recessive syndrome (therefore affects males, transmitted by unaffected females) seen in infancy, manifested by triad of thrombocytopenia (melaena common at onset), eczema and infection (especially otitis media, skin sepsis, diarrhoea and pneumonia). No cause known. IgM low. Treatment of little avail. Transfer factor may help. Lymphoma may develop. Total body irradiation followed by bone-marrow transplantation is curative.

Haemangiomas with Secondary Thrombocytopenia

Association of thrombocytopenia and very large haemangiomas sometimes noticed in newborn period. Theory is that large number of thrombocytes sequestrated in haemangioma. Peripheral blood may demonstrate features of intravascular coagulation.

Purpura from Blood-vessel Disorders

Occurs in cutis hyperelastica, hereditary haemorrhagic telangiectasia, pulmonary haemosiderosis, scurvy, bacterial and other toxins, and anaphylactoid purpura.

Thrombotic Thrombocytopenic Purpura

Very rare condition manifested clinically by fever, a bleeding tendency (commonly haematuria) and terminal neurological signs; haematologically by haemolytic anaemia and thrombocytopenic purpura; pathologically by widespread fibrin deposition on vessel walls, sometimes with severe coagulopathy. Affects older children or adults (*see* DIC, p. 423).

Chapter 134   # *HENOCH–SCHÖNLEIN SYNDROME (Anaphylactoid Purpura)*

This syndrome comes into group of so-called collagen diseases which are aetiologically, pathologically and clinically similar.

Other members of the group are: acute rheumatism, acute nephritis, polyarteritis nodosa, disseminated lupus erythematosus, dermatomyositis, rheumatoid arthritis and scleroderma.

Definition
Uncommon disease of childhood manifested clinically by one or more of following features: rash, abdominal pain, haemorrhage from gut or joint involvement. Acute haemorrhagic nephritis most important complication.

Aetiology
1. Cause. Allergic disease. Possible agents concerned: (*a*) *Bacteria*, e.g. β-haemolytic streptococci in one-quarter of cases. (*b*) *Drugs or foods*, e.g. eggs, chocolate, wheat or beans.
2. Age. 4–15 years.
3. Sex. Boys twice as commonly affected as girls.

Haematology
Capillary resistance test (of Hess), bleeding time, clotting time, platelet count, bone-marrow—all normal. Sometimes polymorphonuclear leucocytosis occurs.

Pathology
Skin lesions have characteristic histological picture: acute inflammatory reaction occurs around small vessels of corium, with out-pouring of polymorphonuclear leucocytes and erythrocytes, occasional eosinophils.

Clinical Features
May present with one or more of following manifestations:
1. Rash. Commonest manifestation. *Character.* Discrete, urticarial, purpuric, maculopapular eruption, which later may coalesce. Appear in crops. In relapses spots not always urticarial. *Colour.* At first pink, but later becomes dusky red and purplish. Several days later the spot turns brown and gradually fades. *Distribution.* Roughly symmetrical. Following sites commonly involved: (i) Extensor surfaces of leg, ankle and foot. (ii) Backs of elbows and extensor surfaces of arms. Papules over tip of elbow characteristic. (iii) Lower back and buttocks. (iv) Points of pressure; for instance, sitting on bed-pan may produce ring around buttocks; stroking skin will sometimes produce rash which appears in that site the following day.
2. Abdominal pain and haemorrhage from gut. Part of syndrome described by Henoch; rarely first or only manifestation. Character of pain: intestinal colic. Probably due to haemorrhage or urticarial effusion into gut wall. Pain sometimes very severe. Few hours after attack of pain, melaena may occur.
3. Joint involvement. Part of syndrome described by Schönlein. May be first manifestation, but rash usually appears soon after. Joints are painful and tender, with periarticular swelling. No haemorrhage into joint. Large joints principally involved. Arthritis may flit from joint to joint.
4. Bizarre oedema. Occasionally occurs, e.g. back of feet, hands or scalp.

Progress
Rash fades in 1–6 weeks, but any of the manifestations, especially the rash, may recur many times. Abdominal pain is a particularly distressing symptom, since it is often acute and may last a long time.

Complications
1. Intracranial oedema and haemorrhage. Occurs in first few weeks only but uncommon.
2. Acute haemorrhagic nephritis. Most important complication. May commence at any time during course of disease.
3. Intussusception. Initiated by haemorrhage into, or swelling of, intestinal wall; bowel perforation, rare.
4. Oedema of epiglottis.

Prognosis
Relapses uncommon. Complete recovery occurs apart from cases with nephritis. This complication carries poorer prognosis than with usual acute nephritis.

Differential Diagnosis
1. Rash. Sometimes mistaken for other forms of purpura, but character and

distribution are characteristic.

2. Abdominal pain. May be difficult to differentiate from intussusception, especially as this very occasionally complicates the disease. *Points of resembl-ance:* (*a*) Frequent attacks of colicky abdominal pain. Child may be shocked. (*b*) Passage of red blood per rectum. *Points of difference:* (*a*) Age incidence: intussusception uncommon after 18 months except in chronic form. Henoch–Schönlein syndrome rare before 3 years. (*b*) In Henoch–Schönlein syndrome some other manifestation, i.e. joint pain or rash, almost always present. (*c*) Abdomen guarded in anaphylactoid purpura.

3. Joint pain. May be mistaken for acute rheumatism.

Rare Special Forms

1. Purpura fulminans. Severe condition associated with large haemorrhages. Usually occurs in children under 2 years. May be difficult to distinguish from Waterhouse–Friderichsen syndrome (*see* p. 97).

2. Gangrene. Very severe purpura which may progress to gangrene with eventual loss of fingers, toes, nose or even a limb.

Treatment

Symptomatic. Steroids may help severe abdominal pain.

Chapter 135   *COAGULATION DEFECTS*

Haemophilia A

Definition

Uncommon disease occurring in males but transmitted by females. Manifested clinically by life-long tendency to excessive haemorrhage and haematologically by reduction of Factor VIII coagulant activity.

Aetiology

1. Inheritance. By sex-linked recessive gene, i.e. disease occurs only in males and is transmitted by females. Theoretically possible for female to be affected but this is excessively rare. Condition sometimes occurs without family history. Reasons for this may be:

> 1.1 Affected gene has been present in previous generations, but disease has not been manifested because there have not been any males.
>
> 1.2 Condition has arisen by mutation, i.e. normal gene has in some way been altered so that in future it transmits haemophilia. Said to account for 20% of cases.

2. Age. Can be manifest at birth, but usually becomes obvious later, e.g. if baby is circumcised, or when he begins to walk and sustains minor injuries. Usually presents before 3 years. Prenatal diagnosis possible.

3. Cause. Production of an abnormal Factor VIII which is functionally incompetent.

Haematology

1. Factor VIII level low, from 0 to 25 % of normal activity.
2. Clotting time prolonged in severe cases.
3. Bleeding time is normal.

Must be distinguished from Factor IX deficiency and von Willebrand's disease.

Clinical Features

1. General

1.1 Haemorrhage initiated by trauma, which may be obvious, e.g. tooth extraction; slight, e.g. knock resulting in extensive bruising; or unnoticed, e.g. twist of joint.

1.2 Haemorrhage characterized by persistence rather than severity.

1.3 Tendency to haemorrhage comes in cycles. At times child able to take risks which at other times would result in multiple bruises or haemarthrosis.

2. Psychological factor.
Of great importance. Affected children always boys, who tend to be protected from injury, are not allowed to play with other children, and have to have frequent injections. They may rebel and become 'behaviour problems'.

3. Common forms of haemorrhage

2.1 *Following Circumcision.* May be first indication of disease.

3.2. *Bruising.* Always due to trauma. Bruise may be small, or very large, resulting in obvious swelling of limb and sudden fall in haemoglobin. Absorption of blood usually occurs without difficulty.

3.3 *Haemorrhage into Joint (Haemarthrosis).* Very characteristic and important. Joint suddenly becomes painful, tender, hot, red and swollen. Resembles acute infective arthritis. Temperature often raised. Re-absorption of blood often slow and fibrous ankylosis can result.

3.4 *Haemorrhage from Teeth.* May occur after accident to teeth, following extraction, and especially when milk teeth drop out around 6 years of age.

3.5 *Retroperitoneal Haemorrhage.* May simulate acute abdominal catastrophe.

Diagnosis

Given by:

1. History of excessive bleeding from minor accidents.
2. Presence of many bruises.
3. Family history of haemophilia in brothers, uncles, or male cousins on mother's side common but not invariable.
4. Low Factor VIII level in blood.

Differential Diagnosis from Thrombocytopenic Purpura

Note:

1. In haemophilia bleeding time normal but clotting time is prolonged. Factor VIII always low.

2. In thrombocytopenic purpura—bleeding time prolonged but clotting time and coagulation factors normal.

Prognosis
1. For life—severity varies in different individuals. After puberty may be some improvement.
2. Disability: (*a*) Haemarthrosis may result in ankylosis and contractures. (*b*) Psychological.
3. Factor VIII level indicates severity.

Management
1. Boys should be shielded from trauma, especially during 'bad periods'. When condition temporarily better, however, relaxation of restrictions should be allowed for psychological reasons.
2. Teeth must be carefully preserved to avoid risk of extraction later. Fluoride should be given if water content insufficient.
3. Genetic counselling: sister of case may be carrier (50%) and her sons may be haemophiliac (50%).

Treatment of Haemorrhage
1. Principle. Factor VIII level must be increased by intravenous injections of Factor VIII concentrate (cryoprecipitate or lyophilized powder) to raise level to about 50% of normal—should be 70–100% for surgery or if only one injection is given for haemarthrosis. Desmopressin (DDAVP) sometimes helpful: indications not yet clarified. Cyklokapron may limit mucous membrane haemorrhage, especially helpful in dental surgery.
2. Complications of therapy. Occasionally inhibitors develop which are IgG antibodies to Factor VIII. If bleeding severe in a patient with inhibitors, he must be given massive doses of Factor VIII or exchange transfusion. Avoid venepuncture of deep veins at all times. Viral hepatitis possibly leading to chronic liver disease. AIDS.
3. When required:
        3.1 Haemarthrosis.
        3.2 Rctroperitoneal haemorrhage.
        3.3 Intracranial haemorrhage.
        3.4 Very severe or prolonged bleed.
4. Parents—and the patient himself—can be trained to give i.v. Factor VIII. Note: If parent presents to doctor saying boy needs injection, wise to assume that he does. *Parent knows best.*
5. Aspiration of a haemarthrosis is of dubious value. Local pressure and cold helpful for some bleeding points.

Haemophilia B (*Christmas Disease*)

Cause is deficiency of Factor IX. Clinically similar to haemophilia A. Differentiated by specific factor assay. Can be treated by fresh frozen plasma or Factor IX concentrate. Heterozygote carrier may have bleeding tendency.

Disseminated Intravascular Coagulation (DIC)

DIC manifests in many different ways, e.g. haemolytic uraemic syndrome, thrombotic thrombocytopenic purpura, meningococcal septicaemia or haemorrhage in newborn. Occasionally bleeding from lungs, into skin, gut or CNS is due to a severe coagulation defect caused by removal (consumption) of certain essential factors—so-called 'consumption coagulopathy'. Underlying pathological process initiating coagulation may be cardiovascular collapse, severe acidosis, hypoxia, septicaemia or haemolysis. Consumed factors include fibrinogen, II, V, VIII and platelets. Fibrin-degradation products are liberated and can be detected in plasma. Diagnosis can be made by appropriate screening tests including kaolin cephalin clotting time, thrombin clotting time and platelet count; if abnormal, individual factor assay and fibrin-degradation product level should be estimated.

Treatment is that of underlying cause. Heparin together with fresh blood or plasma transfusion advocated by some.

Rare Haemorrhagic Diseases

1. Haemophilia C
A mild disease due to deficiency of Factor XI or Plasma Thromboplastin Antecedent (PTA). An autosomal dominant.

2. Congenital Fibrinogenopenia
Non-sex-linked. Clotting time and prothrombin time prolonged.

3. Von Willebrand's Disease
Hereditary disease of simple dominant type, affects both sexes. Clinically: tendency to bleed, especially epistaxis and after tooth extractions, or operations. Markedly cyclical. Haematology: prolonged bleeding time and reduced content of Factor VIII protein and clotting activity. Cryoprecipitate or fresh frozen plasma corrects bleeding.

Chapter 136 # HAEMORRHAGIC DISEASE OF NEWBORN

Definition
Uncommon disease, completely preventable, occurring from second to fourth day of life, due to hypoprothrombinaemia from lack of vitamin K-dependent factors (II, VII, IX, X) which are depressed in cord blood and drop considerably in first 2–4 days then slowly rise over next 3 months. Manifested clinically by haemorrhage, usually from gut but occasionally occurring elsewhere.

Pathogenesis
Poor neonatal synthesis of vitamin K-dependent clotting factors. Breast milk poor in vitamin K—also inhibits gut bacteria which synthesize vitamin K.

Clinical Features
Bleeding occurs during first week of life from gastrointestinal tract, i.e. stomach or per rectum (melaena neonatorum). Bleeding starts suddenly and may be profuse, even fatal.

Other causes of gastrointestinal bleeding in neonate, e.g. stress ulcers, swallowed blood (*see below*), infection, severe obstructive jaundice. *Note*: phenytoin and warfarin pass placenta and can cause haemorrhage.

Prevention

Completely preventable by vitamin K_1 (phytomenadione BP) 1·0 mg given routinely to all newborn infants. May be repeated once only. Larger doses cause kernicterus (*see* p. 406). Groups at risk and for whom vitamin K_1 is mandatory include abnormal deliveries and pre-term babies.

Treatment

1. *Vitamin K_1* 1·0mg (phytomenadione, B.P.) i.m. or orally.
2. *Blood transfusion*. For severe melaena neonatorum. Baby may die from simple haemorrhage into gut before any quantity of blood appears per rectum. Essential to gauge severity by pallor, pulse rate and degree of shock and not by quantity of blood passed. Blood transfusion restores blood volume and corrects anaemia.

'Swallowed Blood' Syndrome

Melaena neonatorum may be due to maternal blood which baby has swallowed during birth.

Test to distinguish maternal from fetal blood in infant's stool is based on the fact that fetal blood pigment more resistant to denaturation with alkali than adult's blood.

Method. Blood-containing stool (must be red, not tarry) mixed with water to lyse erythrocytes. Centrifuge. 5ml supernatant fluid mixed with 1ml sodium hydroxide (1%). Colour read after 2min. Adult haemoglobin: changes from pink to brown-yellow. Fetal haemoglobin: colour remains pink.

Chapter 137   # THE LEUKAEMIAS

Definition

Not uncommon malignant disease; fatal unless treated; manifested clinically by anaemia, haemorrhages, enlargement of spleen and often lymph nodes; haematologically by proliferation of leucocyte precursors with appearance of primitive forms in peripheral blood.

Aetiology

Cause. Unknown. Predisposing factors include:

1. Certain immune deficiency diseases, e.g. agammaglobulinaemia; chromosomal abnormalities, e.g. Down's syndrome (risk 20 × that of population); Bloom's syndrome.

2. Virus aetiology still actively pursued. The leukaemic cells have reverse transcriptase—an enzyme thought to come from a virus. Burkitt's lymphoma which is considered to be EB virus induced may end in leukaemia. Clustering of cases suggests viral cause.

3. Some evidence to suggest that maternal radiation during pregnancy may cause increased risk to fetus.

Note:
1. More common in siblings, especially twin.
2. One of few diseases which is more common in higher social classes.
3. Abnormal chromosome—Philadelphia chromosome Ph_1—which is chromosome No. 21 with deleted long arm—present in myeloid leukaemia.
Age groups. May occur at any age, more common before 5 years. Maximum incidence at 3 years. Males more than females.
Types. Following occur in children:
   1. Acute Leukaemia. Usually lymphoblastic (80% cases); some however, may be myelogenous (15%) or monocytic.
   2. Chronic Myelogenous Leukaemia. Very rare in young children.
   3. Other Types. Reticulum cell, monocytic, megakaryocytic and erythroid very rare.

Acute Leukaemia

Initial Manifestations
Onset: Child usually brought to doctor because of progressive pallor and lassitude. May have fever, weight loss, fatigue, infections of skin, lung, mouth, gums or throat. Sometimes bruising and haemorrhage may be first symptom. Condition may present with limb pain, or central nervous system abnormality. On examination child usually pale. May have petechial rash, haemorrhages into skin, retinae or from mucous membranes. Lymph nodes, liver and spleen, together with testes and kidney, often enlarged. Occasionally child may present with intracranial haemorrhage. Deafness, haematuria, haemorrhagic diarrhoea, skin deposits occur rarely.

Haematology
1. *Red blood cells*. Normocytic, normochromic anaemia almost constant feature, rarely macrocytic. Haemoglobin usually low but may be normal in aleukaemic phase.
2. *White blood cells*. Total may vary from very low, in aleukaemic phase, to very high. Half cases have count in normal range.
3. *Differential count*. Primitive cells (blasts) found, often in large numbers. May be difficult to decide type of cell; staining by PAS and Sudan black helpful. Lymphoblasts are PAS positive and Sudan black negative; myeloblasts opposite.
4. *Platelets*. Usually reduced, except in chronic myeloid type.
5. *Bone marrow*. The diagnostic investigation. Many primitive cells found. Marrow sometimes megaloblastic; may be difficult to diagnose from aplastic anaemia. Sample other sites.

Pathology
Infiltration with leukaemic tissue occurs in all organs, especially liver, spleen, lymph nodes, kidneys, testes, bones and central nervous system.

Radiology of Bones
Lifting of periosteum, especially near epiphyses, sometimes seen due to leukaemic deposit under it. Bones may show patchy rarefaction at metaphyses or osteosclerosis.

Clinical Course

At first, condition usually responds well to treatment. Lymph nodes and spleen regress. Blood picture returns to normal. This state may continue for weeks or months. Toxic effects of various drugs may be more prominent during remissions. About three-quarters of patients with lymphoblastic leukaemia have long remission which may be 5 years or more. This can be counted as a cure. Others have exacerbations at intervals and fail ultimately to respond to treatment. Outlook for myeloid leukaemia poor.

Differential Diagnosis

1. Other diseases with high white cell counts

> *1.1. Infectious Mononucleosis (Glandular Fever).* Cell of infectious mononucleosis characteristic in appearance. No anaemia or thrombocytopenia present. Paul–Bunnell test positive.
> *1.2. Pertussis.* May be high lymphocytosis up to $100000/mm^3$, but cells are mature. Other features of disease, e.g. cough, make diagnosis obvious.
> *1.3. Acute Infectious Lymphocytosis*
> *1.4. Tuberculosis.* Rarely may have very high white cell count but other haematological and clinical features of leukaemia absent.

2. Haemorrhagic diseases. Thrombocytopenic purpura or agranulocytosis may resemble aleukaemic leukaemia. Diagnosis made by examination of bone marrow.

3. Rheumatic diseases. Bone pains simulate rheumatoid arthritis, rheumatic fever, brucellosis, osteomyelitis.

4. Leukaemic xanthomatosis syndrome. Café-au-lait spots, xanthoma, normal cholesterol and monocytic or monomyeloid leukaemoid picture.

5. Non-Hodgkin's lymphoma. See p. 431. About one-quarter of children with treated non-Hodgkin's lymphoma develop leukaemia.

6. Familial myeloproliferative disease. Recurrent respiratory infection, protruberant abdomen, retarded growth, hepatosplenomegaly. Acute course. Marrow similar to myeloid leukaemia. Occasional recovery.

7. Metastatic malignant disease, e.g. neuroblastoma.

Treatment

> 1.1 Treatment is specialized and should be administered at regional centres. Actual drug regime varies because of trials which are in operation continuously to determine the optimum therapy.
> 1.2 Combination of drugs superior to individual drugs.
> 1.3 Treatment should be on out-patient basis whenever possible.
> 1.4 Patient's resistance lowered by leukaemic process as well as by drugs and so opportunistic organisms may cause problems, e.g. septicaemia. Organisms encountered include Gram-negative organisms, staphylococci, *Pneumocystis carinii*, fungi and cytomegalovirus.

2. Drugs

> *1.1 Remission.* Many drugs will induce a remission in acute lymphatic leukaemia. In remission the patient is symptom-

free, the peripheral blood and bone marrow are normal cytologically and organ enlargements disappeared. Remission is induced by drugs which often have a profound but limited effect. Remission is maintained by other drugs which have capacity to keep many patients disease-free.

1.2 Induction brought about by prednisone and vincristine. Other drugs capable of inducing remission: asparaginase, thioguanine, cytosine arabinoside, cyclophosphamide, 6-mercaptopurine, adriamycin. The rapid lysis of abnormal cells leads to high uric acid load. Uric acid nephropathy with renal failure is eliminated by concomitant administration of alkalis, allopurinol and adequate fluids. Watch for hyperkalaemia.

1.3 Maintenance Therapy commenced after about 6 weeks—often using combinations of 6-mercaptopurine, methotrexate, cyclophosphamide or cytosine arabinoside. Other drugs used for maintenance—vincristine, thioguanine.

3. Spinal prophylactic radiation should be given early in course of treatment to eliminate nests of leukaemic cells in CNS, which are inaccessible to drugs; long-term consequences—if any—not yet known. Careful screening of organs essential.

Manifestations of toxicity of anti-leukaemic drugs
1. 6-Mercaptopurine

1.1 Nausea and vomiting—omit drug until symptoms disappear, then recommence at lower dosage.
1.2 Neutropenia and/or thrombocytopenia—if not due to leukaemia, reduce dosage.

2. Methotrexate

2.1 Oral ulceration ± diarrhoea ± gastrointestinal haemorrhage—omit until cleared, then recommence at reduced dosage.
2.2 Nausea and vomiting—as 1.1 *above*.
2.3 Neutropenia and/or thrombocytopenia—as 1.2 *above*.
2.4 Anaemia, if not due to leukaemia—omit and recommence with lower dosage when haemoglobin rising.
2.5 Toxic hepatitis (should be confirmed by liver biopsy)—do not use methotrexate again.

3. Cyclophosphamide

3.1 Lymphopenia—ignore.
3.2 Neutropenia and/or thrombocytopenia (as 1.2 *above*).
3.3 Haemorrhagic cystitis—omit drug till cleared, then recommence at 70% previous dose.
3.4 Epilation—ignore if in relapse. Decrease dose if in remission.
3.5 Sterile cystitis—push fluid intake.

4. Vincristine

4.1 Constipation and/or abdominal cramps—if not readily reversed by purgation or enemas, dosage should be decreased.

4.2 Neuritic pains and paraesthesiae—if not severe, non-progressive, and limited to hand and feet, can be ignored.

4.3 Motor abnormalities, e.g. loss of deep reflexes, muscle weakness or wasting, ptosis, diplopia—reduce dosage.

4.4 Oral ulceration—reduce dosage.

4.5 Encephalopathy, convulsions or personality changes—reduce dosage.

4.6 Epilation, almost invariable—ignore.

4.7 Anaemia or neutropenia—if not due to the leukaemia process (bone marrow may be required to distinguish)—reduce dosage.

Parent and child counselling very important. Parents should be informed of diagnosis and likely outcome. Cautious optimism now possible. Child often learns diagnosis by one route or another and should have discussions with experienced sensitive counsellor. Children may be very disturbed.

Chapter 138   *MALIGNANCIES*

Non-Hodgkin's Lymphoma

Definition
A malignant disease of lymph nodes, occurring at any age, affecting boys more than girls. Aetiology unknown, but antibodies to EB virus are present in patients. Increased incidence in children with immunological defects.

Clinical Features
Usually presents with painless enlargement of glands of neck, axillae or inguinal regions. Sometimes starts in thorax and causes mediastinal or respiratory obstruction. This may constitute an acute emergency. May also present with retroperitoneal mass shown by abdominal enlargement. Systemic symptoms, such as weight loss, fever, fatigue, are rare at time of presentation. In 25%, acute lymphoblastic leukaemia develops, with anaemia, haemorrhages and characteristic blood picture. Infiltration of CNS often follows.

Diagnosis
By gland biopsy, possibly marrow biopsy.

Treatment
Local radiotherapy, followed by steroids and chemotherapy as in acute lymphoblastic leukaemia.

Prognosis
Poor except when disease localized.

Burkitt's lymphoma
A variety of childhood lymphoma particularly common in some parts of Africa amd New Guinea. Predilection for jaws and gonads. High titre of EV virus antibody. Cyclophosphamide may induce remission after 1–2 doses.

Hodgkin's Disease
Very rare disease in children. Cause unknown. Manifested clinically by enlargement of lymph nodes, spleen and pathologically by replacement of normal

structure of lymph node or spleen by proliferation of reticuloendothelial tissue with or without giant cell formation. For details, *see* textbooks of adult medicine.

Congenital Disorders

Cystic Hygroma (*Cystic Lymphangioma*)
Not uncommon. Usually presents as soft, poorly defined mass, most commonly in posterior cervical triangle or axilla. May transilluminate. Contains clear colourless or xanthochromic fluid. May increase in size rapidly if haemorrhage occurs into tumour. Similar tumour may occur in mediastinum or mesentery.

Treatment
Surgical removal if possible.

Chylous Ascites

Two Forms Occur
1. True chylous ascites caused by anomaly, injury or obstruction of thoracic duct. If anomaly present, ascites found soon after birth but true chylous appearance is not present until infant takes milk. If child given Sudan III by mouth and paracentesis performed soon after, fat will be found to be stained red.
2. Pseudo-chylous ascites. Milky fluid with high fat content found in some cases of peritonitis. Sudan III test negative.

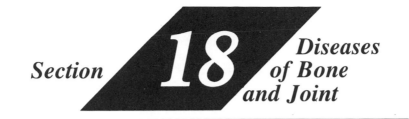

| Chapter 139 | *GENERALIZED ABNORMALITIES OF BONE* |

Osteogenesis Imperfecta (*Fragilitas Ossium*)

Osteogenesis imperfecta is an uncommon systemic disease caused by congenital abnormality of tissues formed by mesenchyme. Inheritance is usually dominant with variable expression; some members of the kindred may show blue sclerae or deafness only. The prognosis varies with severity.

1. Antenatal Cases
During delivery a large number of fractures occur (100 or more) and frequently the child is stillborn. The limbs are short, thick and deformed. If the baby survives, the condition in later life resembles postnatal cases. Extreme deformities are common.

2. Postnatal Cases
Fractures may not develop until the end of the first year of life. They are then caused by minor trauma. Healing occurs readily by callus formation. In some cases there is a tendency for fractures to decrease after puberty.
Blue sclerae. Sclerae of newborn and young babies are always bluish, but in children with osteogenesis imperfecta, colour much darker. Described as indigo (blue-violet).
Deafness. Does not develop until adult life. Due to otosclerosis or labyrinthine disturbance.
Ligaments. May be lax, resulting in dislocation of joints.
Teeth. First dentition often translucent, but permanent teeth usually better.

Renal Osteodystrophy (*Renal Rickets; Renal Infantilism*)

This is a rare complication of chronic renal failure. The bone shafts are osteoporotic and the metaphyses may have a cystic appearance. The epiphyses resemble severe rickets and deformity with considerable bowing may be present. Vicarious (metastatic) calcification sometimes occurs in the soft tissue. Renal

433

tubular insufficiency results in decreased ability to make ammonia and excrete acid urine; phosphate retention occurs; calcium therefore excreted in urine in excess; results in tendency to low serum calcium; this causes parathyroid hyperplasia, which leads to osteoporosis. Epiphysial changes resemble severe rickets. Other factors are failure of kidney conversion of 25-hydroxyvitamin D to 1,25-dihydroxyvitamin D.

Histiocytosis X (Eosinophilic Granuloma of Bone; Hand–Schüller–Christian Syndrome; Letterer–Siwe Disease)

Definition
Uncommon group of diseases of unknown aetiology manifested pathologically by histiocytic granulomas and clinically by varied clinical syndromes of differing severity. Younger children tend to have more widespread lesions. *Note:* Called 'X' to signify unknown aetiology. Non-familial; occurs in any race. Principal age group: 2–7 years.
Cause. Granulomatous deposits develop which may occur anywhere especially bones (75%), skull, spine, femur, ribs. Result in bone absorption and in skull pressure effects on pituitary.

Pathology
Bone, lung, liver, skin, lymph nodes, bone marrow may have granulomatous deposits which contain numerous large histiocytes. Electron microscopy shows typical cytoplasmic 'X bodies' or racket bodies. Proliferative, destructive, xanthomatous and sclerosing features may all be present in the same lesion. May be localized, or widespread throughout all tissues (especially in Letterer–Siwe syndrome).

Eosinophilic Granuloma
Clinical features. Approximately one-third of all cases, mostly aged 4–14 years usually gives rise to no generalized symptoms, but sometimes to spontaneous fracture or localized pain and tenderness over affected bone.

Condition may be discovered on routine radiological examination: Clear-cut area of bone absorption seen, occurring most commonly in skull, vertebrae, pelvis or mandible.

Prognosis
Mortality less than 1% if confined to bones.

Hand–Schüller–Christian Syndrome
Rare disease with some bony and some generalized visceral manifestations: diabetes insipidus, absorption of bones of skull and exophthalmos. Classical triad

of diabetes insipidus, exophthalmos and skull deposits occurs in 10 % of all cases, but chronic relapsing type seen in 30 % cases.

Clinical features

1. *Diabetes Insipidus.* Early symptoms sometimes associated with other evidence of pituitary dysfunction, e.g. dwarfism.

2. *Bony Lesions*

    2.1 Defects caused by xanthomatous deposits in skull can sometimes be palpated. Radiograph shows map-like areas of resorbed bone often involving petrous temporal and sella turcica as well as others. Subjective symptoms, e.g. headache, may occur.

    2.2 Exophthalmos, uni- or bilateral, may occur from mass pushing eye forward.

    2.3 Fractures may develop through rarefied areas of bone.

3. *Otitis Externa.* Common and often early sign.

4. *Skin.* Rashes and rarely xanthomas.

5. *Gums.* Gingivitis with loss of teeth rare.

6. *Lung.* Diffuse lipidosis leading to fibrosis with miliary mottling of lungs and honeycomb appearance on X-ray.

7. *Liver and Spleen.* Not usually enlarged.

Prognosis. Variable, may remain, burn out, or become generalized and death occur. Diabetes insipidus once present, is permanent.

Treatment

1. *Diabetes Insipidus. See* p. 465.

2. *Xanthomatous Lesions.* Disappear with deep X-ray therapy and bone regenerates, but lesions may reappear.

3. *Triple Chemotherapy.* Vinblastine 0·1–0·3 mg/kg i.v. weekly (or Vincristine or Vindesine). Cyclophosphamide 3 mg/kg/day orally reducing to 2 mg/kg/day. (Chlorambucil an alternative.) Prednisone 3 mg/kg/day.

This combination given for 6 weeks, interval of 4 weeks then course repeated. Intervals between courses extended as disease comes under control.

Letterer–Siwe Disease

Incidence 25–30 % all cases, often in infancy, may be congenital.

Clinical features. Child is very ill with:

1. Rash—generalized scaly petechial eruption. Tends to be moist and denuded in areas around groin, axilla, ears and neck. Mouth often extensively involved. Gingivitis and ulceration common.

2. Liver, spleen and lymph nodes palpable.

3. Marrow involvement, with marrow failure; anaemia and purpura.

4. Lungs: infiltrated. Radiograph shows miliary pattern.

5. Bones: lesions occur but are not prominent.

6. Secondary infection occurs terminally.

Immunology. Standard testing of immunological competence by electrophoresis skin testing and lymphoblastic proliferation normal. It appears that there are cytotoxic lymphocytes and autologous erythrocyte antibody with deficiency of suppressor T-lymphocytes. Treatment with calf thymus extract and chemotherapy as above may be helpful.

Mortality. 65 %.

Chapter 140	*ABNORMALITIES MAINLY AFFECTING LIMB BONES*

Congenital Bony Abnormalities

Polydactyly
Extra finger or toe. May be associated with Laurence–Moon–Biedl syndrome. Trisomy 13 (*see* p. 16).

Syndactyly
Fusion or webbing of fingers or toes. Associated abnormalities common. May be familial.

Arachnodactyly
Abnormally long fingers and toes. Often part of Marfan syndrome.

Sprengel Shoulder
The scapula is higher than normal, the lower angle points towards the spine.

Marfan Syndrome
Is a rare disorder with a dominant inheritance. Principal features are: abnormally long fingers and toes, excess height, but weight below average owing to lack of subcutaneous fat, joints often hyperextensile. Long narrow skull, high palate, prominent or sunken sternum.

Some of the following are commonly reported in addition:

1. Skeletal
Prominent supra-orbital ridges; kyphosis; scoliosis; pigeon-chest; spurring of os calcis; elevation of patella.

2. Ocular
Small pupil; dislocation of lens.

3. Cardiac
Various congenital heart lesions (especially atrial septal defect) and aortic aneurysm.

4. Pulmonary
Vestigial lobes of lungs and other abnormalities; propensity to pneumonia.

Achondroplasia (*Chondrodystrophia*)
This is a well-known, but uncommon disorder inherited as a Mendelian dominant

with high mutation rate. Both the arms and legs are short and chubby. There is loose skin present which has extra creases as though the subcutaneous tissue has grown to normal length but had to accommodate itself to the abnormal short bones. Full extension of the elbow joint is not possible. The hands have a characteristic trident shape—the fingers are not parallel. The forehead is prominent and the bridge of the nose flattened. The gait is waddling partly due to laxity of ligaments. Mentality is normal unless hydrocephalus is present. The expectation for life is normal.

The basic histological defect is an abnormality of endochondrial ossification. Cartilage cells are few in number, not formed in orderly parallel rows and are irregular in size. Intercellular matrix is fibrinous, not hyaline in character. Periosteal bone growth is normal but often transverse strip of fibrous tissue grows in from periosteum obstructing normal growth. If this occurs on one side of bone only curvature may result.

Chapter 141	# ABNORMALITIES MAINLY AFFECTING SKULL

Anencephaly

A condition in which the bony vault of the skull is defective. The brain is underdeveloped or absent. The cause is unknown; females much more frequently affected than males. Mother often has hydramnios during pregnancy; may produce more than one anencephalic. Condition can be diagnosed by antenatal radiograph. Other CNS malformations may occur in same family.

Craniostenosis (*Premature Synostosis; Stenocephaly*)

A heterogeneous group of conditions in which, if fusion of one or more sutures takes place early, abnormal shape of skull results. For instance:
1. *Scaphocephaly*. Elongation of skull anteroposteriorly.
2. *Plagiocephaly*. The forehead is prominent on one side and occiput prominent on the other. Mild degrees of skull asymmetry commonly occur in normal babies from lying on one side, but in this case the sutures are normal.

Craniostenosis must be distinguished from microcephaly due to mental retardation. Here the skull is too small and the sutures may fuse early but this is because the brain is small and underdeveloped. Surgical opening of the sutures does not help.

Oxycephaly (Tower Skull)
This is an uncommon condition in which the head is tall and rounded. The fontenelle is closed and the coronal sutures fused. There is often exophthalmos with oblique palpebral fissure with outer end depressed.

Associated Defects
Apert's syndrome is oxycephaly and syndactyly and sometimes other abnormalities.

Clinical Complications
The child develops headaches, squint, nystagmus; even blindness due to optic atrophy. Mentality usually normal at first, but because brain cannot expand secondary mental deficiency may occur.

Radiology of Skull
Shows fusion of some or all sutures. Evidence of raised intracranial pressure.

Treatment
Early surgical opening of sutures advised to prevent blindness and mental deterioration. Teflon placed between cut edges of bone, otherwise fusion will occur again. Results of early operation encouraging.

Hypertelorism

Anatomical Defect
Imbalance between enlarged lesser wings of sphenoid bone and greater wings which are relatively small.

Clinical Picture
Increased distance between eyes with broadening of root of nose.
   Child may be mentally retarded. With mild degrees, which are common, the mentality is normal.

Lacuna Skull (*Craniofenestria*)

An anatomical defect in which there is poor development of frontal or parietal bones resulting in multiple shallow depressions or complete holes. Inner surface lined by dura; bone around lacunae abnormally thick. Total weight of skull reduced.
   Usually there is no associated symptoms although the bony defects can sometimes be palpated. Radiograph of the skull has a characteristic appearance. Lacuna skull may be associated with such defects as hydrocephalus, spina bifida, or meningomyelocele.

Cleidocranial Dysostosis

An uncommon defect with dominant inheritance in which the clavicles are either completely absent or present only at sternal ends. Muscles arising from clavicles are poorly developed or absent. There is delayed development of the membranous bones of the skull. Fontanelles have anterior prolongation and remain patent until adult life. Compensatory bosses appear over frontal, occipital and parietal bones. Often deficient growth of maxilla resulting in maldevelopment of sinuses and high arched palate. Irregular dentition.

Chapter 142	ACUTE INFECTION OF
	BONES AND JOINTS

Acute Osteomyelitis

This condition is commonest in boys aged 5–10 years, but can occur at any age. The organism is usually *Staphylococcus aureus*. Fundamentally, the condition is that of a septicaemia or pyaemia in which the infection settles in a bone. The sequence of events is that blood-borne organisms from septic focus, such as a boil, are arrested by capillaries in bone at metaphysis—possibly in small haematoma caused by trauma. Infection slowly works to surface of bone and up medullary cavity. Periosteum stripped from bone as pus occludes blood vessels in bone, with resulting necrosis and sequestrum formation.

In older children the condition commences suddenly with rigors, generalized aches and pains, toxaemia, headache and sometimes delirium. Pain at site of bone infection, but may not be accurately localized for day or two, but soon affected limb becomes very tender and movement causes pain. If bone is near surface, e.g. tibia, skin may be reddened and affected part feels hot. Considerable swelling may occur. However, if the bone is deeply placed, e.g. femur, this may not be obvious.

Occasionally in babies the condition may be surprisingly benign.

Prognosis
With adequate treatment prognosis is excellent even in very acute cases, complete cure usually resulting within a few weeks. Relapses may occur and if weight-bearing is allowed too early a fracture may follow.

Treatment
Treatment must be commenced immediately. Appropriate antistaphylococcal antibiotics should be given in full dosage i.v. Limb should be immobilized by sandbags or plaster back-splint.

Surgical treatment is rarely required.

Chapter 143	OSTEOCHONDRITIS JUVENILIS

This is a not uncommon group of diseases occurring mainly in children, manifested pathologically by arrest of epiphysial development followed by irregular growth and sclerosis of epiphysis. Clinical manifestations depend on site of lesion.

Following epiphyses especially involved: *(1) Hip:* Perthes' disease (pseudocoxalgia; coxa plana). *(2) Vertebral Bodies:* Scheuermann's disease. *(3) Tubercle of Tibia:* Osgood–Schlatter's disease. *(4) Apophysis of Os Calcis:* Sever's disease. *(5) Tarsal Scaphoid:* Köhler's disease.

Of these the commonest is Perthes' disease.

For differential diagnosis *see Table* 143.1, *over.*

Table 143.1.   Differential diagnosis of pain in hip

	Age	Sex	General condition of child	Clinical appearance	Radiological changes
Transient synovitis	13–10	Mainly boys	Child well	Limp, pain, limitation of movement	Nil
Tuberculosis	2–15	Equal	General malaise	Leg, flexed, abducted or adducted. Movement resented	Early stages: osteoporosis Later: joint space narrowed
Perthes' disease	5–10	Mainly boys	Child well	Limitation of abduction, otherwise movement good	Fragmentation and flattening
Slipped epiphysis	10–15	Equal	Child well	Leg held in adduction, limitation of abduction	Little seen in early stages
Acute pyogenic arthritis	Any age	Equal	Child very ill	Leg a little flexed and abducted. Movement resented	Little seen in early stages

Mild or severe pain in a hip joint is common in children. There are many possible causes, some of which are given in *Table* 143.1. In addition, juvenile rheumatoid arthritis, bone tumours and acute leukaemia may affect the hip joint or give rise to pain referable to it.

Transient Synovitis of Hip
('Irritable' Hip)

Commonest condition affecting hip in childhood. Possibly due to trivial injury causing synovitis. Age 3–10 years. More common in boys. Unilateral.

Clinical Features

Sudden or insidious onset of pain and limp. On examination: muscle spasm and limitation of movement.

Congenital Dislocation of Hip

Aetiology
Sex. Girls more frequently affected than boys.
Heredity. Familial incidence occasionally noticed. Often breech delivery, usually left side.

Clinical Features
Condition latent until infant starts to walk, but should be diagnosed and treated at birth for best results.

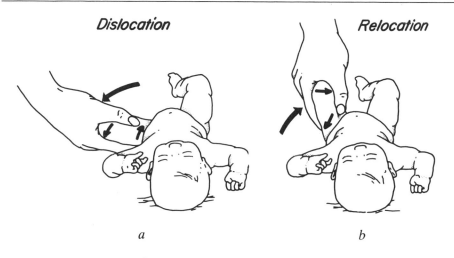

Dislocation   *Relocation*

a   *b*

Fig. 143.1. Ortolani test *a*, for dislocation relocates head of femur. *b*,
Barlow test redislocates femur.

1. Diagnosis in newborn

    1.1 Ortolani's test (*Fig. 143.1*). With baby lying on back
and legs flexed at hips, normal thigh can be rotated outward
almost to a right angle. If hip dislocated this movement is
limited and femur can be felt by finger over greater
trochanter to jump back into acetabulum.

    1.2 *Barlow's test. Reverse procedure dislocates femur* and
movement is felt by thumb.

    Note: These signs should be looked for routinely in every
newborn.

2. Diagnosis in young child. Walking often delayed.

    2.1 Signs in unilateral cases:

    2.1.1 Leg appears short; great trochanter prominent.

    2.1.2 Abduction restricted. 'Telescopic' movement of leg
may be possible.

    2.1.3 Trendelenburg's sign. When child stands on dislo-
cated leg pelvis on normal side drops.

    2.2 Signs in bilateral cases:

    2.2.1 Waddling gait.

    2.2.2 Marked lordosis; increased perineal gap.

Radiology

1. In infants

    1.1 Ossification of epiphysial centre of femoral head delayed.

    1.2 Roof of acetabulum straight, not rounded as in normal.

    1.3 With legs abducted and internally rotated, femur points
above acetabulum on affected side.

2. In childhood. Shenton's line broken, i.e. line connecting upper part of
obturator foramen with neck of femur.

Treatment
Child should lie with legs flexed and abducted in plaster or in frame.

Prognosis
If treatment started within first few weeks of life, walking need not be delayed. If started after walking has commenced, treatment required for many years.

Chapter 144   *JUVENILE RHEUMATOID ARTHRITIS (Still's Disease)*

Aetiology
Autoimmune disease.

Pathology
Disease generalized and affects all mesodermal tissues.
1. *Joints*. Synovial membrane thickened by pannus formation. Synovial fluid increased in amount. Cartilage normal or may be pitted. Bone surrounding joint osteoporotic. Capsule shows periarticular fibrosis. Ligaments fibrosed.
2. *Nodules*. Usually larger than those of acute rheumatism. Contain area of central necrosis surrounded by mononuclear cells.
3. *Muscles and nerves*. May be affected.
4. *Heart*. Endocarditis very rare. Pericarditis may be found at postmortem.
5. *Amyloid disease*. Juvenile rheumatoid arthritis is commonest cause of amyloid in children.

Clinical Features
1. *Age*. Rare under 1 year. Early onset worsens prognosis.
2. *Sex*. Female preponderance less marked than in adults.
3. *Onset*. Three distinct modes of onset:

> *3.1 Polyarticular*. Simultaneous involvement of four or more joints. Usually symmetrical, affecting knees, ankles, feet, hands and wrists. Affected joint warm and swollen but not necessarily red or painful although movement restricted. Apophysial joints between cervical vertebrae often affected, leading to limitation of movement, and head projects forwards. Mandible often recedes. Systemic manifestations usually present—lassitude, anorexia, low grade fever, weight loss, lymphadenopathy, splenomegaly. May be characteristic transient, pink, macular, truncal rash. Nodules rare.
>
> *3.2 Pauciarticular*. Larger joints—knee, hip, elbow, ankle. Up to three joints affected, usually one. Onset usually insidious, symptoms mild. Joint slightly swollen, stiff, slightly painful. May be limp with little objective abnormality. Systemic features uncommon, mild, *except for ocular involvement*—iridocyclitis which can lead to blindness via band keratopathy and cataract. Laboratory investigations frequently normal.

3.3 Acute Febrile Onset. May be minimal joint symptoms, arthralgia only. Systemic manifestations predominate—lassitude, irritability, fever (often high grade for long time, many weeks), weight loss, lymphadenopathy, splenomegaly, myocarditis, pericarditis, pleurisy, rash. Striking leucocytosis, elevated ESR, moderate normochromic, normocytic anaemia.

Investigations

Erythrocyte sedimentation rate. Raised during active stage of disease, even after temperature has returned to normal. *Haemoglobin.* Usually low. *Polymorphonuclear leucocytosis.* Common at onset, may be high; rarely, in very severe cases, leucopenia occurs later. *Rheumatoid factor.* Serological tests using sensitized sheep cells or latex fixation not often positive.

Course and Prognosis

Polyarticular form. Tends to relapse and remit. Occasionally progresses to joint deformity and amyloid disease. Growth failure usually prominent.
Mono/pauciarticular form. Also tends to remissions and relapses, with involvement of other joints, but occasionally progresses to polyarticular disease. Ocular disease may continue insidiously.
Acute febrile form. Fifty per cent suffer recurrent attacks, eventually subside without permanent sequelae. Remainder develop polyarticular course.

Differential Diagnosis

1. Acute rheumatic fever. Characteristically flitting. May be evidence of carditis; ESR, antistreptolysin titre (AST) raised.
2. Systemic lupus erythematosus (SLE). Difficult to distinguish from rheumatoid in early months if no rash or LE cells.
3. Brucellosis. Fever, sweating, low white count and ESR; agglutination test diagnostic.
4. Leukaemia. Blood picture may be confusing at first. Bone marrow may help.
5. Serum sickness
6. Drug reaction
7. Rubella arthritis
8. Mycoplasma pneumoniae arthritis
9. Anaphylactoid purpura
10. Agammaglobulinaemia/hypogammaglobulinaemia
11. Kawasaki disease

Treatment

1. General. Rest in bed during active stages of disease.
2. Local

2.1 Affected limbs require rest but should be moved passively through full range once each day. Plaster back splints help to prevent contractures. If deformity present serial plasters can be applied until deformity corrected.
2.2 Heat, wax baths and massage may be of help.

3. Drug therapy

3.1 Acetylsalicylic acid is drug of choice for all forms, in high, individualized dosage.

3.2 Systemic corticosteroids indicated only when life or vision threatened—myocarditis, vasculitis, iridocyclitis. Dose should be kept to minimum effective. Other drugs, e.g. indomethacin, gold, Brufen may help.

Chapter 145   # POSTURAL DEFORMITIES

Spinal Defects

Lordosis or scoliosis. Can be either:

1. Primary
Condition mainly affects adolescents. May be improved by physiotherapy but sometimes requires surgery. Can lead to serious lung disease.

2. Secondary, due to:
2.1 Bone lesions, congenital or acquired, hemivertebrae or mucopolysaccharidosis.
2.2 Disease of muscle or cerebral palsy.
2.3 Intrathoracic lesions, e.g. resolving pleural effusion.

Congenital Torticollis

Clinical Features
Not uncommon condition, cause uncertain, usually noticed within first few months of life. Owing to shortening of sternomastoid, head is turned to one side so that occiput approximates to shoulder of same side.

Prognosis
Untreated case said to lead to asymmetry of face, but asymmetry is primary condition and involvement of sternomastoid associated defect.

Flat-foot
Normal in children up to 2 years of age.

Pigeon Toe
Very common. Usually of no significance.

Knock-knee
Mild cases not significant. Severe cases may follow rickets.

Bow Legs
Usually physiological, but occasionally due to rickets or Blount's syndrome in which tibiae bowed and inner cortex thick. The upper medial tibial epiphysis is often fragmented. No treatment needed and usually resolves.

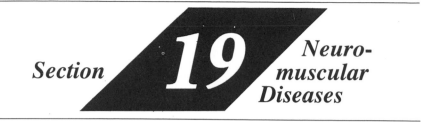

Chapter 146 **CONGENITAL ABSENCE OF MUSCLE**

May be generalized as in arthrogryposis multiplex congenita (*see* p. 454) or involve single muscles.

Muscles Involved
1. Pectoralis major (sternal portion). Muscle most commonly involved. To demonstrate: tell child to press hands together. Normally lower portion of pectoralis major seen as oblique ridge running down from shoulder. If lower part of muscle is absent, the inferior border runs transversely, either unilateral or bilateral. May be associated lesions of ribs. May be part of Poland anomaly with syndactyly and possibly hypoplasia of arm.
2. Serrati, trapezius or quadriceps. May be absent.
3. Abdominal muscles ('Prune belly syndrome'). Absence very rare but important. Almost only in males. Death may occur in infancy as a result of associated urogenital abnormalities, i.e. bilateral hydronephrosis with dilated ureters and bladder, leading to renal failure.

Chapter 147 **MUSCLE ATROPHY**

Classification
Note: Often uncertain which diseases are primarily nervous with secondary muscle atrophy and which primarily muscular with secondary nervous degeneration. For example, arthrogryposis multiplex congenita (*see* p. 454).
1. Primary nervous lesion with secondary muscle degeneration. (*a*) Due to central nerve lesions (*see* Chapter 94). (*b*) Due to generalized lesion of spinal cord, e.g. infantile hypotonia (*see below*); and probably peroneal muscular atrophy (*see* p. 447).
2. Primary diseases of the muscular system. Muscular dystrophies (*see* Chapter 148).
3. Diseases in which muscle atrophy is only one symptom, e.g. myotonic dystrophy (*see* p. 451).

The Floppy Baby Syndrome
(Infantile Hypotonia)

Causes
1. Cerebral. Many forms of mental retardation, e.g. Down's syndrome; Cerebral

palsy—hypotonic or cerebellar varieties; Prader–Willi syndrome, cerebral lipidoses, Lowe's syndrome.
2. Spinal cord. (*a*) *Trauma*, e.g. with breech delivery. (*b*) *Motor Neurone.* Spinal muscular atrophy: acute, chronic and benign.
3. Peripheral nerve. Familial dysautonomia, congenital sensory neuropathy and polyneuritis.
4. Neuromuscular junction. Myasthenia gravis.
5. Muscle diseases. Muscle dystrophies, central core disease, glycogen storage disease, nemaline and mitochondrial myopathies, polymyositis.

Spinal Muscular Atrophy *(Werdnig–Hoffmann Disease; Amyotonia Congenita)*

Classification
1. Infantile spinal muscular atrophy (acute Werdnig–Hoffmann disease). Death usually occurs in first year.
2. Chronic generalized spinal muscular atrophy of infancy and childhood (arrested Werdnig–Hoffmann disease). Death in late childhood.
3. 'Benign' spinal muscular atrophy (Kugelberg–Welander disease). Death in adulthood.

General Consideration
All three have distinct autosomal recessive inheritance.

Incidence
1. Infantile form about second commonest fatal recessive disease.
2. Benign form same as infantile.
3. Chronic form, far less common.

Pathology
1. Atrophy of anterior horn cells and demyelination of nerves.
2. Secondary atrophy of muscles supplied by these nerves. Diaphragm and extra-ocular muscles not affected.

Clinical Features
1. Infantile form. Muscular weakness from birth. Mother may say she did not feel fetal movements. No paralysis. Extreme hypotonia of muscles. If baby lifted by hands placed in axillae, arms shoot upwards and body may slip through hands and fall. Limbs can be placed in extraordinary positions. Lies in frog position. Reflexes absent. Muscular fibrillation of tongue diagnostic.
2. Chronic form. Fetal movements normal. Progressive in a stepwise fashion. Chest movement and cough very weak. Marked chest deformity develops. Usually die of respiratory infection. Weakness and wasting are progressive, muscles being affected in following order: (*a*) Trunk, especially muscles of respiration with indrawing of ribs. Shoulder-girdles. Scoliosis marked. (*b*) Centrifugal spread in limbs. May develop congenital dislocation of hip. Gross

contractures. (*c*) Lastly muscles supplied by bulbar nerves. Rapidly progressive. Reaction of degeneration can be demonstrated.

3. Benign form. Muscle weakness takes longer to appear and disability not so great. Reflexes weak. Child often able to walk and function normally.

Differential diagnosis from pseudohypertrophic muscular dystrophy by: (*a*) Coarse irregular tremor of hands. (*b*) Muscular fasciculation. (*c*) Walk flat-footed, feet everted, whereas dystrophy children walk on toes, with waddling lordotic gait. (*d*) Genetic inheritance. Autosomal recessive. Dystrophy—sex-linked recessive.

Management
Physiotherapy; schooling for older children; genetic counselling.

Peroneal Muscular Atrophy (*Progressive Neuro-muscular Atrophy; Charcot–Marie–Tooth Type*)

Definition
Very rare hereditary disease characterized clinically by wasting of muscles of leg, especially peroneal group. Subsequent condition involves thigh muscles transversely. Other muscle groups involved later. Characterized pathologically by lesions in cord, peripheral nerves and secondary muscle atrophy.

Aetiology
Dominant inheritance, but sporadic cases occur. Age of onset 5–15 years but may occur later.

Clinical Features
Onset. Classically weakness and wasting of peronei; sometimes small muscles of feet affected. Wasting of peronei leads to talipes deformity; wasting of small muscles of feet leads to claw-foot. Always symmetrical. Muscular fibrillation occurs: sensation may be diminished.

Progress
Spreads up the thigh, affecting muscles transversely, up to junction of middle and lower third. This gives rise to 'inverted champagne bottle' appearance. Later—often after years—may involve arm. Spreads as in leg, but muscles above elbow spared. Claw-hand develops.

Prognosis
Although progressive, disease may be arrested. Compatible with long useful life.

Chapter 148   ## MUSCULAR DYSTROPHIES (*Myopathies*)

Definition
Not uncommon hereditarily determined diseases in which lesion is in the muscles. Nerves normal.

Pathology
Lesions are confined to muscles. Stages:
1. *Pseudohypertrophy*. Size of muscles due to: (*a*) Increased deposition of fat between muscle fibres—main cause. (*b*) Increased size of muscle fibres with *true increase* in number of sarcolemma nuclei—unimportant cause.
2. *Atrophy*. Fibrosis with *apparent increase* in sarcolemma nuclei. No real increase. Appearance is due to crowding together of atrophied fibres.
3. Eventually contractures develop.
   Note: Serum levels of aldolase and creatine kinase increased.

Clinical Types
(1) Pseudohypertrophic muscular dystrophy; (2) Facioscapulohumeral type; (3) Limb girdle muscular dystrophy; (4) Ocular myopathy; (5) Distal myopathy; (6) Congenital muscular dystrophy.

1. Pseudohypertrophic Muscular Dystrophy (Duchenne Type)

Commonest type.

Aetiology
Heredity. Sex-linked recessive—transmitted by female, manifested in males.
Age. Usually diagnosed 1–3 years, but often history of delay in learning to walk.

Onset
Gradually increasing difficulty in walking, especially climbing up stairs. Child easily pushed over. Found to have large, powerful-looking lower limb muscles, which are actually weaker than normal (pseudohypertrophy). These muscles undergo atrophy during course of years. Some muscles never show initial hypertrophy, but atrophy later.
Muscles most commonly showing pseudohypertrophy: Calves, quadriceps, glutei, deltoids, infraspinati. Less commonly, triceps, supraspinati, biceps, masseters, serratus.
Muscles which show no hypertrophy but later atrophy. Latissimus dorsi, sternal portion of pectoralis major (may appear early in disease).
Cardiomyopathy present but rarely causes symptoms.

Fully Developed Case
Stance lordotic, with kyphosis on sitting. Gait waddling, with head erect. Characteristic feature is method of rising from supine position. Child rolls over into prone position, raises himself on to hands and knees, then hands and feet, and finally 'climbs up his own legs' (Gower sign) to reach erect position. Reflexes are diminished, later lost; fibrillation is not seen. Sensation normal. Mild intellectual impairment not uncommon.

Diagnosis
1. Serum enzymes—creatine phosphokinase (CPK) raised, especially in early stages. Test can also be used to locate carrier, mother or sister.
2. EMG shows myopathic changes.

3. Muscle biopsy—variation in size of muscle fibres, replacement of fibres by fat.

Becker variety is similar to Duchenne but milder. Has later onset, e.g. adolescence—and slower course.

Prognosis
Progressive condition with increasing muscular atrophy leading invariably to weakness and contractions. Death by the age of 20 years, often from respiratory infection.

Treatment
As child will inevitably develop contractures it is important that these should occur with the limbs in the most advantageous position for later comfort and nursing. Best for child to be in sitting position as later life will be mainly in wheelchair.

2. Facioscapulohumeral Type
(Landouzy–Dejérine Type)

Aetiology
Very rare.
Age. From birth.
Sex. Usually equal but may be confined to girls in some families.
Heredity. Autosomal dominant.

Onset
May commence with difficulty in sucking and in closing eyes or with difficulty in raising arms. Later complete lack of facial expression noted.

Muscles affected: Orbicularis oris and oculi are affected alone at first. Later, shoulder-girdle muscles, trapezius, serratus anterior, latissimus dorsi, pectorals, biceps, triceps. Later still, condition may spread to pelvic girdle muscles.

Progress and Prognosis
Disability usually slight. Slowly progressive, may live 30–40 years.

3. Limb Girdle Type (Scapulohumeral Type; Juvenile Muscular Type; Erb's Type)

Aetiology
Rare.
Age. 10–25 years.
Sex. Equal.
Heredity. Autosomal recessive.

Onset
Wasting of shoulder-girdle muscles; 'winging' of scapula and difficulty in raising arms above head.

Muscles affected: Serratus anterior, trapezius, pectoralis major, latissimus dorsi. Later, muscles of upper arm affected, following by involvement of pelvic girdle. Face not involved. Some muscles show initial pseudohypertrophy.

Occasionally pelvic girdle is first affected and progress is more rapid. Wasting of quadriceps may be the only abnormality.

Prognosis
Slowly progressive. May have normal life span.

4. Ocular Myopathy

Onset
Progressive bilateral ptosis and external ophthalmoplegia, pupils spared. Later face and trunk may be involved. Rare. Differentiate from myasthenia gravis and cerebral tumour.

5. Distal Myopathy

Onset
Small muscles of hand and feet—slowly spreads proximally.

6. Congenital Muscular Dystrophy

Autosomal recessive. Onset: in fetal life, presents with widespread muscular weakness (as a floppy baby) and later develops contractures similar to arthrogryposis multiplex congenita. May die early or survive long time.

Other Myopathies

Central Core Disease
Benign autosomal recessive disease of muscles with widespread hypotonia and delay in walking—often not until age of 4. Biopsy: large muscle fibres with non-functioning core.

Nemaline Myopathy
A diffuse congenital myopathy including the face. Some stigmata of Marfan's syndrome. Histology shows non-specific nemaline rods—which are degenerated Z bands of muscle fibres—underneath sarcolemma.

Myotubular Myopathy
Children show facial diplegia, external ocular palsies and small muscles. Biopsy shows fetal myotubules. Autosomal dominant, variable severity.

Mitochondrial Myopathies
Appearance as limb-girdle dystrophy. Biopsy reveals large numbers of morphologically and functionally abnormal mitochondria.

Glycogen Storage Disease of Muscle (p. 165)
(McArdle's disease) type IV—patient has muscle pain and stiffness increasing on

exercise. Myoglobinuria may occur. Similar illness can be caused by absence of phosphofructokinase and acid maltase.

Carnitine Deficiency
Rare congenital metabolic disease. Lipid vacuoles present in muscle fibres. Fatty liver. Prednisolone may be useful in treatment.

Myotonias

Dystrophia Myotonica (*Myotonic Dystrophy*)
Transmitted as an autosomal dominant.

Clinical Features
    1. When mother suffers from the illness an affected infant presents with: (*a*) diminished movements *in utero*, and (*b*) as a floppy infant once born; may have hypotonia or muscle atrophy and arthrogryposis or contractures at birth. Sucking diminished as are facial movements and there is bilateral ptosis. This manifestation is often accompanied by mental retardation.
    2. Where father transmits disease, the onset is later. Weakness affects cranial nerves and distal part of limbs—causing weak hands and wrists together with foot drop.
    3. Myotonia develops after weakness apparent; seen in hands; patients cannot release grip. Demonstrated by percussing thenar eminence, when adductor pollicis has a sustained contraction; tongue and deltoid similar.
    4. Later, both sexes develop cataracts but males become bald over forehead prematurely and testicles atrophy.
    5. Increased incidence of diabetes and cardiac conduction defects.

Myotonia Congenita (*Thomsen's Disease*)

Definition
Very rare genetically determined condition, cause unknown; manifested pathologically by enlarged muscle fibres and clinically by hypertrophy of muscles (especially of limbs and trunk); prolonged tonic contraction and retarded relaxation of muscles following voluntary movement. Difficulty most marked in initial contraction so performance improves after a few minutes. Chill and excitement make myotonia worse. Child may fall if he attempts sudden movement. May be noticed in childhood or not until adult life.

Chapter 149   # MYOSITIS

Classification
1. Parenchymatous myositis: (*a*) *Infective.* (*b*) *Non-infective:* (i) Dermatomyositis. (ii) Myositis fibrosa. (iii) Myositis from drugs.
2. Interstitial myositis. Myositis ossificans.

Infective Myositis

Abscess formation in muscles very uncommon. May be primary or secondary to necrotizing agent, such as following intramuscular injection of drug. Generalized myositis can occur with virus infection (e.g. Coxsackie, influenza), or toxoplasmosis, trichinosis, trypanosomiasis, schistosomiasis, or staphylococcus.

Dermatomyositis

Definition
Rare progressive collagen disease characterized clinically by inflammation of skin, subcutaneous tissue and muscles, leading to gross wasting and contractures, and pathologically by inflammatory reaction and degeneration of muscles.

Pathology
Initially
   Skin. Oedematous with round-cell infiltration.
   Muscle. Pale yellow, swollen with serum.
Later. Parenchymatous degeneration and atrophy with increase of interstitial fibrous tissue. Calcification may occur in muscles and subcutaneous tissue.

Clinical Features
Onset. Cause unknown. Any age from 5 years upward. May be acute, with general malaise and fever. More commonly chronic. Either dermatitis or myositis may be initially more prominent.
1. Dermatitis. Oedema, especially of eyelids and face, with dusky, purplish erythema. Telangiectasis of nail-bed may occur.
2. Myositis. Muscles affected are weak and tender. Atrophy and secondary contractures ensue rapidly in acute cases.

Complications
Calcification may develop in muscles and tendons. Sometimes also occurs in places where trauma has occurred, e.g. site of intravenous injection. If well marked, condition known as calcinosis universalis.

Differential Diagnosis
   1. Generalized scleroderma (very rare in childhood). May be difficult as conditions closely related, intermediate types occur. Classically in scleroderma skin white, firm, feels waxy.
   2. Focal scleroderma (morphoea) commoner. No general disturbance.
   3. Scleredema adultorum. Skin only involved. No general disturbance.

Prognosis
Usually progressive. Remissions and relapses occur.

Treatment
In early stages steroids may be of value.

Myositis Fibrosa

Very rare condition. May commence in infancy, commoner in adults. Characterized by progressive fibrosis of muscles. May mimic muscular dystrophy or dermatomyositis. *Note*: Localized fibrosis of quadriceps may follow intramuscular injections in infancy.

Myositis Ossificans

Definition
Very rare disease of infancy and childhood, cause unknown. Characterized clinically by localized swellings due to inflammation of muscles and fibrous tissue, which progress to bone formation and secondary skeletal deformities.

Myopathy from Drugs

Muscle weakness can occur with fluorinated adrenal steroids, especially triamcinolone, vincristine, chloroquine and guanethidine.

Chapter 150 **EPIDEMIC MYALGIA**
(Bornholm Disease; Epidemic Pleurodynia)

Definition
Uncommon disease occurring in small epidemics, manifested clinically by fever and pain of pleuritic type. Probably same disease as acute, benign, dry pleurisy.

Aetiology
Infection with Coxsackie B virus.
Age. Children and growing adults. Many of the cases recorded have been in young adults associated with children, e.g. nurses, etc. in children's hospitals.

Clinical Features
1. In older children and adults: General malaise; mild abdominal pain; pyrexia; pain in chest on breathing. Pleural rub common. May be pericarditis. Disease runs its course in a few weeks. Relapses often occur.
2. In young children: Abdominal pain main symptom; may mimic appendicitis. Pleural element minimal although pain may be made worse by breathing. Very difficult to make certain diagnosis except in epidemic. Disease milder in children.

Investigations
Radiological examination of chest usually normal. May be slight leucocytosis. ESR sometimes raised.

Differential Diagnosis
1. *Appendicitis* and other causes of abdominal pain.
2. *Pneumonia*
3. *Fractured rib*
4. *Tuberculous pleurisy*
5. *Trichinosis*

Prognosis
Spontaneous recovery. Recrudescences and relapses common.

Treatment
Symptomatic.

Chapter 151   *OTHER DISEASES OF MUSCLE*

Myasthenia Gravis

Very rare condition in childhood, but may occur at any age.

Varieties
1. Transient neonatal. Mother has the illness. Infant weak and hypotonic. May die in a few hours but recovery usual if treated—lasts about 6 weeks.
2. Persistent neonatal. Mother not affected. Persists for life. May recur in family.
3. Juvenile. Presents same as adult disease. Confirm diagnosis by use of edrophonium chloride. Exclude thymoma.

Endocrine Myopathies

Occur with thyrotoxicosis—a proximal myopathy with ptosis and facial weakness. Note reflexes increased, cf. absent in other myopathies. Hypothyroid children have weak muscles, which are slow to contract and relax and are hypertrophied (Debré–Semelaigne syndrome). Hyperparathyroidism may be associated with weakness and hyporeflexia.

Periodic Familial Paralysis

Definition
Very rare familial disease, probably caused by derangement of potassium metabolism; characterized clinically by recurrent attacks of flaccid paralysis often occurring on waking in morning, in cold and after heavy carbohydrate meal. Serum potassium may be low or raised.

Arthrogryposis Multiplex Congenita
(Amyoplasia Congenita)

Rare congenital syndrome. Mixed aetiology. Possibly neurogenic. (1) Marked abnormalities of muscles a feature but individual muscles may be normal, small and fibrotic, or absent. If one group is contracted antagonists will be absent. (2) Secondary ankylosis in extension of knees and elbows, and in flexion of wrists, fingers and ankles. Joints may appear fusiform; patella may be fixed. But joint capsule always normal. (3) Skin thickened. Other congenital abnormalities frequently associated. Child may be mentally retarded.

Treatment
Physiotherapy. Night plasters may help.

Myoglobinuria

Varieties
Type I. Recurrent, familial, mild—follows exercise.

Type II. Sporadic, may follow injury or usually no known cause. High mortality from renal failure. Malignant hyperthermia occurs with myoglobinuria.

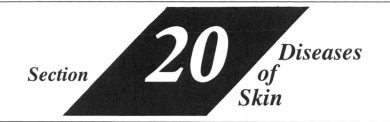

Section **20** *Diseases of Skin*

Chapter 152

NAEVI (Birthmarks) AND GENERALIZED CONGENITAL ABNORMALITIES

Port-wine Stain
May be small or very extensive. Site and colour vary. Occasionally associated with neurological lesions, e.g. Sturge–Weber syndrome (*see* p. 309) or extensive vascular hamartoma.

Strawberry Mark
Small, raised, red patch which appears during first 3 months of life. If left alone disappears spontaneously at about 5–8 years of age without scarring. Lesions near mucous membranes should be carefully watched as they may increase rapidly in size.

Pigmented Naevi
Colour varies: often almost black; may be hairy.

Haemangioma
May be very small or very extensive. If large the affected limb may be larger than fellow owing to increased blood supply. Thrombocytopenia may occur.

Adenoma Sebaceum (see Epiloia, p. 311)
The diagnosis is made by finding 'ashleaf' depigmentation areas on skin of trunk and limbs (seen best under Wood's lamp); by adenoma sebaceum on older child or division of optic disc.

The diagnosis is difficult to make unless the adenoma are present, but these may not appear until after the fits have occurred.

Chapter 153

NAPKIN (DIAPER) RASH AND MEATAL ULCER

Napkin rash and meatal ulcer are caused by the excoriation of the skin by ammonia. The sequence of events is:

1. Urine containing urea which is acted upon by enzyme urease, converting it into ammonia.

2. The urease is produced by *Alcaligenes ammoniagenes*. This lives in colon and easily grows on urine-soaked napkin.

3. *Alc. ammoniagenes* requires alkaline medium for growth. Therefore grows poorly if the contents of colon are acid—as in breast-fed baby, but more readily if contents alkaline, as in artificially fed baby.

Napkin rash is common. It occurs particularly in artificially fed babies especially when the stools are loose and the napkin is soiled for a long time. It is made worse if the napkin is washed in an alkaline soap powder.

The rash is confined to an area of skin covered by the napkin, except sometimes on the back where the urine may soak up through the clothes. The folds and flexures are not affected. In mild cases fiery red erythema occurs which may desquamate on healing; in severe cases large blisters form, which burst leaving raw areas and tags of skin. Secondary infection may occasionally follow.

Ammoniacal dermatitis must be distinguished from fungal dermatitis caused by *Candida* (monilia) *albicans*. Fungal dermatitis involves the creases, anal and labial margins and skin. It may be pseudomembranous or vesicular. Skin condition is often associated with oral thrush lesions. Scrapings reveal *Candida albicans* and the condition does not respond to simple anti-ammonia measures.

Meatal Ulcer

Ammoniacal dermatitis may occur on a glans exposed by circumcision. A small, very tender ulcer appears on the glans penis. Scab may form, occluding the meatus and leading to retention of urine. The possibility of a meatal ulcer is a major reason for advising against of circumcision.

Perianal Dermatitis

Not uncommon condition in newborn infants, in which there is reddening of skin immediately surrounding anus. Affected area may be up to 4 cm in diameter and in severe cases is exudative or even ulcerated. Cause uncertain. More common in bottle than in breast-fed babies, possibly due to alkaline nature of stool of bottle-fed babies. May occur in cystic fibrosis infants given large doses of pancreatic enzymes.

Chapter 154   # VESICULAR ERUPTIONS

Pemphigus Neonatorum

Is caused by haemolytic staphylococcus infection. Thin-walled bullae form on the skin. These rupture easily and condition spreads. The base of the blister is red. The prognosis is poor if the condition is extensive, but with modern antibiotic therapy disease is no longer the scourge it once was.

Chapter 155   # PARASITIC INFECTIONS OF SKIN

Scabies

Is quite common in children, the condition is the same as that found in adults except that in infants the face may be involved.

Pediculosis Capitis (*Nits*)

Are very common in children. They are often found on routine examination, for example when the child is admitted to hospital. Condition is mildly irritating, and if the child scratches secondary infection may take place. Impetiginized lesions of scalp are often preceded by pediculosis capitis and treatment of infective lesion will not be successful until the underlying cause has been removed. Mild degrees of infection are common and lymph nodes in posterior triangle of neck often enlarged.

Chapter 156   # BACTERIAL INFECTIONS OF SKIN

Impetigo Contagiosa

Is a staphylococcal infection of the skin which may follow insect bites or scabies. Usually affects face, but may be found anywhere on the body. Very contagious.

Chapter 157   # TOXIC AND DRUG ERUPTIONS

Drug rashes are common:
Penicillin. Morbilliform.
Sulphonamide. Morbilliform, rarely leads to exfoliative dermatitis.
Atropine, Phenobarbitone. Morbilliform or scarlatiniform. Rarely exfoliative dermatitis.
Iodides and Bromides. Acneform.
Morphine. Erythematous.

Erythema Multiforme

Group of diseases of unknown aetiology manifested by rashes which appear in various patterns, e.g. erythema iris. Sometimes constitutional disturbances present, such as fever, headache, joint pains, etc. Eruption may fade within a few hours or last days or weeks.

Stevens–Johnson Syndrome
(*Erythema Exudativum Multiforme*)

In this condition the child may become very ill with a temperature up to 40°C. The skin lesion, which is generalized, commences as an erythema, but rapidly forms bullae which burst and may become secondarily infected. The mucous membranes of the lips, mouth, pharynx are all covered with bullae which later ulcerate. A purulent conjunctivitis develops. Less commonly, urethritis and balanitis occur and may result in retention of urine. The cause is unknown in many instances although long-acting sulphonamides have been incriminated.

The condition improves spontaneously in 7–10 days, although it may be several weeks before the rash is completely gone. Corneal ulceration is an unpleasant sequel. There is no specific treatment.

Scleroderma

In children generalized scleroderma is far less common than the localized form (morphoea). For further details *see* textbooks on adult medicine.

Focal Scleroderma (*Morphoea*)

Uncommon condition in children, but more common than in adults. Age of onset: 2 weeks to 12 years; average, 5 years. Ratio girls to boys: 3 : 1.

Clinical Features
May be history of preceding local trauma.
Stage I. Discrete, sometimes elevated, waxy-coloured, non-tender plaques appear. Occasionally have violaceous halo.
Stage II. Area undergoes atrophy with scarring.
Stage III. Scarring leads to secondary deformity; muscle contracts, fixing joints and stunting growth of bones.
Areas involved. Face, neck, shoulder, trunk, upper or lower extremities. May be uni- or bilateral, small or large areas. May be multiple.
Result. Often serious scarring and deformity. No visceral involvement.

Chapter 158   # DISEASES OF SUBCUTANEOUS FAT

Sclerema Neonatorum

Subcutaneous fat becomes hard. Skin over affected areas purple and fixed. Limbs may become immobile. Occurs in babies who are very ill. Condition often fatal either from sclerema or the precipitating cause.

Subcutaneous Fat Necrosis

Not uncommon condition which usually follows trauma, e.g. in area where forceps have been applied. Fat lobules larger than normal and contain needle-shaped crystals which resemble cholesterol. Lesions feel firm and thickened; not tender.

Prognosis
Gradual improvement over weeks or months.

Lipodystrophy

Uncommon condition manifested by a progressive loss of subcutaneous fat giving the child a gaunt, emaciated appearance. The condition is usually more marked in the upper part of the body. The cause is unknown. The onset is about 10 years; girls are more affected than boys. Lipodystrophy is progressive but not life threatening.

Chapter 159	DERMATITIS AND ECZEMATOID LESIONS

Atopic Eczema (*Infantile Eczema*)

Term 'atopic' indicates a conditional predisposition characterized by:
1. Heredity with high incidence of asthma, hay fever and topic eczema.
2. Eosinophilia in affected tissues and sometimes in blood.
3. Selective synthesis of IgE antibodies.
4. Hyper-reactivity of skin.
5. Probably abnormal metabolism of cyclic $3',5'$-adenosine monophosphate (cyclic AMP).

Atopic eczema is an allergic skin disease usually commencing during first year of life, manifested by papulovesicular lesions occurring mainly on face, scalp and limbs.

The cause is unknown but there is usually a family history of allergic diseases. Probably caused by food allergens. Note the association with phenylketonuria. Severe, continuing eczema is far less common than in the past, perhaps due to the success of therapy with topical steroids.

Eczema commences as rough, red patches on the cheeks, forehead, scalp, and neck. The lesion progresses from erythema to papules to vesicles which burst or are scratched, resulting in oozing of serum and crust formation. Secondary infection is common. The condition spreads to the flexor surfaces of the arms and legs. It is intensely irritating. Marked remissions and exacerbations occur.

The lesions on the face and body tend to disappear in the second year of life, but the flexural eczema may remain.

Flexural eczema may develop from infantile eczema, or appear spontaneously. It occurs as irritating papules in the antecubital fossa, popliteal fossa and, less commonly, groin. The lesions are scratched with resultant oozing which heals by lichenification. Flexural eczema is a very common chronic condition which lasts for years, with periodical remissions and exacerbations. The child frequently develops asthma about the third year. Acute stage of skin lesion often improves when the asthma is bad and vice versa. Treatment by local emollients, non-halogenated steroids or coal tar ointments. Dietary measures e.g. withdrawing cow's milk may help.

Seborrhoeic Eczema ('Cradle Cap')

This is a very common condition in infants in which crusting or dry scales appear on the head. The mother is often afraid to remove them for fear of damaging the fontanelle. Crust may become infected if not removed.

Toxic Epidermal Necrolysis (TEN; Scalded skin syndrome)

Very rare disease occurring in neonatal period or infancy in which generalized erythema and desquamation of skin occur. Skin comes off in shreds. Cause usually staphylococcal infection. Treat by i.v. antibiotics, fluids including FFP.

Chapter 160

THE PITUITARY AND HYPOTHALAMUS

Action of pituitary gland and hypothalamus intimately connected. Hypothalamus controls pituitary via inhibiting or releasing factors (hormones).

Embryology
Pituitary divided into two parts:
1. Anterior lobe. Derived from downgrowth of forebrain which connects with evagination of stomodeum (primitive mouth). Latter becomes closed pouch (Rathke's), loses connection with mouth and develops into anterior lobe of pituitary.
2. Posterior lobe. Derived from infundibulum of diencephalon. Embryologically, histologically and functionally two parts remain separate.

Physiology
Hypothalamic factors:
  1. Corticotrophin-releasing factor (CRF).
  2. Thyrotrophin-releasing hormone (TRH) stimulates thyrotrophin and prolactin.
  3. Gonadotrophin-releasing hormone (GnRH) stimulates both LH and FSH.
  4. Growth hormone-releasing hormone (GHRH)
  5. Somatostatin—a growth hormone release inhibiting factor. Also found in brain and pancreas.
  6. Prolactin release inhibiting factor (PIF).
1. Anterior lobe. Secretes following hormones:

  1.1 Growth Hormone. Works via production of intermediary hormones—somatomedins secreted in response to stress, exercise, sleep, hypoglycaemia, L-dopa and arginine.
  1.2. Gonadotrophic Hormones. Luteinizing hormone (LH) promotes luteinization of the ovary and Leydig function of testes. Follicle stimulating hormone (FSH) stimulates follicle development in ovary and gametogenesis of testes. Under control of GnRH.
  1.3 Thyrotrophin (Thyrotrophic Hormone; TSH) increases thyroxine formation and release, stimulated by TRH and inhibited by T_4 and T_3.
  1.4 Adrenotrophic Hormones—corticotrophin (ACTH), stimulated by CRF.

1.5 Prolactin (HPr)—initiates and maintains lactation; primes ovary and testis to respond to gonadotrophins.
2. *Posterior lobe*. Excretes arginine vasopressin (AVP) and oxytocin.

Hypersecretion of Anterior Pituitary

Pituitary Gigantism
Excess growth hormone causing tallness in children very rare—but raised levels occur in diabetes, congenital heart disease and renal failure, although tallness is not a feature of these conditions.

Cerebral Gigantism (*Sotos' Syndrome*)
Head big, eyes slant downwards, broad forehead. Height increased in early childhood but then stabilizes and are not big adults; clumsy; behaviour problems and often reduced IQ.

Pituitary Dwarfism

Aetiology
Growth hormone deficiency child often has normal birth weight and progress for first year—more common in boys, rarely familial; may follow obstetric complications, e.g. breech. Usually no cause found—may be isolated or with other pituitary hormone deficiencies—may follow craniopharyngioma or cranial irradiation. Also can occur with Turner's syndrome, congenital rubella, Fanconi's anaemia and optic nerve hypoplasia. Partial deficiency exists.

Clinical Features
1. *Age of onset*. Primary cases usually develop normally until about second or third year. Secondary cases develop normally until later.
2. *Physical characteristics*. In isolated GH deficiency very short relatively fat child with round face and head seems large compared with rest of body. Bridge of nose sunken. Milk teeth survive longer than normal, larynx small, voice shrill. Genitalia remain small and sterility is common. Mentality usually normal. In panhypopituitarism, short stature associated with slender build, narrow rather than round face and evidence of other endocrine deficiencies.

Diagnosis
Essential only to treat cases which are likely to benefit as treatment is prolonged and GH is difficult to procure (at present prepared from autopsy material from human pituitary).

Tests
1. Skull and wrist X-ray.
2. Chromosome analysis.
3. Screening tests for: (i) Malabsorption, e.g. blood picture and folate; consider jejunal biopsy. (ii) Renal disease, e.g. urea. (iii) Thyroid, e.g. TSH, T_4.
A child less than 3rd centile for height and one year velocity less than 25th centile should be investigated, i.e. less than 5 cm/year.

4. GH assay following one of following— exercise, or sleep screening tests. If screening test shows GH <20 i.u./l proceed to specific insulin-induced hypoglycaemia or arginine or L-dopa or clonidine stimulation. Normally peak levels exceed 20 m.u./l after adequate hypoglycaemic reaction (<2·5 µmol/l).

Treatment
Treatment is with human growth hormone (hGH). Three injections per week. Other hormones, e.g. thyroid, adrenal and gonadotrophin deficiencies may need correcting.

Result of treatment in correct case may be very striking—17·5 cm growth in 3 months recorded.

Difficulties of treatment with GH
1. Must be started before epiphysial maturation too far advanced.
2. Child may develop antibodies to natural GH or impurities in pituitary extract after prolonged therapy. Less likely with synthetic GH.

Chapter 161   # DISEASES OF POSTERIOR PITUITARY AND HYPOTHALAMUS

Diabetes Insipidus

Pathogenesis
Posterior pituitary produces antidiuretic hormone (arginine vasopressin, AVP) which acts on kidney to control volume of urine excreted. If deficient, kidney excretes large quantities of dilute urine.

Causes
1. Congenital. May be inherited as Mendelian dominant or X-linked.
2. Acquired. Lesions of the supra-optic and paraventricular nuclei of the hypothalamus, hypophysial stalk, e.g. fractures, meningitis, tumours, xanthomatosis, histiocytosis. May occur in newborn after streptococcal meningitis, or DIC, or intraventricular haemorrhage.

Clinical Features
Onset. In congenital cases polydipsia and polyuria and fever may be noticed in infancy. If condition is not recognized and fluids are restricted symptoms as seen in nephrogenic diabetes insipidus occur (*see over*).

In acquired condition child presents with excessive thirst and polyuria and/or enuresis.

Up to 10 litres of urine may be excreted per day. Specific gravity rarely above 1·007 even after withholding fluids.

Apart from inconvenience caused by thirst and passage of large quantities of urine there are normally no signs or symptoms. On restriction of fluids headache, fatigue, dehydration and collapse occur. Other clinical features of cause may be present. Some children lack thirst response to excessive hyperosmolarity.

Differential Diagnosis

1. Primary polydipsia (compulsive water drinking). Child drinks excessively and therefore passes large quantities of urine of low specific gravity, but if water withheld urine becomes concentrated. Child usually has an abnormal psychosocial background or personality.

2. Chronic renal failure. Diagnosis made by tests for renal function, raised blood urea, hypertension, etc.

3. Diabetes mellitus. Urine contains sugar and, in untreated cases, ketone bodies.

4. Hypercalcaemia or *hypokalaemia*

Diagnosis

1. On withholding fluids, in true case, distress, dehydration and urine osmolality reaches 850 m.osmol/l; serum osmolality rises to 300 m.osmol/l. *Note*: Water deprivation test should be performed under carefully controlled conditions in full recognition of possible danger.

2. Serum vasopressin level.

3. Therapeutic trial with vasopressin (DDAVP) used intranasally, intravenously or intramuscularly.

4. Radiograph skull.

Treatment

1. Of cause—*see* under appropriate headings.

2. Of diabetes insipidus. Polyuria can be controlled by administration of vasopressin as liquid DDAVP instilled into anterior nares. Allow child to drink sufficient water.

Nephrogenic Diabetes Insipidus (*Renal or Vasopressin-resistant Diabetes Insipidus*)

Definition

Very rare genetically-determined disorder, characterized by symptoms of diabetes insipidus not controlled by vasopressin. Usually X-linked but may be dominant.

Clinical Features

Presents in infancy. Bouts of fever, hypotonia, constipation, vomiting and polyuria occur. Polydipsia may be present or may be masked by anorexia. Untreated, the child fails to thrive and mental deficiency develops. Findings in infant: raised serum osmolality, electrolytes and urea: often in absence of dehydration. Urine osmolality low.

Treatment

Give adequate fluids. Low osmotic load diet (i.e. diet low in protein and minerals). Breast milk fulfils these requirements and infant may not present whilst breast fed.

AVP excess or inappropriate secretion of antidiuretic hormone, causes water retention and hypo-osmolality and hyponatraemia. Occurs with any type of brain disease; lung conditions, e.g. pneumonia, TB and CF; certain tumours; postoperative and various endocrine deficiencies. Found in about 1% pre-term infants with hypoxia, artificial ventilation, meningitis or intraventricular haemorrhage.

Disorders of Hypothalamus

Fröhlich's Syndrome (*Dystrophia Adiposogenitalis*)
Very rare condition, manifested by generalized obesity with failure of development, including sexual development, and caused by destructive lesion—most often suprasellar cyst (*see* p. 342)—involving hypothalamus. Main point of difference from simple obesity is that in Fröhlich's syndrome child is fat and short, in simple obesity fat and tall.

Laurence–Moon–Biedl Syndrome
Very rare hereditary condition, manifested by symptoms of Fröhlich's syndrome combined with retinitis pigmentosa, polydactyly or syndactyly, mental deficiency and diabetes insipidus.

Chapter 162   # THE ADRENAL MEDULLA

Neuroblastoma and Ganglioneuroma

Note: Tumours of autonomic nervous system may occur in adrenal medulla or sympathetic nervous system in abdomen, thorax and elsewhere.

Pathology
1. *Neuroblastoma*. Not uncommon. Very malignant. Usually occur as large, hard, haemorrhagic tumour in retroperitoneal tissues of abdomen. Occasionally commence in posterior thorax. Composed of small round cells, sometimes arranged in characteristic rosettes.
   Metastasizes mainly to: (*a*) *Liver*. Especially if adrenal on right side involved. (*b*) *Bones*. Occurs if right or left adrenal involved. Following bones affected: (i) Skull. Deposits may occur in orbital region, rsulting in exophthalmos. (ii) Long bones. Characteristic rosette cells may be found in bone marrow.
2. *Ganglioneuroma*. Rare. Relatively benign. Encapsulated tumours of slow growth. Occur most commonly in chest or abdomen. Microscopically: nerve cells and nerve fibres seen.
3. *Intermediate forms*. These occur and development of one type into the other occurs.

Clinical Features of Neuroblastoma
Found in children usually under 5, sexes equal.
Presentation. (*a*) Primary tumour may present as abdominal swelling, but usually child already obviously ill with poor appetite, loss of weight, lethargy and pallor. Abdominal pain may be a feature. Sometimes jaundice or diarrhoea. (*b*) Secondary deposits around orbit or long bones may be first manifestation. Child has limb pains which mimic rheumatoid arthritis or osteomyelitis. May present with anaemia mimicking leukaemia.

Signs. On palpation firm, fixed, often nodular mass can be felt. Often crosses midline in contradistinction to Wilms's tumour.

Clinical Features of Ganglioneuroma
Causes pressure symptoms, sometimes diarrhoea.

Investigation of Neuroblastoma
1. Radiological examination of abdomen. Calcification may occur—usually as uniform stippling. *Ultrasound* shows mass.
2. Intravenous pyelography. (*a*) If tumour arises from adrenal: Renal pelvis displaced downward but not distorted. (*b*) If arising from sympathetic chain: Ureter usually displaced.
3. Raised excretion of breakdown products of adrenaline and noradrenaline (3-methoxy-4-hydroxy-mandelic acid (VMA) and homovanillic acid) in urine.
4. Bone marrow for malignant cells.

Table 162.1   Differential diagnosis of some renal swellings

	Onset	Haematuria	Uni- or bilateral	IVP	Meta-stases	Character of mass
Wilms's tumour	Abdominal swelling; child well	Uncommon	Unilateral very rarely bilateral	Distortion of pelvis	Lung	Firm; rounded lobulated
Neuroblastoma	Child ill; mass palpable	Rare	Unilateral but may spread over midline	Displacement of pelvis	Liver or bones especially orbit	Nodular, fixed, indeterminate outline
Hydronephrosis	Abdominal swelling; child well	Uncommon	Often bilateral	Enlargement of pelvis or no secretion	—	Tensely cystic, may transilluminate
Polycystic kidney	Renal failure; mass palpable	Common	Usually bilateral	'Spider pelvis'	—	Nodular; cystic

Prognosis
1. Neuroblastoma. Still usually fatal in older children but occasionally tumour retrogresses and disappears with or without treatment (approximately 3%). Outlook better for infants in first year, and when primary in chest. Some chemotherapy and autologous bone marrow transplantation promising.
2. Ganglioneuroma. Good.

Treatment of Neuroblastoma
   1. Surgical removal of as much tumour as possible.
   2. Radiotherapy, accompanied by chemotherapy; various drugs tried but still have limited success.

Phaeochromocytoma
Small, very rare, benign tumour of adrenal medulla or organs of Zückerkandl which produces adrenaline or noradrenaline.
Note: May be associated with neurofibromatosis.

Clinical Features
Intermittent or persistent hypertension. Periodical exacerbation in which headache, sweating, palpitations and polyuria occur. Tumour rarely palpable.

Diagnosis
By estimating noradrenaline and adrenaline, VMA and metanephrines in 24-h urine.

Treatment
Surgical removal of tumour. Very careful operative and postoperative care needed to maintain normal blood pressure.

Some Causes of Hypertension

Persistent
1. Renal—chronic nephritis, microcystic disease, bilateral hydronephrosis.
2. Cardiovascular—coarctation of aorta, renal artery stenosis.
3. Essential hypertension.
4. Rare forms of adrenal hyperplasia and Cushing's syndrome.

Transient
Acute nephritis, haemolytic-uraemic syndrome, dysautonomia, steroids, hyper-calcaemia, intracranial hypertension, polyneuritis and poliomyelitis, Stevens--Johnson syndrome, hypernatraemia, leukaemia.

Chapter 163   **THE ADRENAL CORTEX**

Physiology and Pathology
The adrenal cortex is mesodermal in origin. Adrenal cortex produces following main hormones:
1. Corticosteroids (glucocorticoids). Regulated by adrenocorticotrophic hormone (ACTH) produced in zona fasciculata and corticotrophin releasing factor (CRF).

> 1.1 Cortisol (Hydrocortisone; Compound F). 12–13 mg/m^2/day for *all* ages. Major action on carbohydrate, protein and fat metabolism in body tissues. Amino acids converted into carbohydrate (gluconeogenesis). Also has anti-anabolic effect as amino acids are used for synthesis of carbohydrate and fat rather than protein. Also causes Na retention and K loss, suppression of inflammatory response, involution of thymus, and psychological effects.
>
> 1.2 Corticosterone (Compound B). Effect similar to cortisol except more salt-retaining and less anti-inflammatory action.

2. Aldosterone (mineralocorticoid). Formed in zona glomerulosa. Promotes Na retention and K loss. Controlled by renin–angiotensin via cholesterol desmolase.
3. Androgens. Little produced before puberty.

Hormone Synthesis

Each stage is performed by specific enzyme. Enzyme deficiency leads to:

1. Absence of end-product—the specific hormone.

2. Build-up of substances produced earlier in the metabolic pathway. Some have unwanted physiological actions.

3. Failure to inhibit pituitary by feed-back mechanism, hence continued adrenal stimulation and adrenal hypertrophy. Note paradox: adrenal hypofunction with hyperplasia of gland.

4. Results are adrenal insufficiency and altered sex characteristics from excess androgenic hormones produced by pituitary stimulation.

Effects of Enzyme Deficiencies

1. Absence of mineralocorticoids (aldosterone) and excess of 17-hydroxyprogesterone results in salt-losing type of congenital adrenal hyperplasia.

2. Excess androgens produced by build-up in metabolic pathway results in:

      2.1 Secondary sex characteristics appearing early.

      2.2 Accelerated growth, but early fusion of epiphyses leads to eventual small adult.

      2.3 In *females*—heterosexual development; pseudo-hermaphroditism.

      2.4 In *males*—isosexual precocious puberty.

Congenital Adrenal Hyperplasia
(*The Adrenogenital Syndrome*)

Presentation

Varied; including ambiguous genitalia, salt-losing crisis shortly after birth; unexplained early death, hypertension, precocious puberty, virilization, amenorrhoea and operative collapse.

Genetics

Autosomal recessive.

Features of Individual Enzyme Defect

1. 21-Hydroxylase defect. Commonest type. About 30% are salt-losers.

2. 11β-Hydroxylase defect. Not salt-losers. Ambiguous genitalia, cryptorchidism. Have hypertension and hypernatraemia.

3. Beta-hydroxysteroid dehydrogenase deficiency. Very rare. Always salt-losers. *Note*: In this type, because biosynthesis of androgens is impaired there is imperfect formation of genitalia in male, but as only hormone gland can make is dehydroepiandrosterone (DHA), females are masculinized: hypospadias, small penis, bifid scrotum in male; big clitoris, fused labia in female.

4. Defective C20, 22-desmolase (lipoid hyperplasia). Cholesterol accumulates in cortex. Absence of androgens in fetus allows complete feminization of male fetus. Presents with Addisonian crises shortly after birth and with pigmentation, gammaglobulins raised. Usually die.

Other Causes of Female Pseudohermaphroditism

If mother has received synthetic progesterone or some oestrogens during

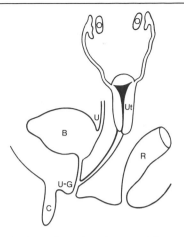

Fig. 163.1. Anatomical configuration in pseudohermaphroditism. B, bladder; C, clitoris; O, ovary; R, rectum; U, ureter; U-G, urogenital sinus; Ut, uterus.

pregnancy, female offspring may show mild or moderate pseudohermaphrodite picture but not progressive postnatal virilization.

Anatomy of Commonest Type of Genitalia Abnormality (*Fig. 163.1*)
1. Ovary, tubes, uterus and vagina. Normal, although small.
2. Urogenital sinus. Persists with vaginal opening about 1 cm above meatus.
3. Genital tubercle. Hypertrophies and becomes large clitoris, which resembles penis with perineal hypospadias.
4. Labioscrotal folds. Fuse in midline to form empty scrotum.

Investigations
1. Urine. Excess or deficiency of steroid precursors or their metabolites found, *see Table 163.1*. Most useful test is raised 17-OH progesterone or pregnanetriol excretion. 11-Oxygenation ratio helpful because it can be performed on a small amount of urine.

2. Blood 17-OH progesterone raised—normally up to (32 nmol/l) 1 µg/dl: ACTH levels increased. Serum Na low, serum K high, urea high and glucose low in crisis.

3. Chromosome studies should be performed when genitalia ambiguous.

4. Radiological studies. In ambiguous genitalia, vaginogram via urogenital sinus demonstrates presence of a vagina.

Differential Diagnosis
May be difficult to distinguish female pseudohermaphrodite from perineal hypospadias. Two types of perineal hypospadias: (*a*) Variety associated with 3-hydroxysteroid dehydrogenase and 20, 22-desmolase deficiency (*see above*). (*b*) Congenital variety. *Note*: Following points important in differentiation between hypospadias and pseudohermaphroditism.
   In pseudohermaphroditism:
1. Vagina usually present and vaginogram demonstrates uterus and tubes.

Table 163.1 Varieties of adrenal gland enzyme defects

Adrenal enzyme defect	Urine steroids	
	Increased	*Decreased*
20, 22-desmolase	Nil	17-OS; 17-OGS; 17-OHCS corticosteroids
3β-hydroxysteroid dehydrogenase	17-OS; 17-OGS; 17-OHCS; DHA; 3β-21-dihydroxypregn-5-ene-20-one	THE; THF; aldosterone
17α-hydroxylase	Pregnenolone	17-OS; 17-OCS; 17-OHCS THE; THF
21-hydroxylase	Plasma 17, hydroxy progesterone 17-OS; 17-OGS; 17-OHCS; Pregnanetriol (Pregnanetriolone)	Aldosterone when 21-hydroxylation of progesterone defective
11β-hydroxylase	17-OS; 17-OGS; 17-OHCS; 11-deoxycortisol; Tetrahydro-11-deoxycortisol	THE; THF
18-hydroxylase 18–oxidase	Corticosterone; Tetrahydrocorticosterone; 11-dehydrocorticosterone; Tetra-hydro-11-dehydrocorticosterone	Aldosterone

17-OS = 17-oxosteroids; 17-OGS = 17-oxogenic steroids, 17-OCHS = 17-hydroxycorticosteroids; THE = tetrahydrocortisone; THF = tetrahydrocortisol; DHA = dehydroepiandrosterone.

2. Ovary or ovotestis very rarely present in scrotum or inguinal canal. Biopsy distinguishes.

In hypospadias:

1. Testes may be palpable in scrotum or inguinal canal.
2. Penis has ventral groove.

Special Features of Adrenocortical Insufficiency, 'Salt-losing Type'

Clinical Features
1. Onset. Usually insidious, within first week or two of life.
2. Symptoms. Vomiting, failure to gain weight and sweating. May have attacks of hypoglycaemia. Pigmentation may occur. Vomiting becomes more marked, collapse with dehydration occurs, diarrhoea may develop, untreated child lapses into coma and dies.

Biochemistry during Crisis
Plasma sodium and glucose low, potassium and urea high; acidaemia.

Differential Diagnosis
Pyloric stenosis, meningitis, urinary infection, etc.

Treatment of Adrenogenital Syndrome
Aims
1. To depress pituitary overactivity.
2. To substitute for missing hormones.
3. To correct anatomical defects.
4. To support parent and child psychologically.
Practice
1. To depress pituitary activity steroid therapy must be used. Hydrocortisone acetate given in sufficient dose to maintain appropriate growth centile and bone maturation. Split cortisol to mimic normal circadian rhythm. Biochemical

monitoring varies according to enzyme defect but aims at getting appropriate metabolite approximately within physiological ranges and with circadian rhythm—judged usually by 17-OH progesterone or ACTH.

Note: Dose must be increased two to tenfold during conditions of stress, such as infection or operations and given i.m.

2. Salt losers. (*a*) In crisis: Infant requires i.v. normal saline and hydrocortisone. (*b*) For maintenance: (i) Salt supplements to diet 1–4 g/day, for up to 3 years and then let patient have salt *ad lib*. (ii) Salt-retaining hormone: 9α-fluorohydrocortisone needed for life. Dose 0·05–0·2 mg daily by mouth. This compound may cause hypertension, so blood pressure must be watched carefully.

3. Surgery. (*a*) Clitoris—reduce size but leave glans if possible. *Time*: When steroid dosage stabilized, and early in infancy. (*b*) Refashion vagina. Should be performed much later.

4. Psychological management of parents and, later, of child.

Adrenal Insufficiency

Causes
1. Neonatal. Permanent or transient hypoplasia in newborn. Renal tubular insensitivity to mineralocorticoid. Adrenal haemorrhage. Often associated with birth trauma. Salt-losing type of adrenogenital syndrome (*see* p. 470). ACTH deficiency.
2. Later childhood. Septicaemia. Usually, but not always meningococcal. (*See* Waterhouse–Friderichsen syndrome, p. 97.) Corticotrophin deficiency from hypothalamic or pituitary failure. Bilateral removal of adrenals. Removal of adrenal tumour (unilateral) due to compensatory atrophy of contralateral adrenal. Rapid withdrawal of therapeutic steroid.

Addison's Disease

Very rare in children. Sometimes associated with Schilder's disease.

Cushing's Syndrome

Very rare condition caused by overexcretion of cortisol and to lesser extent androgens. Clinical features similar to those found in adults. May be due to pituitary or adrenal lesion or prolonged steroid therapy.

Chapter 164   *THE THYROID GLAND*

Hypothyroidism (*Cretinism; Congenital Aplasia or Hypoplasia of Thyroid Gland*)

Classification and Causation of Hypothyroidism

Congenital
1. Deficiency of thyrotrophin releasing-hormone (TRH).
2. Deficiency of thyrotrophin (TSH).

3. Inadequate thyroid gland tissue. Dysgenesis (athyrotic cretinism; sporadic cretinism). Commonest type of cretinism in those parts of the world where iodine supply is inadequate. Thyroid tissue may be malplaced and/or inadequate, e.g. midline base of tongue, subhyoid. Mother does not usually have thyroid disease but often family history of thyroid disorders. Thyroid tissue rarely found in child without technetium or ^{123}I scan. Congenital condition but often no abnormality noted for some weeks or months if not picked up by screening.

4. Inadequate synthesis of thyroid hormone: (*a*) Enzymatic deficiency. Seven different, genetically transmitted defects of thyroid hormone synthesis are known, e.g. iodide trapping defect, iodide organification defect, iodotyrosine coupling or de-iodination defects. These may give rise to: (i) Familial cretinism. (ii) Enlargement of thyroid gland (goitre) either at birth or later with little or no evidence of hypothyroidism (presumably hyperplasia of gland succeeds in compensating for enzyme lack). (*b*) Iodine deficiency. If there is insufficient naturally occurring iodine in diet for synthesis of thyroid hormone, thyroid gland enlarges in endeavour to supply needs of body. This may be: (i) Adequate. Child has goitre but no hypothyroidism. (ii) Inadequate. Child has goitre and cretinism. *Note*: It is possible that iodine lack may exacerbate pre-existing enzyme deficiency in some instances. (*c*) Antenatal ingestion of antithyroid drugs by the mother. Drugs such as propylthiouracil given for maternal thyrotoxicosis may cross the placenta or be excreted in breast milk. Infant may be born normal, or born with an enlarged thyroid and some evidence of hypothyroidism. After birth condition improves spontaneously but can be quickened by giving thyroxine. Breast feeding should not be permitted.

Acquired. (*a*) Surgical removal of thyroid either for therapy, e.g. thyrotoxicosis, or in error, e.g. removal of ectopic thyroid which is the sole functioning gland. (*b*) Ingestion of antithyroid drugs. (*c*) Hashimoto's disease, occurs rarely in older children.

Clinical Picture

Neonatal period. Typical appearance usually take some weeks to develop but may be present at birth. May be prolonged physiological jaundice in *large* baby. (More commonly prolonged jaundice occurs in *small* babies.)

Note: Cretinism can commence prenatally even though mother normal, indicating that thyroid hormone does not cross placenta in adequate amount. Classic signs listed below in advanced hypothyroidism not seen nowadays because of neonatal screening.

1. Anatomical. (*a*) *Stature.* Dwarf, infantile proportions with large head, short arms and legs, hands broad, supraclavicular pads of fat. (*b*) *Skin.* Coarse, dry, cool. Pale from poor circulation and anaemia and with characteristic yellow colour due to carotinaemia. (*c*) *Hair.* Coarse, scanty, and brittle. Hairline extends down on to forehead. (*d*) *Facies.* Eyes far apart, bridge of nose depressed, palpebral fissure narrow, eyelids puffy. Tongue large and protruding. Dentition delayed. (*e*) *Umbilical Hernia.* Almost invariable in infants. (*f*) *Bones* (i) Osseous development retarded. Shown by delay in radiological appearance of epiphyses (= delayed 'bone age') clinically by large posterior fontanelle. (ii) Epiphysial dysgenesis shown on radiography as 'stippled epiphyses'; affects all centres which would normally have ossified during span of life when thyroid deficient.

2. Physiological. (*a*) Pulse slow; pulse pressure small, 20 mmHg or less;

temperature subnormal. (*b*) Basal metabolic rate low. Child sluggish and sleeps more than normal. This may be noticed before other stigmata of cretinism arise. Coarse cry, which is slow to come ('flat battery' sign). (*c*) Delayed passage of meconium, later constipation. (*d*) Muscle power poor and child hypotonic. Rarely muscle hypertonia with pseudohypertrophy (Kocher–Debré–Semelaigne syndrome).
3. Mental. Mental retardation often present. Milestones passed late.

Investigations
1. Low T_4 and T_3 in blood. With treatment rise to normal levels (normal, *see* Appendix 1).
2. TSH high when defect is in gland; low when defect in pituitary.
3. *Radioactive iodine* (^{123}I). Uptake low. This investigation is questionably justifiable in child, especially any child who is likely to have normal thyroid tissue. Technetium scan will show thyroid position.
4. When goitre present, complicated tests needed to evaluate specific defect.
5. *Radiology.* (*a*) Retarded ossification. Bone age, *see* Appendix 6. (*b*) Stippled epiphyses may occur especially during recovery on therapy. (*c*) First or second lumbar vertebra may be hypoplastic (beaked).

Differential Diagnosis
1. *Gargoylism.* Superficial resemblance with coarse features, dwarfism and mental retardation. Constipation not a feature. Enlarged liver and spleen, corneal opacities, and radiograph of spine gives diagnosis.
2. *Perthes' disease.* Fragmentation of femoral epiphysis may occur in both conditions, but Perthes' disease is usually unilateral and painful.
3. *Chondrodystrophy.* Bears superficial resemblance only to cretinism. Mental development normal.

Prognosis
Depends on: (*a*) Time in ante- or postnatal life that disorder commenced. the earlier, the greater the mental damage. (*b*) The severity of the deficiency. (*c*) Age of child before adequate treatment commenced. *Note*: Obvious gross cases often started on treatment earlier than milder cases as diagnosis easier to make but prognosis worse because disease is more severe. In cases diagnosed early, child becomes normal in appearance. Mental condition also improves, often becomes normal.

Treatment
1. *Initial Therapy.* Sodium-L-thyroxine 6–18 µg/kg/day in newborn, dropping to 2·5 µg/kg/day in older child, should be given at first. Given as single dose once daily. Larger doses often not well tolerated when treatment first commenced. T_3 may be used initially because of quick action. Monitor treatment to obtain correct dose, aim to keep T_4 at high normal level or TSH normal.

Goitre

Definition
A goitre (or 'struma') is any enlargement of the thyroid gland.

Classification and Causation of Goitres

Hy = Hypothyroidism, i.e. decreased thyroid excretion; Eu = Euthyroidism, i.e. normal thyroid excretion; Th = Thyrotoxicosis, i.e. excessive thyroid excretion.

1. Inadequate synthesis of thyroid hormone:	
1.1 Enzymatic deficiency	Hy or Eu
1.2 Iodine lack (endemic goitre)	Hy or Eu
1.3 Antithyroid drugs, prenatal or rarely, postnatal	Hy or Eu
1.4 'Simple' (puberty) goitre	Eu
2. Thyroiditis	Eu but later Hy
3. Benign adenoma, cysts, etc.	Eu
4. Carcinoma	Eu
5. Thyrotoxicosis	Th

Endemic Goitre

Occurs in iodine-poor areas—size of goitre varies. Endemic cretinism common when deficiency severe but usually patients euthyroid. T_4 low but T_3 raised to compensate so TSH normal.

Subacute Thyroiditis (*de Quervain's Thyroiditis*)

Common condition commencing just before puberty. More common in girls than boys. Goitre soft, diffuse and only moderately enlarged. May be painful and tender. All tests of thyroid function normal, resolves in few weeks.

Pendred's Syndrome

Congenital deafness—usually severe with goitre—often appearing at puberty. Patients usually euthyroid. There is a thyroid defect of organification. Thyroxine given to stop gland enlarging. Disease is autosomal recessive.

Autoimmune Thyroiditis (*Hashimoto's Disease; Lymphocytic Thyroiditis*)

Very rare condition in childhood, but common cause of thyroid enlargement after puberty in girls.

Thyroid enlarged, diffuse, non-tender. Child usually euthyroid but may be hypo-or hyperthyroid. Occurs in families; in Down's and Turner's syndromes. Thyroid antibodies raised in 60%. Thyroxine may control size.

Thyroiditis

May rarely by suppurative, or due to TB, sarcoid, mumps, Coxsackie and cat scratch disease.

Benign Adenoma, Cysts, etc.

Rare in childhood. If in doubt they should be removed because of risk of carcinomatous change.

Carcinoma of Thyroid

Very rare in childhood. Most cases have followed radiotherapy in infancy for 'enlarged' thymus. However, because of poor prognosis it is important for physician to bear the condition in mind.

Thyrotoxicosis

Uncommon disease in childhood. Girls to boys, 6 : 1. Symptoms may appear at any age. Neonatal cases may be associated with thyrotoxicosis in mother. Disease may follow physical or mental stress. High familial predisposition.

Clinical Features
As for adults but note the following:
1. Behaviour problems, active restless movements often mistaken for chorea. Acute anxiety may be presenting symptoms.
2. Tachycardia, increased pulse pressure, increased peripheral circulation, warm moist skin. Exophthalmos.
3. Accelerated growth in height and bone age common. Craniostenosis may occur in young. Appetite large so that weight often commensurate with height. Vomiting and diarrhoea may occur.
4. Thyroid gland palpable, smooth, diffuse, symmetrical, and bruit common.
5. Menarche may occur early.

Investigations
Blood levels of thyroxine and triiodothyronine increased. Occasionally T_4 normal but T_3 raised—so-called T_3-toxicosis. Other thyroid tests rarely indicated.

Treatment
1. Medical. Antithyroid drugs such as prophylthiouracil and carbimazole (methimazole) can be used.
   Note: (*a*) Initial dose should be fairly high then reduced to maintenance level after 1–3 months. this dose should be continued for from 1 to 3 years. Remission in 75% permanent. (*b*) Dosage is best controlled by serial T_4 measurements. (*c*) Thyroid gland decreases in size initially but if child becomes hypothyroid, it may increase in size again. Addition of thyroxine will reduce size. Some physicians advise combining the two treatments routinely. (*d*) Toxic signs: rashes not uncommon; fever, arthralgia; granulocytopenia rare but occasionally fatal.
2. Surgical. Some cases come to surgery because of unsuccessful medical treatment. Careful preoperative treatment necessary. Risk of postoperative hypothyroidism and/or hypoparathyroidism serious.
3. Radio-iodine therapy. Not advised in childhood.

For Further Reading

Grant D.B. and Hulse J.A (1980) Screening for congenital hypothyroidism. *Arch. Dis. Child.* **55**, 913.

Chapter 165   *DIABETES MELLITUS*

Definition
Uncommon condition in children, caused by diminished insulin secretion or utilization, resulting in hyperglycaemia, glycosuria, ketosis and, in untreated cases, coma and death.

Comparison with Adult Diabetes

In adults two main variants of diabetes mellitus are recognized:

Type 1. Insulin-dependent (Juvenile-onset diabetes) type. Due to lack of insulin. Occurs in young, thin patients.

Type 2. Non-insulin-dependent (Maturity-onset diabetes) type. Cause unknown. Occurs in older, fat patients.

In children only insulin-dependent type occurs.

Pathogenesis

Full pathogenesis unknown. Essential fact is lack of insulin production by islets of Langerhans in pancreas. Anterior pituitary also plays important part.

Aetiology

1. Hereditary factors. Probably multiple distinct types of diabetes exist. Most likely mode of inheritance is autosomal recessive, with gene frequency about 0·30 and lifetime penetrance of about 70% for males and 90% for females. Others consider that it may be dominant. Association with tissue (HLA) types B8/DW3 has been demonstrated. Hereditary element is not always obvious, however, for following reasons:

> 1.1 Diabetes mainly disease of older age groups. In any given family, members destined to have diabetes may not yet be old enough.
> 1.2 Family may be small or members die of other causes before developing diabetes.

2. Age. Uncommon in early childhood. Rare before 3 years of age. UK incidence 10–15 per 100,000 children per year.

3. Environmental factors (e.g. infections, particularly Coxsackie B4) or stress (e.g. pregnancy) may precipitate overt diabetes. Islet cell antibodies are present in 70% newly diagnosed diabetics.

Clinical Features

1. Onset. Usually fairly rapid, symptoms becoming more marked for 1–6 weeks. If these are ignored child may lapse into diabetic coma. In few cases preceding symptoms of very short duration with early coma.

2. Symptoms

> 2.1 Child drinks excessively and passes large quantity of pale urine frequently by day and night. Child sometimes brought to doctor for enuresis.
> 2.2 General malaise, tiredness, lassitude and loss of weight usually occur. Abdominal pain is common in ketoacidosis.
> 2.3 In girls pruritus of vulva may develop, in boys, balanitis.

3. Signs. Loss of weight may be obvious; skin often dry and inelastic owing to dehydration; smell of acetone in breath. In severe cases child in precoma or coma (*see* p. 482).

Investigations
1. *Urine*

    1.1 Sugar. In untreated case glycosuria always present.
    1.2 Ketone Bodies. Acetone often present.
    1.3 Specific Gravity. Raised owing to presence of sugar.

2. *Blood sugar*

    2.1 Fasting blood sugar raised. May be any value from 8 mmol/l (130 mg%) to 20 mmol// (800 mg%) or more, depending upon severity of condition. Usually above 14 mmol/l.
    2.2 After food, blood sugar rises more in diabetic than normal child and the return to initial levels takes much longer.
    2.3 Glucose tolerance curve. To obtain true record patient should be off insulin, and on normal diet for 3 days before test. Usually unnecessary for diagnosis.

3. *Glycosylated haemoglobin* (HbA_{1c}) Elevated in newly-diagnosed and poorly controlled diabetics (normal 5·5–8·5%), falls with good control.

4. *Blood cholesterol*. Raised. Normal below 5·5 mmol/l. Does not run parallel with blood sugar, but persistent high blood cholesterol (i.e. above 10 mmol/l) indicates poor long-term prognosis as complications such as atherosclerosis more liable to occur.

5. *Electrolytes and pH*. Metabolic acidosis and biochemical changes of dehydration present if child is severely ill.

Differential Diagnosis
1. *Of polyuria*

    1.1 Diabetes Insipidus. Urine contains no abnormal substances; is of low specific gravity. Child physically healthy apart from polydipsia and polyuria.
    1.2 Chronic Renal Failure. Urine may contain little or no albumin and no other abnormalities. Specific gravity low and fixed. Blood pressure and blood urea raised; changes may be present in fundi.

2. *Of glucose in urine*. Many causes known, for instance:

    2.1 Renal Glycosuria. If renal threshold low, glucose may be found in urine even when blood sugar within normal limits.
    2.2 Alimentary Glycosuria. Due to such rapid absorption of glucose from gut and slow storage so that blood sugar temporarily rises above renal threshold. Proved by glucose tolerance curve in which rapid, high rise in blood sugar seen. So-called 'lag storage curve'.
    2.3 Neurogenic Glycosuria. Due to stimulation of hypothalamus by tumour, haemorrhage, etc.
    2.4 Endocrine Glycosuria. Occasionally occurs in hyperthyroidism, or with administration of corticosteroids.

3. *Of other reducing substances in urine*

    3.1 Galactose. Due to inborn error of metabolism. Child fails to thrive. Hepatomegaly and congenital cataract may occur (p. 159).

3.2 Pentose. Due to inborn error of metabolism or occasionally from ingestion of pentose-containing fruit. Gives rise to no symptoms.

Complications of Diabetes
1. Those commonly seen in children:
    1.1 Ketosis and diabetic coma (*see* p. 482).
    1.2 Insulin coma (*see* p. 484).
    1.3 Infections, especially tuberculosis (*see* p. 482).
    1.4 Local alterations in subcutaneous fat due to insulin (*see* p. 485).
    1.5 Behaviour problems (*see* p. 485).
2. Those uncommonly seen in children:
    2.1 Retardation of growth and development (*see* p. 485).
    2.2 Xanthomatosis.
    2.3 Hepatomegaly.
    2.4 Hypersensitivity to insulin (*see* p. 485).
3. Those rarely seen in children, but which commonly occur when patient has had disease more than 20 years:
    3.1 Atherosclerosis.
    3.2 Retinal changes.
    3.3 Nephritis—Kimmelstiel–Wilson type.
    3.4 Cataract.
    3.5 Neuropathies.

Prognosis
1. At present time expectation of life almost the same as for healthy child but depends upon:
    1.1 Good medical treatment.
    1.2 Character of diabetes. Sometimes disease stable and easy to control. Sometimes labile and difficult to control as blood sugar fluctuates violently.
    1.3 Parental intelligence.
    1.4 Patient's intelligence and morale; when old enough to conduct his own treatment.

Management
Very important that child should feel that he is normal and the same as other children despite diabetes. He should therefore be encouraged to lead full active life with treatment as flexible as possible. Otherwise he will become rebellious and essential cooperation in therapy will not be obtained.

The Diabetic Balance

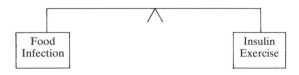

Food
Infection

Insulin
Exercise

Following factors modify day-to-day progress of diabetic:

1. Insulin. Every child with diabetes mellitus requires insulin. Dosage has to be regulated individually. If child is not in ketoacidosis, start with 0·5–1·0 u/kg/day in 3 doses given with main meals, using a short-acting preparation. After a few days in which child and parents learn insulin injection technique, change to a longer-acting preparation as single daily dose. Additional short-acting insulin (admixed) may be necessary if the child has persistent morning hyperglycaemia. Dosage is adjusted according to blood glucose levels.

Note: Insulin requirements usually decrease, sometimes to negligible level, after initial stabilization. This 'honeymoon period' may last up to a year or more but permanent remission is extremely rare.

Insulin types: Many available. Basic requirements include purity and freedom from contaminating polypeptides, suitable duration of action, and simple nomenclature. Highly purified animal preparations or synthetic human insulin should be used.

	Available after (hours)	Maximum effect (hours)	Duration (days)
a. Short-acting (e.g. Actrapid, Velosulin, Neutral soluble insulin, Neusulin, Humulin S)	½	1–3	6–8
b. Medium-acting (e.g. Semitard MC, (Amorphous suspension, Semilente)	½–1	2–4	10–12
c. Long-acting (e.g. Monotard MC, (Isophane) Insulatard, Neuphane, Humulin I)	2	8–10	28–30
d. Mixtures (e.g. Rapitard MC (25% soluble and 75% crystalline); Mixtard 30/70 (30% soluble and 75% isophane) etc	½	4–8	24

All preparations are available in (new) standard strengths of 100 u/ml.

2. Diet. Must be such as to allow normal growth and utilization of all insulin given. Diet should:

2.1 Contain adequate calories for all normal needs of active child, including growth.

2.2 Contain protein not less than 2·2 g/kg body weight/day.

2.3 Contain more carbohydrate than fat. Restrict carbohydrate to 40–60% of total calories, in portions or exchanges of 10g carbohydrate. Usual diet contains at least 100g plus 10g per year of age per day divided into 3 main meals, 2 snacks and a bedtime snack (to avoid hypoglycaemia).

2.4 Provide adequate fibre. High fibre intake reduces speed of carbohydrate absorption and thus controls postprandial hyperglycaemia.

2.5 Ensure vitamin intake.

2.6 Largest meals should be those 'covered' by insulin injection.

3. Physical excercise. Muscular activity utilizes blood sugar and therefore less insulin required. If unexpectedly severe amount of exercise taken, hypoglycaemia may develop. This can be countered by giving sugar.

Note: Child in bed will require more insulin than when he is up and about. When child in hospital for stabilization this fact should be remembered and either:

3.1 Child allowed up in ward most of day; or

3.2 Dosage of insulin reduced slightly on discharge, if accurate stabilization has been attained.

4. Infection. Increases insulin requirements. May precipitate diabetic coma—constant danger in child; commoner cause of coma than dietetic indiscretion. Infection is important complication for following reasons:

4.1 In adults persistent skin infection may be due to underlying diabetes. Children with diabetes, however, seem little more prone to skin infections than normal children.

4.2 If infection does occur, it may precipitate attack of diabetic coma.

4.3 Tuberculosis is a dangerous complication of diabetics. All measures for prevention should be considered, including BCG vaccination.

5. Endocrine, e.g.:

5.1 Girls at puberty may require temporary increase in insulin.

5.2 Administration of steroids dangerous in patients with diabetes.

Monitoring Diabetic Control

Clinical. Regular reviews should include following checks:

General health

Ketoacidosis

Hypoglycaemic episodes

Insulin injection sites (*see* p. 485)

Growth

Hepatomegaly

B.P. fundi

School attendance

Menses (irregular in poor control)

Laboratory tests

Capillary blood glucose (best method, can be managed at home and recorded by parents or child).

Urine glucose, ketone and protein.

24-h urine glucose (inconvenient for routine use).

Glycosylated haemoglobin (HbA_{1c})—indicates overall effectiveness of control.

Complications. Diabetic Coma and 'Precoma' (Ketosis) (*Hyperglycaemia*)

Common Causes

1. Presenting symptoms in unknown diabetic.

2. Infection—common.

3. Too little insulin. Very often child stops eating for some reason, e.g. because of vomiting, and parents or doctor reason that therefore insulin should be stopped. *Fundamental error* as in starvation body stores are metabolized and child still requires insulin.

Clinical Features

Onset. Child feels ill; often has headache. Nausea and vomiting prominent and insulin therefore often omitted. Abdominal pain occurs, maximal over liver (possibly due to stretching of liver capsule as organ undergoes fatty change). Later drowsiness or restlessness occurs, passing into deepening coma.

On examination. Child may or may not be rousable, florid complexion, obviously dehydrated; odour of acetone in breath; marked air hunger with characteristic deep respirations. Pulse thready; blood pressure low; limbs become cold and blue as peripheral circulatory failure develops; oliguria or anuria may lead to fatal termination.

Investigations
1. Urine. Contains sugar and acetone in large amounts. Specific gravity high despite polyuria.
2. Blood sugar. Over 16·5 mmol/l (300 mg %). May be over 25 mmol/l. Hyperosmolar.
3. Plasma bicarbonate low.
4. Plasma ketone bodies. Elevated (Ketostix).
5. Electrolytes. Serum sodium and potassium may be high, normal or low. High sodium occurs in hyperosmolar hyperglycaemic coma without ketosis.
6. Acid–base balance. Usually low arterial pH, metabolic acidosis.
7. Blood urea and haemoglobin. May be elevated due to haemoconcentration.

Prognosis
Very dangerous state. Death inevitable without prompt and adequate treatment.

Differential Diagnosis
1. Ketosis

> *1.1 Due to temporary starvation*: Common in normal children. Ketonuria frequently found in non diabetic children admitted to hospital.
> Causes:
> 1.1.1 Child frightened and eats poorly.
> 1.1.2 Infection often present.
> 1.1.3 Vomiting.
> *1.2 Periodic syndrome*: Vomiting initial and most prominent symptom. Ketosis due to resultant starvation.

2. Other causes of coma in child. Uraemia; poisons; intracranial lesions—haemorrhage, encephalitis, lead encephalopathy.
In every case of coma, specimen of urine should be obtained, by catheter if necessary, and tested for sugar, acetone and drugs.
3. Insulin coma.

Treatment
Immediate investigations. Monitor:
1. Blood glucose
2. Blood urea and electrolytes
3. Blood pH and gases
4. Hb, WBC
5. Cultures: blood, urine
6. ECG

7. Body weight
8. Intake and output

I.v. Fluids
1. If in SHOCK, plasma 10–20 ml/kg
2. Fluid replacement calculated as:
   2.1 Deficit (e.g. 10% dehydration) plus
   2.2 Maintenance (60–80 ml/kg/day) plus
   2.3 Supplemental (for fever, tachypnoea) plus
   2.4 Continuing losses (check intake/output)
3. Use 0·9% (normal) saline; ⅓ in first 4h, ⅓ in next 8h, ⅓ in next 12h.
4. When blood glucose falls to 12–14 mmol/l change to 0·18% saline in 4% dextrose.

Electrolytes
1. Potassium 3·5 mmol/kg/day. Start with 20 mmol/l.
2. Bicarbonate. *Rarely required*. If pH <7·0 and in shock give i.v. over 2h according to the formula: 12—observed HCO_3 × body wt (kg) × 0·6 mmol.
3. Oral KCl supplements will probably be required later.

Insulin
Use only *short-acting* insulin i.v.
1. 0·25 u/kg stat.
2. 0·10 u/kg/l or 2 u/h by continuous i.v. infusion.
3. Double rate if no decrease in blood glucose after 2–4h.
4. Titrate infusion rate against blood glucose change.

Later, use s.c. insulin on sliding scale according to blood glucose, e.g. >20 mmol/l = 0·5 u/kg, 15–20 = 0·4 u/kg, 12–15 = 0·3 u/kg, 10–12 = 0·2 u/kg, 8–10 = 0·1 u/kg.

Subsequent: Once oral intake has been established, give s.c. soluble insulin every 4–6h according to blood or urine glucose concentrations.

Insulin Reaction (*Hypoglycaemia*)

Causes
1. Too large dose of insulin.
2. Too little food.
3. Excessive exercise.

Clinical Features
Onset. Rapid, within a few minutes.
Symptoms. Ascribed to two main causes:

1. Hypoglycaemia: Irritability, incoordination, squint, epileptiform convulsions, drowsiness and coma.

2. Hyperadrenalism due to low blood sugar: Feeling of apprehension, pallor, sweating, tremor, weakness, occasionally vomiting. Symptoms may occur at night or in early morning, especially on delayed-action insulin. Child may then be difficult to awake, be irritable and complain of early morning headache.

Course and Prognosis

Although alarming, condition not usually dangerous if attack short-lived. Spontaneous recovery often occurs within a few hours. Severe hypoglycaemic coma can result in permanent cerebral damage with mental deterioration, fits, and neurological lesions. Child may remain in coma long after blood sugar has returned to normal. Death can occur.

Treatment

Early symptoms can easily be warded off by taking food. If vomiting or stuporose, glucagon 1 mg given subcutaneously. In severe cases intravenous glucose—20 ml of 50 % solution may effect dramatic cure.

Insulin Lipodystrophy and Lipomatosis

Definition

Localized atrophy or increased deposition of fat occurring at sites of insulin injections. Both common occurrences in children of both sexes. Probably due to impurities in insulin; occurs less frequently in adults. Can be treated by injecting highly purified insulin into atrophic sites, when fat reaccumulates. Best prevented by varying sites of injection daily.

N.B. Insulin injected into affected area often less painful. Absorption may be poor, however, resulting in adequate stabilization and apparent increase in insulin requirements.

Behaviour Problems

Common, particularly in adolescents. Correct parental attitude to disease very important. The patient must be helped to accept his/her diabetes as a part of life which will not go away. Contact with other affected children (as at diabetic camps) is often helpful.

Retardation of Growth and Development (*Mauriac's Syndrome*)

Children are dwarfed, obese and have enlarged livers. Most likely to occur with single daily dose of short-acting insulin. Cured by adequate control, with longer-acting preparations. Should never occur with adequate diet and correct insulin dosage.

Hypersensitivity to Insulin

Rare. Changing type of insulin may effect cure. Sometimes desensitization required.

Chapter 166   *HYPOGLYCAEMIA*

Definition

In newborn—two whole blood glucose levels below 1·7 mmol/l (30 mg/dl) in full term and less than 1·1 mmol/l (20 mg/dl) in preterm infants. In infants over 3 days of age whole blood glucose should be more than 2·2 mmol/l

(40 mg/dl). For children a fasting level below 2·8 mmol/l (50 mg/dl) is diagnostic.

Clinical Features
Vary from child to child; even when blood glucose is similar.

Symptoms are sweating, nervousness, fatigue, hunger, pallor, behaviour abnormalities, irritability, confusion coma, convulsions and headache.

Causes
1. Excess insulin, e.g. islets of Langerhans β-cell tumour or hyperplasia: infant of diabetic mother, haemolytic disease of newborn, hypopituitarism, Beckwith's syndrome. Leucine-sensitive children have β-cell hyperplasia. Some teratomas.

2. Liver enzyme defects: glycogen storage diseases, fructose intolerance, pyruvate carboxylase deficiency, galactosaemia, maple syrup urine disease.

3. Endocrine diseases: adrenal hypo- or hyperplasia, Addison's disease, pituitary growth hormone or ACTH deficiency, panhypopituitarism.

4. Drugs: alcohol, salicylates, sulphonylureas, propranolol.

5. Miscellaneous: malabsorption, Reye's syndrome, liver damage in leukaemia and neoplasms.

6. Ketotic hypoglycaemia: accounts for half of all cases in childhood, onset between 2 and 5 years, ceasing by 10 years. Usually boys, often low birth weight—attacks first thing in morning with ketonuria (hence name). May have fits and coma. Associated with infections (occasionally) and relative fasting. Children respond to i.v. glucose but not satisfactorily to glucagon because of glycogen depletion. Patients appear to have poor gluconeogenesis from amino acids (plasma alanine low).

So-called adrenal medullary hyporesponsiveness where children have poor adrenaline response to hypoglycaemia is probably a variant of ketotic hypoglycaemia. Treatment by small frequent feeds, e.g. 5 per day, rich in protein and carbohydrate.

Chapter 167   SHORT STATURE

No agreed definition but term may be used for children less than third centile in height.

Classification and Causes of Short Stature
1. Delayed development
2. Endocrine disorders
        2.1 Pituitary
        2.1.1 Hypothalamic–pituitary growth hormone (GH) deficiency. May occur as isolated phenomenon or as part of panhypopituitarism.
        2.1.2 Low somatomedin, high GH levels (Laron syndrome).

2.1.3 Peripheral unresponsiveness to GH and somatomedin.
2.2 Thyroid—hypothyroidism.
2.3 Adrenal—late result of sexual precocity, congenital adrenal hyperplasia, or Cushing's syndrome because of premature closure of epiphyses.
2.4 Hypoparathyroidism

3. *Genetic disorders*

3.1 Familial short stature
3.2 Chromosomal, e.g. Turner's syndrome or trisomies.
3.3 Skeletal
3.3.1 Osteochondrodystrophies, e.g. achondroplasia.
3.3.2 Rickets; vitamin-D resistant and other late forms.
3.3.3 Osteogenesis imperfecta.
3.3.4 Mucopolysaccharidoses, e.g. Morquio's syndrome.
3.4 Other. Organ or system disease, e.g. cardiac, pulmonary, skeletal, cerebral, etc. Cystic fibrosis. Glycogen storage disease. Russell–Silver syndrome. de Lange (Amsterdam dwarf) and other specific syndromes.

4. *Acquired disorders*. Malnutrition and emotional deprivation. Coeliac disease. Chronic renal disease. Cirrhosis of liver. Iatrogenic—steroids.

5. *Uncertain*. Intra-uterine growth retardation from infections, e.g. maternal rubella or cytomegalovirus, or placental inadequacy. Progeria. Microcephaly. Leprechaunism and others.

Delayed Development

Child small throughout childhood for no apparent reason. Puberty may be delayed until age 16 or later. Ultimately puberty occurs and child catches up with contemporaries although often remaining a small adult. Prognosis depends upon whether bone age is commensurate with height age (good prognosis) or with chronological age (poor prognosis).

Management

1. Medical treatment of no avail except for growth hormone deficiency.
2. Short stature can be a severe disability because of psychological consequences, e.g. made to feel inferior by peers. Counselling required for boys—because of small size and poor athletic prowess, and girls—because of delayed secondary sex characteristics.

Congenital Short Stature

Uncommon condition in which child is below normal weight and length at birth although not premature. Child remains normally proportioned although small throughout life.

Intra-uterine Growth Retardation

Infant born small for dates—usually less than 10th centile. Many causes. Catch-up growth occurs but the extent depends upon the duration of growth inhibition in utero. Growth restriction in utero affects weight, then length, then head

Table 167.1   Some bone disease causes of short stature

	Genetics	Clinical features
Achondrogenesis	Recesive	Deficient calcification: early death
Achondroplasia	Dominant	Large head and short limbs
Cartilage-hair hypoplasia	Recessive	Fine, sparse, hair; scalloped metaphyses
Conradi's syndrome	Recessive	Punctate calcification of epiphyses
Diastrophic dwarfism	Recessive	Limitation of joints; club feet; scoliosis
Ellis–Van Creveld syndrome	Recessive	Chondroectodermal dysplasia with hypoplastic nails and teeth; congenital heart lesions
Hypophosphataemic rickets	X-linked dominant	Poor renal tubular reabsorption of phosphorus needs high dosage of vitamin D
Hypophosphatasia	Recessive	Variable severity; low alkaline phosphatase levels, usually die early.
Metaphysial dysostosis	Dominant	Tibial bowing; splayed metaphyses
Spondylo-epiphysial dysplasia	Dominant and recessive	Several types; deformities become evident after birth
Thanatophoric dwarfism	? Recessive	Short limbs; small chest; all die in neonatal period

circumference in that order. Catch-up growth shown in reverse order. Some idea of duration of poor growth given by examination of extent of retardation in various parameters.

de Lange Syndrome (*Cornelia de Lange Syndrome; Amsterdam Dwarf*)

Rare form of mental retardation and dwarfism. Cause unknown, not apparently inherited but may occur in twins.

Features
Low birth weight, failure to thrive, microcephaly, severe mental retardation, bushy eyebrows which meet in centre, low hair line, characteristic face, hirsuties. Often skeletal malformations. Usually die in first decade.

Progeria

Very rare condition. Cause unknown. Often first noted in second or third year. Child undergoes all the physical effects of ageing throughout life condensed into a few years.

Clinical Features
Combination of dwarfism, sexual retardation, lack of subcutaneous fat, micrognathia, prominent scalp veins, alopecia, prominent eyes, 'horse-riding' stance, thin limb with big joints, thin dry wrinkled skin, beaked nose. Age prematurely.

Prognosis
Death usually occurs before 20 years. Sometimes due to coronary occlusion.

Microcephalic Dwarfism

Mixed group of children notable for mental retardation, dwarfism, microcephaly and bird-like heads. Sometimes familial. May be associated with ring chromosome.

Leprechaunism

Very rare syndrome manifested by: characteristic facies, severe growth failure, enlargement of breasts and external genitalia, ovaries and liver. Mental retardation common.

Russell–Silver Syndrome

Rare syndrome of dwarfism with asymmetry of body, low birth-weight, triangular face, abnormalities of sexual development and abnormal fingers.

Chapter 168   # SEXUAL DEVELOPMENT

Major determinants of child's sexuality include chromosome constitution, presence and function of testes or ovary, state of external genitalia and type of rearing.

Stages of Sex Differentiation

Organizing Factor	Result
1. *Ferilization*: X ovum receives X or Y chromosome from sperm	Determines chromosomal sex
2. *Chromosomal sex*	Determines whether testes or ovaries develop
3. *a. Testes* (only) testosterone which is converted to dihydrotestosterone by 5α reductase	Testosterone acts on Wolffian duct system differentiation and dihydrotestosterone causes masculinization of external genitalia
b. Ovary. Absence of 'organizing substance'	No organization so: (*a*) Wolffian duct system becomes vestigial. (*b*) Müllerian system develops into female genitalia.

Sexual Maturation: Secondary Sexual Characteristics

Stages of development of the secondary sex characters may be recorded. The following standard ratings on a scale of 1–5 may be used. (Taken by kind permission of the publishers from the standard illustrations in *Growth at Adolescence*, 2nd ed., Oxford, Blackwell Sci. Publ., 1962; *see also* Chapter 7 in *Textbook of Paediatrics*, 3rd ed. Forfar J. and Arneil G., Churchill–Livingstone, 1984.)

Boys: genital (penis) development:

Stage 1. Pre-adolescent, testes, scrotum and penis are of about the same size and proportion as in early childhood.

Stage 2. Enlargement of scrotum and testes. Skin of scrotum reddens and changes in texture. Little or no enlargement of penis at this stage.

Stage 3. Enlargement of penis, which occurs at first mainly in length. Further growth of testes and scrotum.

Stage 4. Increased size of penis with growth in breadth and development of glans. Testes and scrotum larger; scrotal skin darkened.

Stage 5. Genitalia adult in size and shape.

Girls: breast development.

Stage 1. Pre-adolescent: elevation of papilla only.

Stage 2. Breast bud stage: elevation of breast and papilla as small mound. Enlargement of areola diameter.

Stage 3. Further enlargement and elevation of breast and areola, with no separation of their contours.

Stage 4. Projection of areola and papilla to form a secondary mound above the level of the breast.

Stage 5. Mature stage: projection of papilla only, due to recession of the areola to the general contour of the breast.

Both sexes: pubic hair.

Stage 1. Pre-adolescent. The vellus over the pubes is not further developed than that over the abdominal wall, i.e. no pubic hair.

Stage 2. Sparse growth of long, slightly pigmented downy hair, straight or slightly curled, chiefly at the base of the penis or along labia.

Stage 3. Considerably darker, coarser and more curled. The hair spreads sparsely over the junction of the pubes.

Stage 4. Hair now adult in type, but area covered is still considerably smaller than in the adult. No spread of the medial surface of thighs.

Stage 5. Adult in quantity and type with distribution of the horizontal (or classically 'feminine') pattern. Spread to medial surface of thighs but not up linea alba or elsewhere above the base of the inverse triangle (spread up linea alba occurs late and is rated stage 6).

Chapter 169   # ABERRATIONS IN SEXUAL DEVELOPMENT

Retardation of the Onset of Puberty

Common condition, more common in boys than girls. Child has usually been slow in physical development throughout childhood (*see* p. 487). Puberty may be delayed until 16 years old or more. When puberty commences may proceed rapidly or slowly. Child may attain full adult height. Any severe constitutional disease such as malnutrition, hypopituitarism, coeliac or Crohn's disease, renal failure, persistent heart failure tends to delay puberty.

Gynaecomastia in Males

Common condition in adolescent boys, possibly due to undue end-organ sensitivity. Occurs in Klinefelter's syndrome, Leydig cell tumours, adrenal tumours and testicular feminization syndrome.

Premature Development of Breasts in Female
(*Precocious or Premature Thelarche*)

Condition in which there is isolated enlargement of breasts in young girl. Slight degrees common. Marked degrees rare. May occur in first two years. Often transient. Exclude premature puberty by finding normal vaginal mucosa for age, and ovarian mass detected either by rectal examination or ultrasonography. Possibility that cause is some oestrogen-containing substance or premature puberty, hence review must always be considered.

Precocious Adrenarche (*Pubarche*)

Occasionally pubic and axillary hair develop long before other signs of puberty, associated with some growth spurt and advancement of bone age. Normal puberty follows. Often in girls and with some brain disease.

Testicular Feminization Syndrome

Genetic male (XY) with testis but female external genitalia, secondary sex characteristics and psychosexual orientation. X-linked recessive inheritance. Thought to be due to target cell failure to respond to androgens in utero. Vagina blind or absent, uterus absent, gonads (testes) may be in labia, vaginal region or abdomen. Often discovered when female has inguinal hernia plus mass which is found to be testis. Treat by orchidectomy at puberty and oestrogen replacement.

Chapter 170   # SEXUAL PRECOCITY

Definition
Appearance of secondary sexual characteristics before age of 10 in boys or 8 in girls. May be:
   1. Isosexual (homologous), when secondary characteristics are those of child's own sex.
   2. Heterosexual (heterologous), when of opposite sex. Invariably incomplete.
   Note: In precocious puberty spermatogenesis occurs in boys and ovulation in girls.

Classification
1. *Cerebral Causes*. Constitutional; Organic (*see* p. 491).

2. Gonadal Causes. (*a*) In boys, Interstitial-cell tumour of testis; adrenal hyperplasia or tumour; arrhenoblastoma. (*b*) In girls, granulosa or theca-cell tumour of ovary; functional cyst in McCune–Albright syndrome; adrenal tumour; oestrogens.

3. Precocious Thelarche (premature development of breasts only). *See* p. 491.

4. Pubarche (premature adrenarche). *See* p. 491.

Constitutional Sexual Precocity

Aetiology
Sex. Girls : boys 4 : 1.
Age. May occur at any age.
Cause. Unknown. Probably hypothalamic in origin. May be familial.

Clinical Features
1. Onset. Once puberty has started it takes same time to mature as normal puberty.

2. Sexual development. Always isosexual. Pattern as normal but more variation in sequence of events, e.g. menarche may occur first. Growth initially rapid but premature fusion of epiphyses leads to ultimate short stature. Libido corresponds to degree of sexual development. Pregnancy has occurred in girls as young as 5½ years.

Investigations
1. Plasma gonadotrophin elevated. Plasma testosterone and oestrogens commensurate with stage of sex development.

2. Bimanual examination and ultrasonography of ovary (*see below*).

Differential Diagnosis
See Table 170.1. Careful search must be made for causative lesions, especially cerebral tumour. Constitutional precocity must be differentiated from granulosa-cell tumour of ovary—in latter palpable tumour is almost always present by time

Table 170.1   Differential diagnosis of sexual precocity

Causes	Age of onset	Type of precocity	Testis in boys	Ovary in girls	17-Oxo-steroid level
Cerebral	0–10 years	Isosexual	Adult size. Spermatogenesis present	Adult size. Ovulation occurs	At or below normal
Gonadal	0–10 years	Isosexual	Small, but tumour present	Palpable tumour present	Raised above normal in boys
Adrenal	Prenatal or 0–10 years	Boys: Isosexual Girls: Hetero-sexual	Small	Small	Greatly increased

precocity occurs. *Bimanual examination of pelvis for tumour (under anaesthetic if necessary) should always be performed, and repeated at intervals. Laparoscopy only required if obvious ovarian abnormality found. Small follicular cysts usually present.*

Treatment
Contraceptive pill for premenstrual tension. Danazol, a synthetic derivative of ethisterone, reduces pituitary gonadotrophins LH and FSH and is useful in treatment. Dosage 100–400 mg daily. Growth spurt not usually affected. Care must be taken to prevent sexual interference.

Organic Cerebral Sexual Precocity

Aetiology
Pathological lesion is in posterior region of hypothalamus. May be due to:
   1. Tumours, e.g. of pineal body pressing on floor of third ventricle or invading hypothalamic region.
   2. Hydrocephalus, tuberous sclerosis, neurofibroma, Russell–Silver syndrome and hypothyroidism.
   3. Following encephalitis or meningitis, especially tuberculous meningitis.
   4. Polyostotic fibrous dysplasia.

Clinical Features
As for constitutional type, with addition of direct symptoms due to causative lesion, e.g. raised intracranial pressure. Early onset before age 3 years but without neurological signs, suspect a hamartoma; later onset, e.g. age 6 years, is associated with CNS signs when cause is neurological.

Interstitial-cell Tumour of Testis
(*Leydig Cell Tumour*)

Extremely rare tumour. Most cases occur under 8 years of age. Usually benign; may be quite small. Unilateral. Diagnosed by finding one testis bigger than the other. Isosexual precocity occurs. 17-Oxosteroids may be greatly increased up to 500 mg/day.

Granulosa-cell Tumour of Ovary

Very rare. Tumour usually benign or low malignancy. By the time sexual precocity occurs, tumour palpable, but may require bimanual examination under anaesthetic. Causes incomplete precocity of isosexual type.

Adrenal Sexual Precocity in Boys
(*Macrogenitosomia Praecox*)

Usually due to adrenal hyperplasia or carcinoma.

Clinical Features
Isosexual precocity occurs, accelerated growth, pubic hair, seborrhoea, acne and deepening of voice. Penis may become very large. Some cases have hypertension which decreases with steroid therapy. Differs from constitutional type in that testes remain small and there is no spermatogenesis. Although growth is rapid, epiphyses fuse early—tall child but short adult.

Adrenal Heterosexual Precocity (Virilism) in Girls

Classification
1. Neonatal type—*see* p. 471.
2. Childhood type—considered *below*.

Childhood Type

Definition
Rare condition caused by hyperplasia or neoplasm of adrenal cortex resulting in pseudo-precocity and masculinization, i.e. heterosexual precocity.

Clinical Features
Hypertrichosis of masculine distribution. Greasy skin and acne vulgaris. Voice becomes deep and muscular development is that of boy. Increased growth and premature fusion of epiphyses occurs, resulting in tall child but short adult. Clitoris enlarges and resembles small penis. Considerable psychological upset may occur.

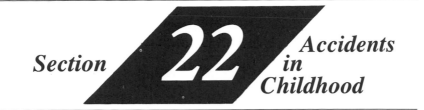

Section **22** *Accidents in Childhood*

Chapter 171   ## POISONING

Incidence
Common accident in age group 1–4 years. Boys : girls, 2 : 1 from age of 12 months upward.

Prevention
1. Storage of drugs in locked or inaccessible cupboards.
2. Childproof containers have reduced incidence of poisoning with drugs but may not be resistant to persevering child, wrapping of individual tablets or capsules helpful.
3. Storage of solvents, paraffin (kerosene), bleach, etc. out of child's reach in clearly marked bottles.

Management
1. Induce vomiting *unless* patient unconscious or poison is corrosive or volatile. Methods: (*a*) Push spoon handle or padded finger down throat. (*b*) Give syrup of ipecac 15 ml followed by 250 ml or more of water or milk. Repeat in 15 min if necessary.
2. If vomiting does not occur, gastric lavage required.
3. Identify drug when necessary. (Write in here telephone number of local poison centre ....).
4. Observation of vital signs.
5. Specific treatment for particular poison.

Iron Poisoning

Source of Iron
In majority of cases iron ingested is in form of sugar-coated tablets which have been prescribed for mother.

Clinical Features
Half to 1 h after ingestion: vomiting and bloody diarrhoea followed by cardiovascular collapse; acidosis and coma may precede death within 4–6 h or gradual improvement. Relapse after 8–16 h not uncommon, when coma and convulsions are prominent features. If child recovers, severe gastrointestinal scarring and liver disease may be delayed problems.

Investigations
Serum iron raised according to quantity ingested. Radiograph may show tablets in abdomen. Ferrous salts in vomit demonstrated by Prussian blue test.

Treatment
Very urgent.
1. Immediate administration of emetic or stomach wash-out with 1 % sodium bicarbonate.
2. Sodium bicarbonate should be left in stomach to convert soluble ferrous sulphate into insoluble forms of iron.
3. Intravenous plasma may be required to correct dehydration and counteract shock.
4. Desferrioxamine: (*a*) 0·5–1·0g i.m. immediately (before lavage). (*b*) Further 5g can be given via gastric tube at end of lavage. (*c*) 15mg/kg/h i.v. if patient collapsed (maximum dose 80mg/kg/24h).

Lead Poisoning

Aetiology
Majority of cases associated with *pica*, especially chewing paint which contains lead. Therefore almost non-existent in countries with adequate legislation to prohibit use of lead paints.

Pathology
Lead is either:
1. Deposited in bone—comparatively innocuous; or
2. Free in circulation—exerts effects principally on brain, kidneys and liver.
Post-mortem. Macroscopically: oedema of brain, and petechial haemorrhages. Microscopically: characteristic eosinophilic inclusion bodies in liver and renal tubules.

Pathological Physiology
Lead acts like calcium, i.e. factors which aid deposition or excretion of calcium do so for lead.

Clinical Features (*Table 171.1*)

Table 171.1. Comparison of classic findings in lead poisoning in children and adults

	Children	*Adults*
Constipation	Common	Common
Vomiting	Common	Rare
Encephalopathy	Common	Rare
Colic	Less common	Common
Blood changes	Common	Common
Bone changes	Invariable	Not seen
Lead line on gums	Rare	Common
Peripheral 'neuritis'	Rare	Common

1. Onset. History of general malaise, irritability, vomiting, constipation, perhaps abdominal pain, over 3–6 weeks.
2. Course. Condition may: (*a*) *Recover*, only to relapse again if source of lead not removed. (*b*) *Progress to Encephalopathy*. Child becomes increasingly

irritable, then lapses into coma. Muscle twitching and convulsions occur. Ocular palsies common. Pulse becomes rapid, full and bounding; may be intense vasodilatation. Systolic blood pressure rises but diastolic may fall.

Fundi: Papilloedema not common in infants, but may occur in older children.

Investigations

1. Urine. Contains coproporphyrin and Δ-aminolaevulinic acid. Fluoresces in ultraviolet light. Albuminuria, glycosuria and amino aciduria common, due to tubular damage. Urine lead elevated (normal up to 50 µg/l).

2. Blood picture. Moderate to severe haemolytic anaemia. Punctate basophilia prominent, but not pathognomonic.

3. Blood lead levels elevated (normal up to 40 µg/dl (1·93 µmol/l)). Toxic levels almost always exceed 80 µg/dl (3·86 µmol/l).

4. CSF. Usually under increased pressure during encephalopathy. Protein and sugar may be raised.

5. Radiography. (*a*) *Bones.* Increased density from lead deposition, maximal at sites of rapid bone growth. In long-standing cases, may be several rings of increased density parallel to epiphysis. (*b*) *Abdomen.* Rarely particles of lead may be seen in abdomen.

Differential Diagnosis

Recurrent abdominal pain and/or vomiting; diabetes; tuberculous meningitis.

Prognosis

Mortality from encephalopathy high. Cases which recover from encephalopathy often show residual mental defect varying from mild to severe. Optic atrophy may occur. Chronic nephritis may be late effect.

Treatment

Object is to remove lead from blood and soft tissues as rapidly as possible.

1. To assist deposition of lead: (*a*) Keep urine reaction neutral. (*b*) Large doses of calcium: given as calcium lactate and milk by mouth. (*c*) Vitamin D.

2. To promote excretion of lead: Calcium ethylenediaminetetra-acetic acid (Ca EDTA), i.m. or i.v. (never orally), in combination with BAL or penicillamine. Undigested lead in gut removed by purgatives and enemas.

3. Symptomatic treatment: Endeavour to reduce cerebral oedema: (*a*) Intravenous glucose, 10–20 ml of 50% solution. (*b*) Magnesium sulphate, per rectum, 100–200 ml of 25% solution. (*c*) Cautious removal of CSF. (*d*) Intravenous calcium gluconate, 5 ml of 10% solution. May cause dramatic temporary recovery. (*e*) In cases which do not respond rapidly, surgical decompression should be considered.

Mercury Poisoning
(Pink Disease; Acrodynia; Erythroedema)

At one time very common disease following ingestion of mercury in 'teething' powders. Manifested by pink hands and feet, photophobia and hypotonia.

Methaemoglobinaemia

Very rare cause of cyanosis occurring almost exclusively in infancy.

Aetiology

Age. Usually within first 2 months of life.

Main causes

1. From ingestion of nitrates in water. Usual history: water contaminated with nitrates (often from shallow well) used in preparation of artificial feed. Sequence of events: nitrates converted into nitrites by bacteria in bowel, nitrites absorbed, oxidize haemoglobin to methaemoglobin.

2. Aniline. Used in marking linen or as crayons. Can be absorbed through skin.

3. Sulphonamides.

4. Rare autosomal recessive condition with inability to reduce methaemoglobin.

Clinical Features

Child appears cyanosed, but no cause can be found. In severe cases vomiting, diarrhoea and even death occur.

Diagnosis

By spectroscopic examination of blood.

Treatment

1. Remove cause.
2. Injection of methylene blue 1–2 mg/kg body weight i.v. Very effective.
3. Ascorbic acid. Slow action.
4. Exchange transfusion may be necessary for very severe cases.

Barbiturate Poisoning

Depth of Coma

Best guide of depth is response to deep pain:

1. Mild coma. Child withdraws stimulated part.

2. Moderate coma. Child restless and grimaces during painful stimulus.

3. Severe coma. No response to stimulus.

Management of Child in Coma

1. Airway. If no cough reflex present, cuffed endotracheal tube inserted before stomach aspiration.

2. Stomach aspiration. With normal saline. Of little value theoretically if more than 6 h after ingestion of poison, but important for legal reasons.

3. Eyes. Cellulose drops instilled. Lids taped shut.

4. Circulatory system. I.v. fluids to replace insensible fluid loss (*see* p. 134). If blood pressure falls below 13·3 kPa (100 mmHg) give dopamine i.v. Osmotic diuresis may be induced with mannitol to induce urinary excretion. Alkalinization of urine with sodium bicarbonate also helpful.

5. Respiratory system. Child turned frequently to avoid lung collapse. Intermittent positive-pressure ventilation may be required.

Note: Analeptic drugs (picrotoxin, Megimide) may be dangerous.

Salicylate Poisoning

Clinical Features
Early signs are hyperventilation and drowsiness, leading to coma. Urine contains salicylates and ketones. Dehydration and hyperpyrexia may occur, occasionally bleeding tendency from hypoprothrombinaemia.

Investigations
1. *Acid–base balance.* Early respiratory alkalosis giving way to metabolic acidosis.
2. *Serum salicylate.* Mild poisoning, without symptoms—less than 40 mg/dl. Severe poisoning, usually lethal—more than 120 mg/dl.
3. *Urine.* Phenistix or ferric chloride test produces violet colour.

Differential Diagnosis
Diabetic ketosis.

Treatment
1. Induce vomiting or gastric lavage.
2. Stimulate diuresis with oral fluids or i.v. dextrose saline (100–150 ml/kg/24 h).
3. I.v. sodium bicarbonate if severe metabolic acidosis.
4. Treat hypoprothrombinaemia with vitamin K.

Poisoning with Tricyclic Antidepressants

Drugs include imipramine, amitriptyline. Fatal dose of imipramine for 18-months-old child 350 mg. Severe symptoms in small children can follow 75–100 mg.

Clinical Features
Loss of consciousness, ataxia, nystagmus, hypertonicity, increased tendon reflexes, convulsions and cardiac irregularity, often with hypotension.

Diagnosis
Significant blood level 1 mg/l.

Treatment
1. Gastric lavage if more than 150 mg swallowed.
2. Maintain respiration, support circulation, control convulsions.
3. Sodium lactate i.v.
4. For cardiac dysrhythmia, prostigmine by repeated injection, 1 mg i.v. at first, later i.m., judging dose by response on monitor.

Kerosene (Paraffin) Poisoning

Common in rural areas and developing countries where kerosene is main source of domestic heating and light.

Clinical Features
Initially few but after some hours, cough, dyspnoea and possibly cyanosis may develop. Chest radiograph shows pulmonary oedema.

Treatment
Do not induce vomiting or perform gastric lavage because of risk of aspiration into lungs.
    Treat respiratory complications symptomatically.

Turpentine Poisoning

Essentially similar to kerosene poisoning.

Atropine Poisoning

Sources
Atropine-like drugs (e.g. hyoscine) in travel sickness pills. Berries (e.g. deadly nightshade).

Clinical Features
Skin hot, dry, flushed. Pupils dilated, pulse rapid. Urinary retention. Restlessness, delirium, coma.

Treatment
    1. Gastric lavage or induce vomiting.
    2. Sedation with chlorpromazine.
    3. Reduce pyrexia with fans and tepid sponging.
    4. Pilocarpine 0·1 mg/kg i.m. or pyridostigmine 1 mg/kg 4-hourly by mouth.
    5. Procainamide 10 mg/kg orally every 6 h for cardiac arrhythmia.

Boron Poisoning (*Boric Acid Poisoning*)

Rare cause of poisoning. In past boron used to be given as glycerin and borax to clean mouth or as boric acid externally. Boron and boric acid should not be used in paediatrics. Manifestations: vomiting, diarrhoea; 'boiled lobster' appearance of skin.

Chapter 172   **BURNS AND SCALDS**

For full description, *see* surgical textbooks.

Classification of Burns
Probably best divided into:
1. Superficial
2. Deep
Of greatest importance is area of skin loss. *Special sites*: Eyelids—beware of

exposure damage to cornea. Inhalation of hot air or gases leads to respiratory oedema and obstruction.

Prevention
Almost all burns and scalds are preventable.
Following measures should be enforced:
1. All fires should have adequate guard.
2. Clothing should be fire-proofed.
3. Education of public about means of avoiding home accidents.

Management
1. First aid. (*a*) Immersion of part or child in cold water. (*b*) During rescue cover nose and mouth with damp cloth to reduce inhalational trauma to respiratory tract from hot air.
2. Resuscitation by intravenous infusion of saline and plasma alternately, pending transfer to Burns Unit.
3. Specialist management in Burns Unit if burns are extensive or deep.
4. Other general measures. (*a*) Sedation. (*b*) High-protein diet required during convalescence. Food can be fortified with amino acids. (*c*) Give maximum psychological help to child, his relations and nursing staff. Discussion sessions often of value. (*d*) Prevention of infection, local treatment, skin grafting, etc. *see* surgical textbooks. Injections of gammaglobulin useful for young children initially to resist infection.

Chapter 173   # SUDDEN DEATH

Some Causes of Sudden Death
1. Easily discernible at autopsy:
    - 1.1 Haemorrhage into brain or adrenals.
    - 1.2 Congenital abnormalities of heart, brain, etc.
    - 1.3 Endomyocardial fibroelastosis.
    - 1.4 Fulminating gastroenteritis.
    - 1.5 Asphyxia from aspiration of foreign body. *Note*: Vomitus found in respiratory tract may be agonal and not cause of death.
    - 1.6 Meningitis.
2. Causes sometimes discovered with difficulty, if at all:
    - 2.1 Acute infection, particularly *H. influenzae* septicaemia.
    - 2.2 Poisoning.

Sudden Unexpected Death Syndrome ('cot death')
Young infant found dead in cot. Cause of death not found at autopsy in half the cases. Deaths more common in lower social classes, in winter months and at week-ends. Often some aspiration of vomit occurs. Rare in breast-fed infants.

Incidence
About 3/1000 live births in UK.

Theories of Causation

1. Immunological incompetence in young infant predisposes to fulminating infection or anaphylactic response to antigenic stimulus (e.g. cow's milk).
2. Hypernatraemia and uraemia (observed in some infants post mortem).
3. Hypoglycaemia.
4. Exaggerated apnoeic response to upper airways obstruction e.g. in gastro-oesophageal reflux.
5. Congenital or acquired abnormality of cardiac conduction leading to arrhythmia.
6. Suffocation by pillow (rarely, if ever, responsible).

Prevention

1. Improve social and preventive medical services to families at risk, i.e. lower social classes, and where attendance at infant clinics is poor.
2. Apnoea monitoring, using similar alarm device to those used in neonatal units, may be employed after episode of 'near-miss' or for infants whose parents previously lost a child in this way.

Management

Grief and guilt feelings in parents demand expert, sympathetic help and follow-up.

Chapter 174   # Non-Accidental Injury (NAI; Battered Baby Syndrome)

A syndrome of recurrent injuries inflicted on child by attendant—often mother, less commonly father. Infliction of injury often follows a quite regular, even ritualistic, pattern. Abuse occurs in many degrees and manifested in many ways, physical or emotional. Can be described as neglect, maternal deprivation, inadequate mothering/parenting or maltreatment.

Frequency varies from country to country but probably represents only severe instances which are discovered. Mortality 1·0%—a third are under 6 months, and a third over 3 years. All social groups affected. Higher incidence in families under stress, e.g. single parent, alcoholism. Often only one child in family selected for abuse. Reason may be apparent, e.g. congenital abnormality, premature, only girl; but often reason not obvious.

In year following physical abuse, one-sixth of children show poor physical growth, one-third show 'hard' signs of CNS damage, one-fifth show 'soft' signs of CNS damage.

History of cause of injuries may be difficult to obtain—parents reluctant to give explanation, often account inadequate, e.g. infant banged head against cot, or sibling aged 3 caused the injuries. Accounts by various relatives may conflict. Parents frequently delay seeking medical advice.

A. THE ABUSED CHILD
   1. Average age: under 4 years most under 2.
   2. Average age at death: slightly under 3 years.
   3. Average duration exposure to battering: 1–3 years.
   4. Sex differentiation: none.
B. THE ABUSING PARENT
   1. Marital status: majority married and living together at the time of abuse.
   2. Average age of abusing mother: 26 years.
   3. Average age of abusing father: 30 years.
   4. Abusing parent: father slightly more often than mother.

Diagnosis should be considered when some of following are present

When Parent
   1. Shows loss of control, or fear of losing control, or is detached.
   2. Gives contradictory history.
   3. States cause of injury is sibling or third party.
   4. Delays bringing child for care.
   5. Suggests inappropriate awareness of seriousness of situation (over- or under-reacts).
   6. Complains about irrelevant problems.
   7. Uses drugs or alcohol.
   8. Causes doctor to be worried or suspicious for unknown reasons.
   9. Gives a history which does not explain injury.
   10. Gives a history of repeated injury.
   11. Has no one to help when exasperated by child.
   12. Is reluctant to give information.
   13. Refuses consent for reasonable diagnostic studies.
   14. Moves around from hospital to hospital.
   15. Cannot be located.
   16. Is psychotic or psychopathic.
   17. Has been reared in 'motherless' atmosphere.
   18. Has unrealistic expectations of child.
When Child
   1. Has unexplained injury.
   2. Shows evidence of dehydration and/or malnutrition and/or coma without obvious cause.
   3. Has been given inappropriate food, drink and/or drugs.
   4. Shows evidence of overall poor care.
   5. Is unusually fearful.
   6. Shows evidence of repeated injury.
   7. 'Takes over' and begins to care for parents' needs.
   8. Is seen as 'different' or 'bad' by the parents.
   9. Is indeed different in physical or emotional make up.
   10. Is dressed inappropriately for degree or type of injury.
   11. Shows evidence of sexual abuse.
   12. Shows evidence of repeated skin injuries.
   13. Shows evidence of repeated fractures; subdural haematoma.
   14. Unexplained coma (drugs administered by abuser).
   15. Shows evidence of 'characteristic' radiographic changes to long bone.

16. Has injuries not mentioned in history.

Note: Child often wasted—below 3rd centile for weight but height less depressed.

Examination

Reveals any of the following: (1) Bruises—especially of face (crescentic bruises or cuts suggest human bites); (2) Cuts of frenulum, or around ear, or external genitalia; (3) Poor skin care—napkin dermatitis; (4) Burns from cigarettes or contact with electric fires or hot water; (5) Anxious expression—gaze avoidance; sometimes catatonic postures; (6) Fundal haemorrhages frequent; less common are hyphema, detached retina and dislocated lens. Sight may be permanently lost; (7) Subdural haematoma occurs with or without a fractured skull—due to shaking; (8) Internal abdominal injuries include intestinal haematoma, ruptured viscera (e.g. spleen) and torn mesentery; (9) Malnutrition may or may not be a feature.

Radiology

1. Multiple fractures of almost any bone(s).
2. Fractures are of different dates.
3. Long bone fractures may be of shearing variety—epiphyses torn away by a twist; ribs often fractured posteriorly.

X-rays and photographs should be legally attested in case required as evidence.

Investigations

Essential to rule out any organic cause for bruising, etc. therefore should include (1) Blood count and coagulation studies; (2) Vitamin C level of white cells sometimes useful when scurvy suspected.

Note: occasional children who are injured also may have relevant coexisting illness, e.g. coeliac disease or osteogenesis imperfecta.

Psychological assessment important. IQ may be low because:

1. Mentally retarded children at special risk for abuse.
2. Injuries, e.g. subdural haematoma, may cause damage to brain.
3. Poor environment. Maternal deprivation.

Management

Child must be admitted to hospital immediately to protect him and to allow investigations to proceed. Case conference should be called by Medical Social Worker within 48 h. Attenders should be members of a properly constituted team to include Consultant Paediatrician, Medical Social Worker and representative of local statutory body. In some countries compulsory notification in force.

Best for one paediatrician to be involved with all local cases to establish routine. All members of team need to guard against natural reaction of anger and resentment by remembering that injury likely to have been done in a moment of anger and stress. Sometimes child's behaviour evokes parental outburst.

Parents must be told that injuries are considered to be non-accidental and a case conference will be called to determine best way of helping child and family. If police are involved parents should be told.

Objective:

1. If possible to work with family in hope that child may be returned. Important to review child regularly at home. Outlook for child both physically and emotionally often poor.

2. Child may have to be removed from home, temporarily or permanently. Raises important questions.
a. Which is best for child: adoption, fostering, institutionalization or poor home?
b. What is possible in the particular instance?

Sexual Abuse

Up to 70% of mothers who abuse their children have themselves been the victims of incest when they were children. They do not necessarily sexually abuse their children, they just abuse them.

Note the term perpetrator, referring to fathers, step-fathers, the mother's 'boyfriend', relatives or family friends, also siblings. Note that there is far more in house, than out of house sexual abuse. That is to say, it is usually from people the child knows rather than from complete strangers. Sexual abuse does not necessarily lead onto vaginal intercourse, but includes all sorts of indecent habits, practices which are perpetrated on the child. 50% of the victims are less than 12 years of age and 15% are less than 6 years of age. Sometimes the abuse may continue for as long as over 7 years. These are the cases which are most resistant to later therapy. Apparent 'seductiveness' when the child is seductive, is often because the only way the child can gain attention is by an appearance of sexuality. They must learn to give the message of friendship without the message of sexual availability.

Clinical Pathology in Children: Normal Values

NORMAL BIOCHEMICAL VALUES

B—whole blood; P—plasma; S—serum

[a] These concentrations are age-dependent.

[e] Enzyme activity depends on the method and units used: consult the local laboratory for normal values.

	SI units	Conventional units	Conversion factor
Blood			
Acid-base balance (Astrup, B)			
pH	7·36–7·42	7·36–7·42	—
P_{CO_2}	4·3–6·1 kPa	32–46 mmHg	0·133
Standard bicarbonate	21·3–24·8 mmol/l	21·3–24·8 mEq/l	—
Base excess	−4–+2 mmol/l	−4–+2 mEq/l	—
Amino-acid nitrogen (P, S)	2·1–3·6 mmol/l	3·0–5·0 mg/dl	0·714
Ammonia (Fenton method P)	2–22 µmol/l	3–35 µg/dl	0·587
Bilirubin (P, S)	2–14 µmol/l	0·1–0·8 mg/dl	17·1
Calcium (P, S)	2·25–2·70 mmol/l	9·0–11·0 mg/dl	0·25
Cholesterol (P, S)[a]	2·6–5·7 mmol/l	100–200 mg/dl	0·0259
(lower during first 2 years of life)			
Creatinine (P, S)[a]	25–115 µmol/l	0·3–1·3 mg/dl	—
Electrolytes (P, S)			
Sodium	136–145 mmol/l	136–145 mEq/l	—
Potassium	4·0–5·5 mmol/l	4·0–5·5 mEq/l	—
Chloride	100–110 mmol/l	100–110 mEq/l	—
Fibrinogen (P)	2–4 g/l	0·2–0·4 g/dl	10·0
Folate (P)	16–36 mmol/l	0·71–1·59 µg/dl	22·65
Glucose (specific, fasting)	2·5–5·3 mmol/l	45–95 mg/dl	0·0555
Haptoglobin	0·3–1·7 g/l	30–170 mg/dl	10·0
Haptoglobin-haemoglobin combining power. Significant depletion shown by 0·2 g/l or less. Normally may be zero up to age of 6 m	0·45–0·50 g/l	45–50 mg/dl	—
Iron (S)	11–36 µmol/l	60–200 µg/dl	0·179
Iron binding capacity (S)	45–70 µmol/l	250–400 µg/dl	0·179
Lactate (B)	0·3–0·8 mmol/l	3·1–7·0 mg/dl	0·112
Lead (B)	Less than 1·75 µmol/l	Less than 36 µg/dl	—
Lipid, total (P, S)[a]	4–8 g/l	400–800 mg/dl	0·01
Magnesium (P, S)	0·60–1·0 mmol/l	1·5–2·5 mg/dl	0·411
Non-protein nitrogen (P, S)	14–18 mmol/l	19–25 mg/dl	0·714
5′ Nucleotidase (S)[e]	2–15 iu/l	2–15 iu/l	—
Osmolality (P, S)	275–295 mosmol/kg	275–295 mosmol/kg	—
Phenylalanine (P)	85–300 µmol/l	1·4–5·0 mg/dl	60·5
Phosphatase, alkaline (S)[ea]	8–35 KA units	8–35 KA units	—
Phosphatase, acid (S)[a]	1–4 KA units	1–4 KA units	—
Phosphate (as inorganic P) (P, S)	1·1–1·9 mmol/l	3·5–6·0 mg/dl	0·323
Protein (S)			
Total	63–81 g/l	6·3–8·1 g/dl	10·0
Albumin	36–48 g/l	3·6–4·8 g/dl	10·0
Globulin	23–27 g/l	2·3–3·7 g/dl	10·0

	SI units	Conventional units	Conversion factor
Immunoglobulins[a]			
IgG	5–18 g/l	500–1800 mg/dl	0·01
IgM	0·3–3·5 g/l	30–350 mg/dl	0·01
IgA	0·8–4·5 g/l	80–450 mg/dl	0·01
IgD	0–0·9 g/l	0–90 mg/dl	0·01
IgE	Less than 100–500 μg/l	Less than 100–500 ng/ml	—
T_3 (Triiodothyronine)	1·3–3·5 mmol/l	0·84–2·27 μg/dl	1·54
T_4 (Thyroxine)	55–150 mmol/l	4·26–11·62 ng/dl	12·9
Triglycerides	0·34–2·26 mmol/l	30–200 mg/dl	0·0112
TSH	Up to 5·0 mu/l		
Urate	0·1–0·25 mmol/l	2–3·8 mg/dl	0·0595
Urea	2·5–6·6 mmol/l	15–40 mg/dl	0·166
Urea nitrogen	1·1–3·1 mmol/l	7–19 mg/dl	0·166

Enzymes	Method of determination	Reference values determined at 37°C	
		SI units	Conventional units
Enzymes			
1. Acid phosphatase			
(a) Total	King–Armstrong	Less than 8·2 iu/l	Less than 4·6
(b) Prostatic (Formaldehyde stable)	King–Armstrong	Less than 7·2 iu/l	Less than 4·0
2. Alkaline phosphatase	King–Armstrong	21–100 iu/l	3–14
	Bessey–Lowry	20–50 iu/l	0–3
	Bodansky	8–27 iu/l	1·5–5
3. Amylase	Somogyi	150–340 iu/l	80–180
	Street–Close		9–35
	Dyed substrates		
	Phadebass		70–300
	Amylochrome		45–200
	Dy–Amyl		36–158
4. Alanine transaminase (Ala-T or SGPT)	Reitman–Frankel	5–30 iu/l	
5. Aspartate transaminase (Asp-T or SGOT)	Reitman–Frankel or Karmen	5–30 iu/l	5–40
6 Creatine kinase (CK or CPK)	Oliver (modified) Rosalki	♂ Less than 100 iu/l ♀ Less than 60 iu/l	
7. Hydroxybutyrate dehydrogenase (HBD)	Rosalki-Wilkinson McQueen	150–325 iu/l 80–440 iu/l	
8. Lactate dehydrogenase (LDH)	Wroblewski–La Due McQueen	120–365 iu/l 240–525	250–760
9. γ-Glutamyl transpeptidase (γ-GT)	Szaz	♂ 6–28 iu/l ♀ 4–18 iu/l	
10. 5-Nucleotidase (5-NT)	Persijn	2–15 iu/l	

	SI units	*Conventional units*	*Conversion factor*
Cerebrospinal fluid			
Protein			
Total	0·1–0·25 g/l	10–25 mg/dl	0·01
IgG	0–0·07 g/l	0–7 mg/dl	0·01
Sugar	2·5–4·8 mmol/l	45–85 mg/dl	0·0555
Cells	0–5 lymphocytes/ mm^3		
Urine			
FSH (Radioimmunoassay, 2nd IRP HMG as standard)		Less than 5 iu/24 h	—
Pregnanetriol (prepubertal levels)	Less than 1·75 μmol/l	Less than 0·5 mg/24 h	—
17 oxogenic steroids	1·75–24·5 μmol/l	0·5–7 mg/24 h	—
17 oxosteroids[a]	1·75–21 μmol/l	1–6 mg/24 h	
Total oestrogens	Less than 18 nmol/l	Less than 5 μg/24 h	
Steroid ratio:			
$\dfrac{\text{Pregnanetriol (11 deoxy fraction)}}{\text{Cortisol metabolites (11 oxy fraction)}}$	Less than 0·5		
Urine levels for older children			
Amino acid nitrogen	4–20 mmol/24 h	50–300 mg/24 h	0·071
Ascorbic acid	110–280 μmol/24 h	20–50 mg/24 h	5·7
Calcium	2·5–7·5 mmol/24 h	100–300 mg/24 h	0·025
Creatine	0–400 μmol/24 h	0–50 mg/24 h	7·63
Creatinine	9–17 mmol/24 h	1·2 g/24 h	8·84
Glucose	0–11 mmol/l	0–0·2 g/dl	55·5
HIAA	15–75 μmol/24 h	3–14 mg/24 h	5·23
HMMA	10–35 μmol/24 h	2–7 mg/24 h	5·05
Magnesium	3·3–4·9 mmol/24 h	80–120 mg/24 h	0·04
17 oxogenic steroid	35–70 μmol/24 h	10–20 mg/24 h	3·47
17 oxosteroids	35–85 μmol/24 h	10–25 mg/24 h	3·47
Phosphate	15–50 mmol/24 h	0·5–1·5 g/24 h	32·3
Potassium	40–120 mmol/24 h	40–120 mEq/24 h	—
Sodium	100–250 mmol/24 h	100–250 mEq/24 h	—
Uric acid	3·0–12·0 mmol/24 h	0·5–2·0 g/24 h	5·95
Urea	166–580 mmol/24 h	10–35 mg/24 h	116·6

Clinical Assessment of Gestational Age in the Newborn Infant

(By permission of Lilly Dubowitz and Victor Dubowitz and the publishers of 'Journal of Pediatrics')

SOME NOTES ON TECHNIQUES OF ASSESSMENT OF NEUROLOGICAL CRITERIA (*Figs.* A,B)

Posture. Observed with infant quiet and in supine position. Score 0: arms and legs extended; 1: beginning of flexion of hips and knees, arms extended; 2: stronger flexion of legs, arms extended; 3: arms slightly flexed, legs flexed and abducted; 4: full flexion of arms and legs.

Square Window. The hand is flexed on the forearm between the thumb and index finger of the examiner. Enough pressure is applied to get as full a flexion as possible, and the angle between the hypothenar eminence and the ventral aspect of the forearm is measured and graded according to diagrams. (Care is taken not to rotate the infant's wrist while doing this manoeuvre.)

Ankle Dorsiflexion. The foot is dorsiflexed onto the anterior aspect of the leg, with the examiner's thumb on the sole of the foot and other fingers behind the leg. Enough pressure is applied to get as full flexion as possible, and the angle between the dorsum of the foot and the anterior aspect of the leg is measured.

Arm Recoil. With the infant in the supine position the forearms are first flexed for 5 seconds, then fully extended by pulling on the hands, and then released. The sign is fully positive if the arms return briskly to full flexion (Score 2). If the arms return to incomplete flexion or the response is sluggish it is graded as Score 1. If they remain extended or are only followed by random movements the score is 0.

Leg Recoil. With the infant supine, the hips and knees are fully flexed for 5 seconds, then extended by traction on the feet, and released. A maximal response is one of full flexion of the hips and knees (Score 2). A partial flexion scores 1, and minimal or no movement scores 0.

Popliteal Angle. With the infant supine and his pelvis flat on the examining couch, the thigh is held in the knee–chest position by the examiner's left index finger and thumb supporting the knee. The leg is then extended by gentle pressure from the examiner's right index finger behind the ankle and the popliteal angle is measured.

Heel to Ear Manoeuvre. With the baby supine, draw the baby's foot as near to the head as it will go without forcing it. Observe the distance between the foot and the head as well as the degree of extension at the knee. Grade according to diagrams. Note that the knee is left free and may draw down alongside the abdomen.

Scarf Sign. With the baby supine, take the infant's hand and try to put it around the neck and as far posteriorly as possible around the opposite shoulder. Assist this manoeuvre by lifting the elbow across the body. See how far the elbow will go across and grade according to diagrams. Score 0: elbow reaches opposite axillary line; 1: elbow between midline and opposite axillary line; 2: elbow reaches midline; 3: elbow will not reach midline.

Head Lag. With the baby lying supine, grasp the hands (or the arms if a very small infant) and pull him slowly towards the sitting position. Observe the position of the head in relation to the trunk and grade accordingly. In a small infant the head may initially be supported by one hand. Score 0: complete lag; 1: partial head control; 2: able to maintain head in line with body; 3: brings head anterior to body.

Ventral Suspension. The infant is suspended in the prone position, with examiner's hand under the infant's chest (one hand in a small infant, two in a large infant). Observe the degree of extension of the back and the amount of flexion of the arm and legs. Also note the relation of the head to the trunk. Grade according to diagrams.

If score differs on the two sides, take the mean.

For further details *see* Dubowitz et al., *J. Pediat.* 1970, **77**, 1.

Note: Gestational age assessment using Dubowitz' method gives 95 per cent confidence limit of 15 days. Use of four best physical characteristics—**skin colour, skin texture, breast size**, and **ear firmness** gives 95 per cent confidence limit of 18 days. (Parkin J. M., Hey E, N. and Clowes J. S. (1976) *Arch. Dis. Child.* **51**, 259) Use total from these four items.

Score	Gestational age (d)	(w)
1	190	27
2	210	30
3	230	33
4	240	34½
5	250	36
6	260	37
7	270	38½
8	276	39½
9	281	40
10	285	41
11	290	41½
12	295	42

NEURO-LOGICAL SIGN	SCORE					
	0	1	2	3	4	5
POSTURE						
SQUARE WINDOW	90°	60°	45°	30°	0°	
ANKLE DORSI-FLEXION	90°	75°	45°	20°	0°	
ARM RECOIL	180°	90–180°	<90°			
LEG RECOIL	180°	90–180°	<90°			
POPLITEAL ANGLE	180°	160°	130°	110°	90°	<90°
HEEL TO EAR						
SCARF SIGN						
HEAD LAG						
VENTRAL SUSPEN-SION						

Fig. A. Neurological criteria

EXTERNAL SIGN	SCORE				
	0	**1**	**2**	**3**	**4**
OEDEMA	Obvious oedema hands and feet; pitting over tibia	No obvious oedema hands and feet; pitting over tibia	No oedema		
SKIN TEXTURE	Very thin, gelatinous	Thin and smooth	Smooth; medium thickness. Rash or superficial peeling	Slight thickening. Superficial cracking and peeling esp. hands and feet	Thick and parchment-like; superficial or deep cracking
SKIN COLOUR (Infant not crying)	Dark red	Uniformly pink	Pale pink: variable over body	Pale. Only pink over ears, lips, palms or soles	
SKIN OPACITY (trunk)	Numerous veins and venules clearly seen, especially over abdomen	Veins and tributaries seen	A few large vessels clearly seen over abdomen	A few large vessels seen indistinctly over abdomen	No blood vessels seen
LANUGO (over back)	No lanugo	Abundant; long and thick over whole back	Hair thinning especially over lower back	Small amount of lanugo and bald areas	At least half of back devoid of lanugo
PLANTAR CREASES	No skin creases	Faint red marks over anterior half of sole	Definite red marks over more than anterior half; indentations over less than anterior third	Indentations over more than anterior third	Definite deep indentations over more than anterior third
NIPPLE FORMATION	Nipple barely visible; no areola	Nipple well defined; areola smooth and flat diameter <0.75 cm.	Areola stippled, edge not raised; diameter <0.75 cm.	Areola stippled, edge raised diameter >0.75 cm.	
BREAST SIZE	No breast tissue palpable	Breast tissue on one or both sides < 0.5 cm. diameter	Breast tissue both sides; one or both 0.5-1.0 cm.	Breast tissue both sides; one or both > 1 cm.	
EAR FORM	Pinna flat and shapeless, little or no incurving of edge	Incurving of part of edge of pinna	Partial incurving whole of upper pinna	Well-defined incurving whole of upper pinna	
EAR FIRMNESS	Pinna soft, easily folded, no recoil	Pinna soft, easily folded, slow recoil	Cartilage to edge of pinna, but soft in places, ready recoil	Pinna firm, cartilage to edge, instant recoil	
GENITALIA MALE	Neither testis in scrotum	At least one testis high in scrotum	At least one testis right down		
FEMALES (With hips half abducted)	Labia majora widely separated, labia minora protruding	Labia majora almost cover labia minora	Labia majora completely cover labia minora		

(Adapted from Farr et al. Develop. Med. Child Neurol. 1966, **8**, 507)

Fig. B. External (superficial) criteria

Denver Developmental Screening Test (Cardiff Modification)

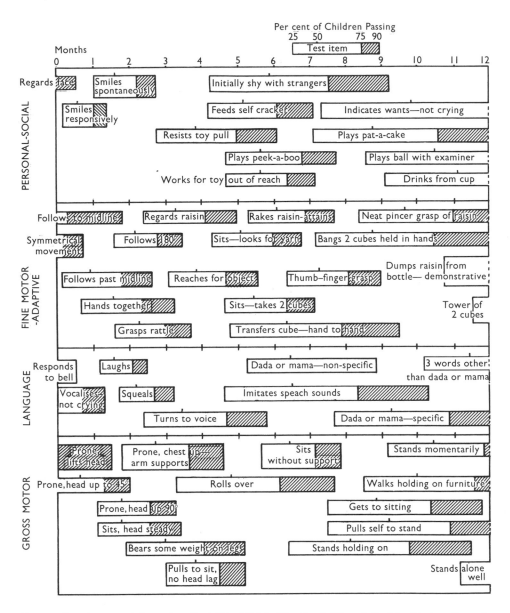

Denver Developmental Screening Test (Cardiff Modification.) (Bryant G. M., Davies, K. and Newcombe R. G. (1974) *Dev. Med. Child. Neurol.* **14**, 482.) (*By permission of Dr G. M. Bryant and the publishers of 'Developmental Medicine and Child Neurology'.*)

Drugs which may Colour Urine or Faeces

The following list is a guide to the more commonly used drugs which may colour urine or faeces in certain patients.

Drugs	Possible colour change Urine	Faeces
Aluminium hydroxide and other antacids		White discoloration or speckling
Amitriptyline	Blue green	
Aspirin		Pink, red or black if internal bleeding occurs
Bismuth preparations		Black
Chloroquine	Rust yellow to brown	
Chlorpromazine (and rarely other phenothiazines)	Pink to red or red to brown	
Danthron preparations (Normax, Dorbanex)	Pink to red in alkaline urine	
Daunorubicin	Red	
Doxorubicin (Adriamycin)	Red	
Indomethacin		Pink, red or black if intestinal bleeding occurs
Iron preparations		Black
Liquorice		Black
Methyldopa	Darker than usual	
Methylene blue	Blue or green	Blue
Mepacrine	Yellow	
Metronidazole	Dark brown	
Niridazole	Brown	
Nitrofurantoin	Rust yellow or brown	
Phenazopyridine	Orange or red	Orange or red
Phenindione	Orange to red brown in alkaline urine	Pink, red or black if intestinal bleeding occurs
Phenolphthalein	Pink or magenta in alkaline urine	
Phenytoin	Pink to red	
Quinine or derivatives	Brown to black	
Rifampicin	Orange to red (also sputum and tears)	
Senna	Brown	Yellow
Sulphasalazine	Orange yellow in alkaline urine	
Triamterene	Pale blue fluoresence	
Viprynium		Bright red
Vitamin preparations containing riboflavine	Bright yellow	
Warfarin (and all oral anti-coagulants)		Pink, red or black if intestinal bleeding occurs

515

Normal Values for Cerebrospinal Fluid (Mean values in brackets)

	First 24 hours	Day 1	Day 7
Red blood cells (mm^3)	0–1070	0–620	0–48
	(9)	(23)	(3)
Polymorphs (mm^3)	0–70	0–26	0–5
	(3)	(7)	(2)
Lymphocytes (mm^3)	0–20	0–16	0–4
	(2)	(5)	(1)
Protein	0·3–2·4 g/l	0·4–1·48 g/l	0·27–0·65 g/l
	(0·6 g/l)	(0·73 g/l)	(0·47 g/l)
	32–240 mg%	40–148 mg%	27–65 mg%
	(63 mg%)	(73 mg%)	(47 mg%)
Glucose	1·8–4·35 mmol/l	(2·1–3·55 mmol/l	2·65–3·45 mmol/l
	(2·85 mmol/l)	(2·65 mmol/l)	(3·05 mmol/l)
	32–78 mg%	38–64 mg%	48–62 mg%
	(51 mg%)	(48 mg%)	(55 mg%)
Chloride (mmol/l and mEq/l)	680–760	680–760	720–760
	(720)	(720)	(720)

Naidoo T. (1968) *S. Afr. Med. J.* **42**, 939.

Bone Age. Average Time of Appearance of Osseous Centres

Age	Radiograph required				
	Shoulder (AP)	Elbow (Lat.)	Wrist and hand (AP)	Knee (Lat.)	Ankle and foot (Lat.)
3 months	Head of humerus		Hamate: epiphysis of radius		
6 months			Capitate		
1 year					External cuneiform; epiphysis of tibia
2 years	Great tuberosity	Capitellum			Epiphysis of fibula
3 years			Triquetrum; epiphysis of phalanges and metacarpals		Internal cuneiform; epiphysis of metatarsals
4 years			Lunatum	Head of fibula	Mid-cuneiform; navicular
5 years		Head of radius	Trapezium; scaphoid	Patella	
6 years		Internal epicondyle	Trapezoid; epiphysis of ulna		
7 years					
8 years					Epiphysis of os calcis
9 years		Olecranon; trochlea			
10 years			Pisiform		
11 years		External epicondyle			Tubercle of tibia

*International Classification of Seizures (ILAE 1981)**

Partial (Focal, Local) Seizures

Clinical seizure type	*EEG seizure type*	*EEG interictal expressio*
A. Simple partial seizures (consciousness not impaired)	Local contralateral discharge starting over the corresponding area of cortical representation (not always recorded on the scalp)	Local contra-lateral discharge

1. With motor signs
  (a) Focal motor without march
  (b) Focal motor with march (Jacksonian)
  (c) Versive
  (d) Postural
  (e) Phonatory (vocalization or arrest of speech)
2. With somatosensory or special-sensory symptoms (simple hallucinations, e.g., tingling, light flashes, buzzing)
  (a) Somatosensory (d) Olfactory
  (b) Visual   (e) Gustatory
  (c) Auditory   (f) Vertiginous
3. With autonomic symptoms or signs (including epigastric sensation, pallor, sweating, flushing, pileoerection and pupillary dilatation)
4. With psychic symptoms (disturbance of higher cerebral function). These symptoms rarely occur without impairment of consciousness and are much more commonly experienced as complex partial seizures
  (a) Dysphasic
  (b) Dysmnesic (e.g., déjà-vu)
  (c) Cognitive (e.g., dreamy states, distortions of time sense)
  (d) Affective (fear, anger, etc.)
  (e) Illusions (e.g., macropsia)
  (f) Structured hallucinations (e.g., music, scenes)		

B. Complex partial seizures (with impairment of consciousness; may sometimes begin with simple symptomatology)	Unilateral or, frequently bilateral discharge, diffuse or focal in temporal or frontotemporal regions	Unilateral or bilateral generally asynchronous focus; usually in the temporal or frontal regions

1. Simple partial onset followed by impairment of consciousness
  (a) With simple partial features (A.1.-A.4.) followed by impaired consciousness
  (b) With automatisms
2. With impairment of consciousness at onset
  (a) With impairment of consciousness only
  (b) With automatisms		

C. Partial seizures evolving to secondarily generalized seizures (These may be generalized tonic-clonic, tonic, or clonic) 1. Simple partial seizures (A) evolving to generalized seizures 2. Complex partial seizures (B) evolving to generalized seizures 3. Simple partial seizures evolving to complex partial seizures evolving to generalized seizures	Above discharges become secondarily and rapid generalized	

Generalized Seizures (Convulsive or Non-convulsive)

Clinical seizure type	EEG seizure type	EEG interictal expression
A. 1. Absence seizures	Usually regular and symmetrical 3Hz but may be 2-4 Hz spike-and-slow-wave complexes and may have multiple spike-and-slow-wave complexes. Abnormalities are bilateral	Background activity usually normal although paroxysmal activity (such as spikes or spike-and-slow-wave complexes) may occur. This activity is usually regular and symmetrical
(a) Impairment of consciousness only		
(b) With mild clonic components		
(c) With atonic components		
(d) With tonic components		
(e) With automatisms		
(f) With autonomic components		
(b through f may be used alone or in combination)		
2. Atypical absence	EEG more heterogeneous; may include irregular spike-and-slow-wave complexes, fast activity. Abnormalities are bilateral but often irregular and asymmetrical	Background usually abnormal; paroxysmal activity (such as spikes or spike-and-slow-wave complexes) frequently irregular and asymmetrical
May have:		
(a) Changes in tone that are more pronounced than in A.1		
(b) Onset and/or cessation that is not abrupt		
B. Myoclonic seizures Myoclonic jerks (single or multiple)	Polyspike and wave, or sometimes spike and wave or sharp and slow waves	Same as ictal
C. Clonic seizures	Fast activity (10 Hz or more) and slow waves; occasional spike-and-wave patterns	Spike-and-wave or polyspike-and-wave discharges
D. Tonic seizures	Low voltage, fast activity or a fast rhythm of 9-10 Hz or more decreasing in frequency and increasing in amplitude	More or less rhythmic discharges of sharp and slow waves, sometimes asymmetrical. Background is often abnormal for age
E. Tonic-clonic seizures	Rhythm at 10 or more Hz decreasing in frequency and increasing in amplitude during tonic phase, interrupted by slow waves during clonic phase	Polyspike and waves or spike and wave or, sometimes, sharp and slow wave discharges
F. Atonic seizures (Astatic) (combinations of the above may occur, e.g., B and F, B and D)	Polyspikes and wave or flattening or low-voltage fast activity	Polyspikes and slow wave

Unclassified Epileptic Seizures

Includes all seizures that cannot be classified because of inadequate or incomplete data and some that defy classification in hitherto described categories. This includes some neonatal seizures, e.g., rhythmic eye movements, chewing, and swimming movements.

*With acknowledgement to *Epilepsia* and Raven Press.

A Scheme for Immunization against Common Infections

Age				
*USA**	*British†*	*Vaccine*	*Dose*	*Route*
3 months	6 months	Triple†	0·5 ml	i.m. or s.c.
		Polio	3 drops	oral
4 months	7½–8 months	Triple†		
		Polio	0·5 ml	i.m. or s.c. Interval of 6–8 weeks after
6 months	14 months	Triple†	0·5 ml	i.m. or s.c. Interval of 6–12 months
		Polio	3 drops	oral
12 months	15–16 months	Measles		
		Rubella (USA)	0·5 ml	i.m. or s.c. Omit if child had disease. Girls and boys
18 months		Triple or D/T (PTAH)†	0·5 ml	i.m. or s.c. School entry
5 years	5 years	Polio	3 drops	oral
	11–14 years	Rubella	0·5 ml	s.c. Girls only
	13 years	BCG	0·1 ml	i.d. Tuberculin negative only
	15–19 years	Tetanus	0·5 ml	i.m. or s.c. School leavers
		Polio	3 drops	oral

Note: Different countries have different immunization schemes, examples are given above.
* American Academy of Pediatrics, 1974.
†*Note*: Because of rare encephalopathy following pertussis vaccine, some British authorities recommend diphtheria and tetanus vaccine alone.

Inherited Metabolic Disorders detected in the Mid-trimester of Pregnancy

Disorder	Diagnostic assay
Lipid disorders:	
Adrenoleucodystrophy	Cholesterol ester (C_{26}) fatty acids
Fabry disease	α-Galactosidase A
Familial hypercholesterolaemia	LDL receptors
Farber disease	Ceramidase
Gaucher disease, type 2	β-Glucosidase
G_{M1}-gangliosidosis:	
type I	β-Galactosidase A, B, and C
type II	β-Galactosidase B and C
G_{M2}-gangliosidosis:	
Tay–Sachs	Hexosaminidase A
Sandhoff	Hexosaminidase A and B
Krabbe disease	Galactocerebroside β-galactosidase
Metachromatic leucodystrophy	Arylsulphatase A
Niemann–Pick disease	Sphingomyelinase
Wolman disease	Acid lipase
Mucopolysaccharidoses and related disorders:	
MPS type IH-Hurler	α-Iduronidase
MPS type II-Hunter	Iduronate sulphatase
MPS type IIIA-Sanfilippo A	Heparin sulphamidase
MPS type IV-Morquio	N-acetylgalactosamine 6-sulphatase
MPS type VI-Maroteaux–Lamy	Arylsulphatase B
Mannosidosis	α-Mannosidase
Mucolipidosis (combined neuraminidase-β galactosidase deficiency	Neuraminidase and β-galactosidase
Mucolipidosis I (sialidosis)	Neuraminidase
Mucolipidosis II (I-cell disease)	Multiple lysosomal enzymes
Mucolipidosis IV	Storage bodies—EM
Carbohydrate disorders:	
Galactosaemia	Galactose 1-phosphate uridyl transferase
Glycogen storage disease:	
type II	α-1,4-glucosidase
type IV	Amylo-(1,4→1,6)-transglucosidase
Pyruvate carboxylase deficiency	Pyruvate carboxylase
Amino acid and related disorders:	
Argininosuccinic aciduria	Argininosuccinase
Citrullinaemia	Argininosuccinate synthase
Cystinosis	^{35}-S-cystine uptake
Glutaric acidaemia type II	Fatty acid oxidation
Homocystinuria	Cystathione-β-synthase
Maple syrup urine disease	Branched-chain α-keto acid decarboxylase

Disorder	Diagnostic assay
Methylmalonic acidemia:	
B_{12} non-responsive	Methylmalonyl-CoA apomutase
B_{12} responsive	Defects in cobalamin synthesis
Non-ketotic hyperglycinaemia	Glycine-serine ratio
Ornithine carbamyl	Ornithine carbamyl
transferase deficiency	transferase (liver)
Propionic acidaemia	Propionyl-CoA carboxylase
Tyrosinaemia type I	Succinyl acetone
Other disorders:	
Acid phosphatase deficiency	Lysosomal acid phosphatase
Acute intermittent porphyria	Uroporphyrinogen 1-synthase
Adenosine deaminase deficiency	Adenosine deaminase
α_1-Antitrypsin deficiency	α_1-Antitrypsin (fetal blood)
Chronic granulomatous disease	NBT reduction (fetal blood)
Congenital adrenal hyperplasia	17-α-hydroxyprogesterone
(21-hydroxylase defect)	
Congenital erythropoietic porphyria	Amniotic fluid porphyrin
Congenital nephrosis	α-Fetoprotein
Cytochrome b_5 reductase deficiency	Cytochrome b_5 reductase
Hypophosphatasia	Alkaline phosphatase
Lesch–Nyhan syndrome	Hypoxanthine-guanine
	phosphoribosyl transferase
Menkes disease	^{64}Cu uptake
Osteogenesis imperfecta	Collagen metabolism
Pituitary dysgenesis	Prolactin
Xeroderma pigmentosum	DNA excision-repair synthesis

Index